The Scientific Bases of
Cancer Chemoprevention

The Scientific Bases of Cancer Chemoprevention

Proceedings of the International Forum on the Scientific Bases of Cancer Chemoprevention, 31 March – 2 April 1996, Bologna, Italy

Editors:

Cesare Maltoni
European Ramazzini Foundation
Bologna, Italy

Morando Soffritti
European Ramazzini Foundation
Bologna, Italy

Walter Davis
Formerly International Agency for Research on Cancer
Lyon, France

1996

ELSEVIER

Amsterdam – Lausanne – New York – Oxford – Shannon – Tokyo

International Congress Series No. 1120
Advances in the Biosciences Volume 96
ISBN 0 444 82453 7

This book is printed on acid-free paper.

Published by:
Elsevier Science B.V.
P.O. Box 211
1000 AE Amsterdam
The Netherlands

Library of Congress Cataloging-in-Publication Data:

In order to ensure rapid publication this volume was prepared using a method of electronic text processing known as Optical Character Recognition (OCR). Scientific accuracy and consistency of style were handled by the author. Time did not allow for the usual extensive editing process of the Publisher.

Printed in the Netherlands

Foreword

Chemoprevention is intended as a pharmacological treatment which can prevent, interrupt, or slow the cascade of biological events that lead to the appearance of clinical cancer, and has in recent years been proposed as a possible tool for controlling some specific types of neoplasia. Chemoprevention should be specifically designed for population groups at risk, and it should aim at a specific target or targets, within the carcinogenic process, particularly during the latent period.

Chemoprevention requires specific activity drugs. To develop these drugs experimental systems and protocols must be established for evaluating their anticancer potential, that are as close as possible to being human equivalent, i.e., capable of providing results that are easily transferable to humans. These experimental systems can also expose unwanted side effects.

Recently, studies have been expanding, particularly those on the molecular biology of the neoplastic process, and on drugs with potential cancer chemopreventive effects. Suitable experimental models to assess these effects are also being developed. In parallel with these developments, there has been an increase in experimental and clinical studies of single drugs as candidates for chemoprevention of specific tumours. Hormones and antihormones, such as antioestrogens, LH-RH agonists-antagonists, progestins and antiaromatase drugs, have been considered as possible chemopreventive agents in the control of mammary cancer in woman.

The aim of the present forum is to bring together experts in the fields of molecular biology and carcinogenesis, epidemiologists, pathologists, experimental and clinical oncologists, to review the basic biological knowledge applicable to chemoprevention, and the available results and ongoing studies in the practical application of potential chemopreventive agents for cancer control. On the basis of the available data, the forum further evaluates the potentialities of these new tools, and indicates future developments for research in this area.

During the forum consideration is furthermore given to the design of clinical trials, to questions of cost/benefit and risk benefit, and to related ethical problems.

Particular emphasis is placed on the chemoprevention of mammary cancer, since this has already attracted the interest of the oncological community, as there are both stimulating experimental data and early clinical results available.

Professor Cesare Maltoni
Conference Chairman

ACKNOWLEDGEMENTS

The organizers gratefully acknowledge the financial support received from the "Europe against Cancer" programme of the European Commission.
In addition, thanks are due to Zeneca, the major sponsor, and to the Bologna Section of the Italian League for the Fight against Cancer,
Ciba-Geigy
Coca-Cola
Fondazione Cassa di Risparmio in Bologna
Leica
Manutencoop
Redwall
Takeda Italia Famaceutici

THE MARIA THERESA CHIANTORE SERAGNOLI MEMORIAL LECTURE

Public health control of cancer. An interim measure pending the discovery of the "magic pill"

Nigel Gray

President, International Union against Cancer, Geneva, Switzerland

Mr Mayor, distinguished guests and colleagues, it is a great honour and pleasure for me to be here in this beautiful hall in this beautiful city to present the inaugural lecture in honour of Maria Theresa Chiantore Seragnoli.

The Public Health approach to cancer control means, essentially, an attempt to control cancer by preventing its development, either directly as in the case of tobacco or slightly less directly by the early detection of such cancers as melanoma and cancer of the cervix.

To illustrate the principles involved it is convenient to go back to the beginning of my career. I started life, after basic training, working for a decade in a 400-bed infectious disease hospital. Such hospitals are no longer necessary, at least for the diseases we cared for in the 1950s and 60s. We had the ability to vary our bed state to match the epidemic of the moment, but always had a specialist ward with specialist nursing staff for treating diphtheria, poliomyelitis, whooping cough, croup, scarlet fever, measles, and, of course, the regular epidemics of winter influenza which brought in their wake epidemics of pneumonia, often requiring the opening of an extra 100 or so beds. Our daily clinical work involved bedside decisions based on clinical experience. They were often urgent and mistakes were often costly for the patient. The ability to tell, by briefly viewing a septic throat, whether we were looking at a streptococcal throat requiring penicillin only; a diphtheritic throat requiring penicillin plus antitoxin; or a glandular fever throat requiring neither, was an everyday necessity. Penicillin in those days produced severe anaphylaxis rarely, but diphtheria antitoxin was a horse serum which produced severe anaphylaxis, sometimes fatal anaphylactic shock, in 5—10% of the patients. These historic diseases, particularly poliomyelitis and diphtheria, were frightening and I hated them.

The response of Public Health authorities to new developments, in those days, was immediate and anything else was unconscionable. The Salk vaccine was produced and introduced as a matter of urgency and vaccination programs for this and the standard vaccines against whooping cough, diphtheria, tetanus and, later, measles were aggressive, free of cost to the patient, and a routine part of postnatal care of children. The message, in simple terms, was that when we got a new weapon we used it, immediately and without half-measures. By the early 1960s, the combination of vaccination, penicillin, sanitation, undercrowding and routine quarantine measures had actually eradicated, not merely diminished, poliomyelitis, whooping cough, diphtheria, scarlet fever, and measles from the Victorian community in which I worked. The contrast between the speed and efficiency with which we attacked these diseases and the apathy and vacillation with which we approached the controllable cancers is both stark and scandalous, as well as a reflection of our poor understanding of the long latent period between intervention and response which characterises cancer.

The successes with infection were an object lesson to me but failed to prepare me for the frustration which accompanies attempts to control cancer.

There are, however, some excuses. Cancer control is immensely complex. It was in the 1960s and it is in the 1990s. Measles antibodies protected against measles, polio antibodies protected against polio, but cancer antibodies do not protect against cancer. They are polyglot and badly behaved antibodies and have not given us any universal vaccines despite several decades of good quality immunological research. Furthermore, treatment has been a disappointment. Despite substantial research efforts over decades we can cure childhood leukaemia, which is rare, but we cannot cure lung cancer, which is common. Slightly less than half the patients with colorectal cancer survive, late-stage breast cancer, cervical cancer and melanoma are all accompanied by high treatment failure rates, and we cannot even claim that we deliver state-of-the-art treatment to every patient in developed countries. In developing countries there are hundreds of millions of people to whom no cancer treatment is available, often including the pain-relieving qualities of morphia.

So, from my point of view, treatment is difficult and a seriously deficient response to a disease which is rapidly becoming the world's most important cause of death. Hence, I turn to prevention, under which heading I include early detection, and will talk about the activities which have occupied my working life for the past 27 years.

In considering prevention, I must enter a most important caveat. To control cancer we will have to continue to do everything we know how to do, and this involves the full spectrum of research into treatment and prevention, but we must also apply a lot more effort to applying the knowledge we already have. By this I mean the Public Health approach to cancer control.

There are, in my view, five cancers which are controllable to a significant degree by a combination of prevention and early detection. They are: cancers of the lung, cervix, breast, skin and melanoma, and, again a personal view, colorectal cancer. Further, to be blunt, there are no excuses for failing to do the maximum to attack cancers of lung, cervix, breast, and skin melanoma.

I will come back to these cancers in some detail but, since this is a conference on chemoprevention, will spend a little time on this issue.

Again, there is a caveat. Despite some significant disappointments, there is no excuse for not continuing to support research in this area.

In considering chemoprevention we again run in to the profound complexities posed by cancer as a biological process. There are four formidable obstacles to the development of chemoprevention. They are:
1. The prolonged nature of the clinical trials necessary to demonstrate benefit.
2. The conflicting nature of some of the evidence.
3. Uncertainty of the size of benefits achievable.
4. The side effects of drugs, our "magic pills", which are effective.

There are, in fact, four potent preventive agents currently available and review of the effects is illustrative of the points made above. They are: tamoxifen, hormone replacement therapy, the contraceptive pill, and the humble aspirin.

Tamoxifen

Tamoxifen is a very promising substance. It prevents breast cancer (though it may increase the risk of uterine cancer), it decreases cardiovascular disease, and decreases osteoporosis. So, it has mixed effects, most of which are beneficial, but the potential for increased risk of uterine cancer and the clinical side effects seen in a proportion of patients mean that its place as a "magic pill" is, on present judgement, uncertain.

Hormone replacement therapy

Such therapy is used widely throughout the Western world. To summarise again, it prevents menopausal symptoms, prevents osteoporosis, it increases – possibly, but not certainly – cancer of the uterus, it decreases heart disease and decreases the chance of a stroke.

The contraceptive pill

Surely one of the most important developments of the last several decades, the various contraceptive pills clearly prevent pregnancy, have, probably no significant effect on breast cancer, appear to decrease ovarian cancer and to decrease endometrial cancer.

Aspirin

Finally, here is a preventive pill which is a friend to us all. It exemplifies my point that, when we have a preventive pill, it is very difficult to discover its effect; and, particularly, to find a pill that has only one effect – that of preventing cancer. Aspirin may well prevent colorectal cancer; but it does prevent coronary occlusion, thromboembolic stroke, and it appears, unsurprisingly, to increase the risk of haemorrhagic stroke and it certainly causes gastrointestinal bleeding. Thus, it causes mixed effects of uncertain size and we have used it for over half a century before discovering its role as a potential cancer preventive agent.

I must ask forgiveness for this brief and somewhat assertive approach to a large body of evidence on the grounds that this lecture has its major focus elsewhere. I will summarise the conclusion by the further assertion that our search for simple preventive agents has not so far provided us with one which everyone can take without hesitation, and that discoveries so far will continue to provide work for epidemiologists for some years to come.

The controllable cancers

There are four eminently controllable cancers: Lung, cervix, breast, and skin melanoma. It is appropriate to draw attention to some of the difficulties and failures in the field of Public Health activity.

There is, however, clear evidence that this approach has worked, or will do so, and that the outcome of our endeavours has led, or will lead, to trends which will reflect a continuing decrease in mortality and morbidity, as well as health costs, over the long term. So we can claim some success.

I will refer largely to Australian data from here on, although, in most cases, the effects are apparent in various countries. Four important points need to be made:

1. We were slow to start applying established knowledge in each case. Papanicolou described his cervical smear in 1928 and it was introduced into medical practice in Australia in 1965. Doll and Hill and Wynder and Graham, described the clear link between cigarettes and disease in 1950, but serious antismoking activity was not apparent until the mid to late 1960s. The HIP study showed, with reasonable certainty, by 1973 that mammographic screening reduced breast cancer mortality, but we awaited the Swedish trials of the mid-1980s before introducing a pilot program and (in the early 1990s) a statewide, well-organised breast-screening program. Finally, it was suspected last century, and progressively established in this one, that sunshine applied to white skins caused skin cancer and melanoma. Such a dilatory approach would never have been acceptable for poliomyelitis. While I must confess to being one of the people responsible I would also claim that Australia did better than many countries which should know better.

2. There were very substantial obstacles to antismoking activities and there still are. They include the tobacco industry and almost universal professional and political apathy. This did not apply to other preventive programs.

3. There is a long delay between social interventions aimed at incidence reduction, and eventual outcome. Antismoking activity begun in the 1960s produced a decrease in smoking prevalence over 10–30 years, but decreases in lung cancer incidence did not appear until between 10 and 20 years later again, i.e., in the 1980s.

4. Interventions aimed at early detection logically lead to quicker results but the delay time is also long. The campaign against sunshine exposure, and for early detection, began, in Australia, at the end of the 1970s; but changes in mortality which may be attributed to early detection appeared only in the 1990s. A decrease in incidence of skin cancer and melanoma can not be predicted until the present, relatively less exposed, generation of young people reach the age of risk which will be, by and large, next century.

I will now go on to describe the evolution of the relevant public health programs (better described as campaigns), and in doing so, illustrate the points I have made.

Lung cancer

Australia has a Westminster style of government consisting of an upper and lower house. Leadership is provided by a cabinet chosen by the dominant party. Only two parties have held power in recent decades. There are six state governments each with two houses and one central federal government which has the major policy and taxing powers, but only those powers ceded to it at the initial federation process last century. Power to control advertising in cinemas, at point of sale, on billboards, by competitions, and to prescribe the legal age for sale, rests with the States, thus providing a wonderful opportunity for the tobacco industry to obstruct legislation by delaying consensus. The Federal Parliament controls electronic media and print media. In such an environment, which is not unusual around the world, the following legislation was achieved over 25 years.

1970	Health warnings — all States.
1975	Ban on television and radio advertising of cigarettes. Federal. Loophole left which permitted continuation of sporting advertising.
1987	Victorian Tobacco Act. Banned all State-controlled advertising, raised tobacco tax, earmarked 5 cents per packet for a Victorian Health Promotion Foundation, thus indirectly funding the antismoking campaign. Two other States followed.
1989	Print media ban. Federal.
1992	Abolition of all forms of tobacco promotion. Federal.

The struggle to control tobacco advertising is reflective of events in most developed countries. Specific programs aimed at reduction of tar content, at increases of a regular nature in price, at the introduction of a smoke-free workplace, at the effective restriction of sales to minors and a wide variety of education programs targeting the various groups who smoke or are at risk of starting to smoke, have all played a part in reducing smoking prevalence and carcinogen dose.

The outcome of all this effort in Australia has been a downturn in the mortality rate from lung cancer in men and in some cohorts of younger women (Fig. 1). Such effects have been seen in Scandinavia, The UK, and some other countries, but mortality continues to increase in central and Eastern Europe.

In general it is reasonable to suggest that there is a relatively clear correlation between antismoking activity and smoking prevalence which leads over time to mortality reduction.

This is what everybody expected, but only in recent years has the outcome become visible and significant.

The tobacco problem remains unresolved in developing countries. Tar content of cigarettes and other indigenous products such as bidi, kretek, brus, cheroots and cigarlike products remains mostly unmeasured in a systematic way and largely uncontrolled. Advertising has become global in nature albeit severely restricted in many countries. However, broadcast of motor sport and other sport reaches huge audiences and overreaches many local prohibitions.

Among the surprises evident among worldwide antismoking programs is the evidence that tobacco tax is popular, often with smokers, and that the smoke-free

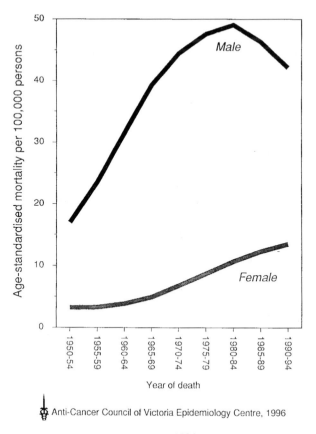

Year of death

Anti-Cancer Council of Victoria Epidemiology Centre, 1996

Fig. 1. Australian cancer mortality: lung cancer 1950–1994.

workplace is also popular with a large number of smokers, as well as nonsmokers.

The diversity of smoking prevalence in Europe is somewhat striking. While about a quarter of men and women smoke in Australia, Sweden and California; male rates in western Europe vary between one third and a half. Smoking among women is even more diverse but there are significantly low rates in, for example, Spain, where the male rate is high and doctors are known to smoke heavily.

Melanoma/nonmelanotic skin cancer

I would now like to spend some time discussing the way in which we have been able to influence Melanoma mortality in Australia in the presumption that in due course the same campaign will influence both melanoma incidence and nonmelanotic skin cancer incidence.

In the North of Australia (Queensland) the incidence of melanoma is approximately double that of the southern States and is the highest in the world. The rate/100,000/annum (Fig. 2), age standardised to the World Standard Population, is

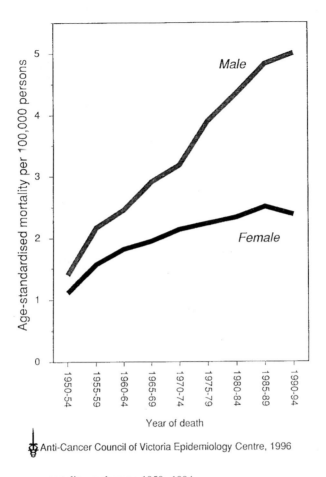

Fig. 2. Australian cancer mortality: melanoma 1950–1994.

for males, 47; for females, 36 in Queensland, while in the south of the country it is for males, 20; females, 19. These differences are striking and consistent with the role attributed to ultraviolet exposure. A similar variation is apparent for nonmelanotic skin cancer, which reaches a high incidence of 1,800/100,000/annum in the north.

Our campaign has two objectives: To decrease population exposure to ultraviolet, and to promote awareness of the problem among the general public and doctors with the expectation of achieving earlier diagnosis. We expected the latter objective to be met more rapidly. The campaign has been a serious endeavour since just before 1980 when modern sunscreens became available and we developed the campaign slogan, "slip (on a shirt); slap (on a hat); slop (on sunscreen)". A cartoon character was developed to accompany the slogan which was built in to a catchy jingle which turned out to be extremely popular with children. Our recent expenditure per head of population in Victoria was approximately 25 cents (300 Lire), which is a significant sum for a Public Health campaign. Specific programs were designed for doctors, children, adults, schools, workplaces, and attempts were made to bring about structural change such as tree planting in schools and kindergarten. A persistent attempt was made to diminish the cultural place of the traditional Australian suntan. The process has been measured by means of a weekly random sample of 150 Victorians through the summers since 1988.

In summary: attitudes to tanning have changed, beliefs about the desirability of suntans have diminished, the association of suntan with being healthy is less and the wearing of protective clothing and hats, and the use of sunscreens is increased. Sunburn persists but is measured as less frequent each year.

The campaign to achieve early detection has obviously been working since the early 1980s as the proportion of melanomas measuring less than 0.75 mm has been of the order of 50% in all registries for many years. The expected outcome of this was a reduction in mortality, which is close to zero in melanoma of this thickness. In 1993 a plateau appeared in male mortality and there was a slight downturn in female mortality and this trend is expected to continue. It is not possible to predict when incidence of melanoma and nonmelanotic skin cancer will occur, but the rate of change in measured public behaviour encourages us to expect it. These measures are not only of self-recorded behaviour, but of behaviour recorded objectively at sporting events over the years.

This experience demonstrates in a stark fashion what can be achieved in a 15-year time frame when the situation is conducive to change and all involved, including relevant industry, is working in the same direction.

Before turning to cervical and breast cancer I wish to point out that there are certain definable characteristics which should apply to population based early detection campaigns. These are:
1. The campaign should be offered to all at risk.
2. Should be organised.
3. Should be registered.
4. Should be regularly analysed.
5. The outcomes should be known.
I am in the unusual position of having had significant responsibility for a campaign aimed at cervical cancer which has resulted in a halving of mortality between 1965 and 1995 and which meets almost none of these criteria.

Based on this experience it was possible to design a breast cancer screening program which meets all of them and is now onstream in Victoria. It is still too early for mortality change to appear.

Cervical cancer

The Papanicolou (Pap) test was introduced into Australia in 1965. A free service was provided, publicity organised, doctors advised of the technique and the benefits, and supportive education was provided by the best means available to us in the 1960s and 70s.

By the mid-1980s it was possible to estimate that about half of the at risk age

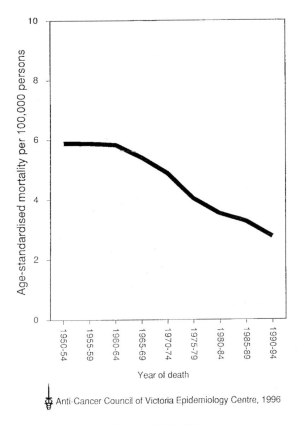

Year of death

Anti-Cancer Council of Victoria Epidemiology Centre, 1996

Fig. 3. Australian cancer mortality: cervical cancer 1950–1994.

groups had experienced at least one Pap test. It then became possible, with the voluntary cooperation of pathologists and a facilitating Act of Parliament, to establish a Pap registry which captured over 98% of tests performed. Using this facility to issue invitations and reminders has now achieved a cover of at least 80% in all the relevant age groups. Mortality, already moving down before the 1980s, is continuing on a downtrend which is expected to continue for some years (Fig. 3). Matching the Pap registry with the cancer registry allows confirmation of results and also accurate estimation of the failures of the program. This has significant implications for quality control.

Breast cancer

Breast screening has now been a reality as an organised program for 3 years in Victoria. The experience gained with cervical screening has been applied to this system. A central registry exists for all mammograms in the program. An invitation list for all women over 50 years is available. A single telephone number can accept bookings for any of the 44 screening clinics in the state. Radiologists contract to keep the recall rate below a set percentage and the biopsy rate similarly. Quality-control interviews record such events as pain. Specialist assessment clinics see most of the patients with suspicious lesions and the biopsy rate is also in accordance with agreed parameters.

While such a program was unthinkable 20 years ago, anything less is unthinkable in 1996.

Conclusions

Despite several decades of good quality research, we have reason to be dissatisfied by the results of both treatment and chemoprevention up to this time. However, the simple but vigorous application of existing knowledge has established an environment in which we can be confident that mortality reduction is set to occur, or continue to occur, for cancers of the lung, cervix, breast and melanoma. While prevention and early detection do not compete with treatment and chemoprevention, their demonstrated potential to create progressive mortality downtrends is much greater than has been anticipated. National governments have no excuses for persistent failure to apply the principles discussed here. Nowhere in this lecture is it suggested that research should be inhibited, but the last point I wish to make is that research which is allowed to lie unutilised might just as well not be done. Failure to implement discovery converts research from one of man's highest endeavours into an intellectual sport.

I thank you for your attention.

Contents

Opening lecture

The potential of chemoprevention in cancer control

Harri Vainio and Paul Kleihues

International Agency for Research on Cancer, Lyon, France

Abstract. Etiological (primary) prevention against the causes of cancer is inherently more effective than any form of prevention which takes place after the exposure to carcinogenic agents has already occurred. However, in practice, one often does not have a choice: exposure has already taken place or there are endogenous risk factors, e.g., genetic susceptibility to cancer. A new approach to cancer control is chemoprevention, which is not a substitute for primary prevention, but an additional element. It is defined as the use of specific natural or synthetic chemical agents to reverse, suppress or prevent carcinogenic progression to invasive cancer. Carcinogenesis is a multistep process characterized by the sequential acquisition of genetic alterations, and often has a long latent period before invasion and metastasis occur. Understanding of the carcinogenic processes should also provide essential elements for the development and appropriate use of effective chemopreventive agents. While clinical chemoprevention is still in its infancy, it has a potential role to play in preventing and suppressing tumour initiation and progression, especially in populations with a high risk of cancer. Sound scientific studies and clinical trials are needed to establish the potential role of chemoprevention in the future scenario for cancer control.

Key words: asbestos, β-carotene, dietary prevention, primary prevention.

Limits of etiological prevention

Primary prevention is defined in public health terminology as etiological prevention, i.e., as prevention directed against the source of disease. Primary prevention contrasts with later forms of prevention that involve the early detection of disease and the treatment of disease to prevent death and reduce disability. Primary prevention, by definition, is inherently more effective than secondary (screening) and tertiary (prevention of death and disability) prevention.

It has been estimated that one-third of all cancers in countries such as the USA and the UK could be avoided by acting on the specific etiological factors identified so far [1]. Tobacco smoke is the major carcinogenic risk factor in industrialized countries, accounting for some 30% of human cancer in those countries [2,3]. In the next few decades, tobacco will continue to be a major cause of mortality in developed countries and will become increasingly so in developing countries [4]. Epidemiological and, to some extent, experimental studies have identified some other specific risk factors, e.g., of occupational origin [5].

Lung cancer is the most frequent cancer worldwide, with some 900,000 new cases estimated to have arisen in 1985 [6]. Around three-quarters of these are due to

Address for correspondence: Dr Harri Vainio, International Agency for Research on Cancer, 150 cours Albert Thomas, 69372 Lyon Cédex 08, France. Fax: +33-72-73-85-75.

tobacco smoking [2]. Primary prevention of lung cancer is thus eminently feasible. Prevention (including cessation) of smoking is, in principle, a major component of cancer-control programs throughout the world. Despite this, the total tobacco usage in the world is now higher than ever before. Given current trends, by the time today's children reach middle age, the number of people killed annually by smoking (now 3 million) will have tripled, the main increase occurring in the developing world.

Asbestos is probably the most important occupational carcinogen worldwide. The first prospective epidemiological study of a population exposed to asbestos, published in 1955, provided unequivocal evidence supporting a causal relationship between exposure to asbestos and lung cancer [7]. Unfortunately, most countries did not take notice of these data at that time and only after hundreds of thousands of workers had been exposed to asbestos, has action been taken during the 1990s in many industrialized countries. Overall, the use of asbestos is decreasing in some in-dustrialized countries. However, in certain areas such as the ex-Soviet Union, only a minimal decrease has taken place and in some developing countries, asbestos use is still on the increase [8]. The cancers occurring today due to asbestos exposure reflect exposures occurring 20–40 years earlier, and models examining time trends indicate that the peak of the mesothelioma epidemic has not yet been reached. But banning the use of asbestos now does not help the people who have already had substantial occupational exposure to asbestos, with high amounts of fibres in their lungs; new approaches are, therefore, essential to prevent lung cancer (or mesothelio-ma) in these people. As a result of the widespread use in the past, there are millions of workers who have had significant exposure to asbestos, e.g., in shipyards, and for whom postexposure preventive measures in the form of chemoprevention would be of great value.

Primary prevention has been quite successful in the field of occupational cancer (for a review, see [9]). Legal initiatives to ban the use of a chemical (such as crocidolite asbestos), setting of stringent exposure limits (in the case of, e.g., vinyl chloride) and improving work practices and hygienic conditions at the workplace have succeeded in either eliminating or substantially decreasing worker exposure to carcinogenic agents. The identification of the chemical and physical hazards responsible for occupational cancers has led to specific preventive measures being taken as part of a wider recognition of the need to improve the working environment through the use of health protection technologies, without waiting for further evidence of health damage.

For cancers other than those caused by smoking, asbestos and other occupational agents, the etiology is more complex and involves interactions between various risk factors, the relative contributions of which may vary from population to population [10]. In particular, the epidemiological literature on the causative role of diet and nutrition is still confusing and contradictory [11,12].

Recently, increased emphasis has been placed on the role of infectious agents — viruses, bacteria and parasites — in human cancer. Viral infections have been estimated to play an etiological role in the induction of some 15% of cancers in humans [13], and probably more in developing countries. At the same time, it is evident that additional endogenous and exogenous risk factors are required for the neoplastic development of these virus-associated cancers. Within the past few years, it has become evident that human hepatitis viruses B and C can play a role in the causation of liver cancer [14]. Specific strains of human papilloma virus have been implicated in the causation of cervical cancer, penile and anal cancer, and some skin cancers [15]. There is also increasing evidence that the bacterium, *Helicobacter pylori*, plays a role in gastric cancer [16]. The infectious agents are uniquely amenable to primary prevention via immunization. Vaccines to prevent infection with hepatitis B are already in use, and many others are under development.

Natural history of carcinogenesis

The process of carcinogenesis often takes 20 or more years before invasion and metastasis occur. Current cancer incidences may reflect preventable exposures which occurred more than 2 decades earlier, including exposure to exogenous factors such as cigarette smoking, occupational exposures (e.g., asbestos fibres), viruses and pharmaceutical agents [10]. The development of fully malignant tumors involves complex interactions between several factors, both exogenous and endogenous (genetic, hormonal, immunological, etc.) (for review, see [17]). In addition, carcinogenesis proceeds through a number of discernible stages [18], often identified as initiation, promotion and progression. In initiation, a carcinogen interacts with DNA to produce a fixed stable genetic alteration after DNA replication. In promotion, which leads to the appearance of premalignant lesions, the initiated cells proliferate. Progression is the phase between a premalignant lesion and the development of invasive cancer.

The main factors determining the progress of carcinogenesis are the rates of the transitions between the successive stages. These transitions can be enhanced or inhibited by various agents. For chemoprevention, there is a high priority, therefore, to develop agents that can block mutagenic carcinogens, prevent cellular hyperproliferation and/or convert premalignant cells back to normal ones. The most efficient preventive agents may, however, turn out to be those that retard the progression of disease. This might be done by converting aberrant genes present in preneoplastic cells back to normal ones.

Chemoprevention based on studies on diet and nutrition

A major impetus for cancer control through chemoprevention stems from studies on diet and cancer. In Doll and Peto's 1981 report to the US Congress on the causes of avoidable cancer, the proportion of cancer deaths attributable to dietary problems was estimated at 35% with a range of acceptable estimates from 10–70% [19]. While the width of this range reflected the scale of uncertainties at that time, we are still, 15 years later, in almost the same situation. Recently, Willett [12] refined these estimates somewhat: the lower boundary is, according to him, well over 10% and the upper boundary is unlikely to exceed 40%. Evidence for the protective role of fruits and vegetables appears to be more consistent than that for other putative carcinogenic or protective dietary factors. In their review of case-control studies of nutrition and cancer, Steinmetz and Potter [20] found that 87% of the studies on raw and fresh vegetables showed a protective effect, as did 61% of the studies on raw and fresh fruits. Carrots were of special interest in many of the case-control studies because of the high levels of β-carotene. In a review of 34 studies on the effect of carrots, Steinmetz and Potter [20] reported that 27 showed a protective effect on cancer risk. Large observational cohort studies have confirmed that high and frequent consumption of fruits and vegetables is consistently correlated with a low risk of cancer (for a review, see [21]).

High blood levels of carotenoid and retinol have been consistently associated in various studies with a low risk of cancer [22]. β-carotene has received particular attention as a disease-preventing antioxidant, with scores of favorable reports in scientific journals and soaring sales of supplement. Observational epidemiological studies have long suggested that people who consume higher dietary levels of fruits and vegetables containing β-carotene have a reduced risk for certain types of cancer, especially lung cancer, and for cardiovascular diseases [23–25]. Proof of its efficacy as a chemopreventive agent has been sought through randomized, placebo-controlled intervention trials. However, the first, large-scale trial from Finland produced unexpected results: it suggested that β-carotene supplementation increased mortality from lung cancer and cardiovascular disease among male smokers [26]. Another large-scale trial among heavy smokers and asbestos-exposed workers in the USA ended prematurely when the researchers similarly recognized an elevated risk of death from lung cancer in the group receiving the β-carotene supplement [27]. The Physicians Health Study followed more than 22,000 US male doctors treated with 50 mg β-carotene or placebo every other day for an average of 12 years. It did not show any reduction in the incidence of cancer or mortality from cardiovascular disease with β-carotene supplementation [28].

The disappointing results with β-carotene demonstrate the difficulty in interpreting ecological or observational studies in terms of single substances, and emphasize the need for intervention trials before drawing conclusions.

Chemoprevention gives another avenue for cancer prevention

A chemoprevention strategy is distinct from a dietary prevention strategy or from chemotherapy. Cancer chemoprevention has been defined as the use of specific chemical compounds to prevent, inhibit or reverse carcinogenesis, whereas dietary prevention involves the modification of foods or dietary patterns [29].

Chemopreventive compounds are drugs and they are developed for clinical use like other pharmaceuticals. Some promising chemopreventive agents such as nonsteroidal anti-inflammatory drugs, for example, are already approved for other purposes.

It is important to note the difference between chemoprevention and chemotherapy. The drugs to be used in chemotherapy are meant for short-term usage in patients with diagnosed malignancies. Those to be used in chemoprevention, on the other hand, are used in "healthy" people for preventive purposes, often for long periods of time. Several types of population may benefit from chemoprevention:

1) Subjects at high risk from acquired risk factors (such as previous heavy exposure to asbestos fibres).
2) Subjects at high risk from genetic risk factors (such as women with breast cancer susceptibility (BRCA1 and BRCA2 genes)).
3) Subjects at high risk due to previously cured cancers (risk of second primary cancers, e.g., contralateral breast cancer).
4) Subjects with precancerous lesions (e.g., subjects with oral leukoplakias).

Intervention in people at high risk because of previous exposures is illustrated by the CARET trial in the US. This involved 18,000 smokers, former smokers and workers exposed to asbestos — all people with an obviously high risk of lung cancer. This trial evaluated combined treatment with β-carotene and retinol for an average of 4 years. The CARET study was interrupted in January 1996 because the intermediary evaluation found a 28% higher incidence of lung cancer in the active treatment group than in the placebo group [27]. Another trial on the effects of β-carotene in workers previously exposed to crocidolite asbestos in Australia began in 1990 but no results have yet been published.

The major advances made in cancer susceptibility testing may bring the subject of chemoprevention to the forefront. If a young woman is born to a family with a high risk for breast cancer and she is found to have a mutation in the BRCA2 gene, what should be done? [30]. It is remarkable that no chemopreventive studies have, so far, been carried out on people with an identified genetic predisposition.

Significant progress has been made in the adjuvant chemotherapy of breast cancer. Tamoxifen, a synthetic nonsteroidal triphenylethylene derivative, has been shown to cause a significant reduction (up to 40%) in the incidence of contralateral breast cancer after it has been used in adjuvant chemotherapy among women with breast cancer [31]. These data have been taken to indicate that tamoxifen would reduce the risk of a first breast cancer in women taking the drug as a purely preventive treatment. However, it is not yet known whether tamoxifen treatment would be preventive among those women who are at high risk for breast cancer because they are carriers of a BRCA1 gene mutation. Because of the potential serious toxicity of tamoxifen [32], such as endometrial and liver cancers and retinopathy, controversy exists over the conduct of intervention trials with tamoxifen [33]. The proponents of this approach consider that potential benefits outweigh the risks, mainly because of the potential beneficial effects on breast cancer, osteoporosis and heart disease. Prevention trials in "healthy" women are in progress in the US and UK.

Conclusions

Chemoprevention is a promising additional cancer control tool, which has a considerable growing database in animal and other experimental studies. The final proof of the safety and efficacy of the potential chemopreventive agents must,

8

however, be obtained in humans. So far, some of the large-scale, randomized, placebo-controlled interventions have produced disappointing results, such as those with β-carotene. With the major advances made in the understanding of the molecular mechanisms of the multistage process of carcinogenesis, chemoprevention must become more specific and less toxic. Chemoprevention has the potential to provide a new tool for people for whom etiological primary prevention has failed.

Acknowledgements

We thank Mrs A. Meneghel for her help in the preparation of the manuscript, and Dr J. Cheney for editing it.

References

1. Peto R. The preventability of cancer. In: Vessey MP, Gray M (eds) Cancer risks and prevention. Oxford: Oxford University Press, 1985;1—14.
2. Parkin DM, Pisani P, Lopez AD, Masuyer E. At least one on seven cases of cancer is caused by smoking. Global estimates for 1985. Int J Cancer 1994;59:494—504.
3. Peto R, Lopez AD, Boreham J, Thun M, Heath C Jr. Mortality from tobacco in developed countries: indirect estimation from national vital statistics. Lancet 1992;339:1268—1278.
4. WHO. Tobacco-attributable mortality: global estimates and projections. Tobacco Alert 1991;1:4—7.
5. IARC. Overall Evaluations of Carcinogenicity: An Updating of IARC Monographs Volumes 1 to 42. IARC monographs on the evaluation of carcinogenic risks to humans Suppl. 7. Lyon: International Agency for Research on Cancer, 1987.
6. Parkin DM, Pisani P, Ferlay J. Estimates of worldwide incidence of eighteen major cancers in 1985. Int J Cancer 1993;54:594—606.
7. Doll R. Mortality of lung cancer in asbestos workers. Br J Ind Med 1955;18:81—86.
8. Pearce N, Matos E, Vainio H, Boffetta P, Kogevinas M (eds) Occupational cancer in developing countries. IARC scientific publications No. 129. Lyon: International Agency for Research on Cancer, 1994;1—191.
9. Swerdlow AJ. Effectiveness of primary prevention of occupational exposures on cancer risk. In: Hakama M, Beral V, Cullen JW, Parkin DM (eds) Evaluating effectiveness of primary prevention of cancer. IARC scientific publications No. 103. Lyon: International Agency for Research on Cancer, 1990;23—56.
10. Tomatis L (ed) Cancer: causes, occurrence and control. IARC scientific publications No. 100. Lyon: International Agency for Research on Cancer, 1990.
11. Riboli E, Cummings JH. Ole Møller Jensen Memorial Symposium on Nutrition and Cancer. Int J Cancer 1993;55:531—537.
12. Willett WC. Who is susceptible to cancers of the breast, colon, and prostate? Ann NY Acad Sci 1995;768:1—11.
13. zur Hausen H. Viruses in human cancers. Science 1991;254:1167—1173.
14. IARC. Hepatitis viruses. IARC monographs on the evaluation of carcinogenic risks to humans, Vol 59. Lyon: International Agency for Research on Cancer, 1994.
15. IARC. Human papilloma viruses. IARC monographs on the evaluation of carcinogenic risks to humans, Vol. 64. Lyon: International Agency for Research on Cancer, 1995.
16. IARC. Schistosomes, liver flukes and *Helicobacter pylori*. IARC monographs on the evaluation of carcinogenic risks to humans, Vol. 61. Lyon: International Agency for Research on Cancer, 1994.
17. Vainio H, Magee PN, McGregor DB, McMichael AJ (eds) Mechanisms of carcinogenesis in risk identification, IARC Scientific Publications No. 116. Lyon: IARC, 1992.
18. Sugimura T. Multistep carcinogenesis: a 1992 perspective. Science 1992;258:603—607.

19. Doll R, Peto R. The causes of cancer: quantitative estimates of avoidable risks of cancer in the United States today. J Natl Cancer Inst 1981;66:1191–1308.
20. Steinmetz KA, Potter JD. Vegetables, fruit, and cancer. I. Epidemiology. Cancer Cause Cont 1991;2:325–357.
21. Hakama M. Why chemoprevention? In: Hakama M, Beral V, Buiatti E, Faivre J, Parkin DM (eds) Chemoprevention in cancer control. IARC Scientific Publications No. 136. Lyon: IARC, 1995;1–5.
22. Willett WC. Nutritional epidemiology. Oxford: Oxford University Press, 1990.
23. Peto R, Doll R, Buckley JD et al. Can dietary beta-carotene materially reduce human cancer rates? Nature 1981;290:201–208.
24. Sporn MD, Roberts AB. Role of retinoids in differentiation and carcinogenesis. Cancer Res 1983;43:3034–3040.
25. Moon RC, Mehta RG, Detrisac LJ. Retinoids as chemopreventive agents for breast cancer. Cancer Detect Prev 1992;16:73–79.
26. The Alpha Tocopherol, Beta Carotene Cancer Prevention Study Group (ATBC Study). The effect of vitamin E and beta carotene on the incidence of lung cancer and other cancers in male smokers. N Engl J Med 1994;30:1029–1035.
27. Omenn GS, Goodman GE, Thornquist MD et al. Effects of a combination of beta carotene and vitamin A on lung cancer and cardiovascular disease. N Engl J Med 1996;334:1150–1155.
28. Hennekens CH, Buring JE, Manson JE et al. Lack of effect of long-term supplementation with beta carotene in the incidence of malignant neoplasms and cardiovascular disease. N Engl J Med 1996;334:1145–1149.
29. Schatzkin A, Kelloff G. Chemo- and dietary prevention of colorectal cancer. Eur J Cancer 1995;31A:1198–1204.
30. Friend SH. Breast cancer susceptibility testing: realities in the postgenomic era. Nature Genet 1996;13:16–17.
31. O'Brian CA, Liskamp RM, Solomon DH et al. Inhibition of protein kinase C by tamoxifen. Cancer Res 1985;45:2462–2465.
32. IARC. Some pharmaceutical drugs. IARC monographs on the evaluation of carcinogenic risks to humans, vol. 66. Lyon: International Agency for Research on Cancer, 1996.
33. Jordan VC. An overview of considerations for the testing of tamoxifen as a preventive against breast cancer. Ann NY Acad Sci 1995;768:141–147.

The scientific bases of
cancer chemoprevention (1)

1996 Elsevier Science B.V.
The Scientific Bases of Cancer Chemoprevention.
C. Maltoni, M. Soffritti and W. Davis, editors.

Importance of genome modifications in carcinogenesis

Alain Sarasin and Leela Daya-Grosjean

Laboratory of Molecular Genetics, Institut de Recherches sur le Cancer, Villejuif Cedex, France

Abstract. Tumor cells contain numerous genetic rearrangements that have an important selective role during development of cancers. Among the sequence of events that occur there are initiating genetic alterations which are found in pretumoral cells and other genetic modifications which can allow tumor progression and the acquisition of metastatic properties. These mutational events take place over a long period of time after the action of a genotoxic agent, correlating with long latent periods for tumor development. Several hereditary syndromes associated with a high predisposition to cancer are due to mutations of either repair genes or tumor suppressor genes. Defects in repair pathways lead to an aggravated genetic instability whose outcome is the rapid formation of cancers.

Key words: cancer, DNA repair, mutagenesis, p53, ultraviolet.

The relationship between genetic instability and cancer has been put forward by scientists for a long time, but practical proof has only recently been made available. The genetic analysis of human tumor cells has shown the existence of a number of genetic modifications varying from point mutations to multiple chromosomal aberrations. These include chromosome rearrangements, ploidy changes and karyotypic alterations by chromosome loss or gain. It is evident that carcinogenesis is a multistep process whereby the accumulation of multiple genetic modifications in target cells result in a sequence of events that lead to neoplastic transformation. In fact, it has been estimated that the mutation frequency in the target tumor cell is significantly higher than that measured in cells using in vitro model systems [1]. It has been suggested that this high mutation rate is due to the acquisition of a generalized "mutator" phenotype [2] by the target cell resulting in progeny cells presenting numerous genetic alterations. In fact, the majority of the mutations tend to be lethal but the expression of certain mutations which provide selective advantage for proliferation allows the build-up of genetically unstable clonal cell populations.

Some mutations are acceptable and even necessary for variability and evolution, but cells are placed under strict controls in order to survive. The major control points operate at the DNA replication level ensuring that fidelity of replication is kept high (Fig. 1). A second important checkpoint occurs at G_2 where chromosome integrity is controlled before mitosis occurs. A number of genes, including the tumor suppressor

Address for correspondence: Alain Sarasin, Laboratory of Molecular Genetics, Institut de Recherches sur le Cancer - IFC1 - CNRS, BP. No. 8-94801 Villejuif Cedex, France. Tel.: +33-1-49583420. Fax: +33-1-49583443. E-mail: sarasin@lovelace.infobiogen.fr

14

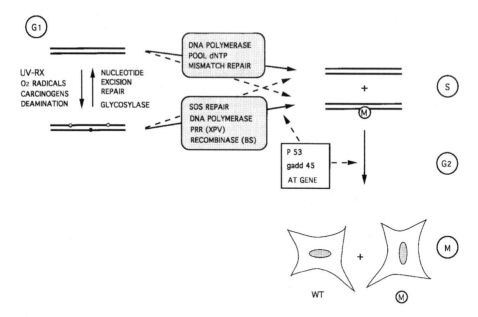

Fig. 1. Regulation of genetic stability through the cell cycle. Cellular DNA in G_1 should be replicated with high fidelity to avoid the appearance of mutation (M) in duplicated DNA (S Phase). Several repair pathways are able to repair the DNA before or after replication. (PRR: postreplication repair deficient in "XP" variant (XPV); BS: Bloom's syndrome). Several gene products can act as a "guardian of the genome" either at the G_1/S or G_2/M boundary (the p53 tumor suppressor gene, the Growth Arrest DNA damage gadd 45 or the ataxia telangiectasia gene). All these regulatory pathways give rise to normal cells (wt), or to mutated cells (M) if one of the pathways is not working well.

genes (e.g., p53) code for proteins which ensure the regulation of the cell cycle. In fact, these proteins integrate DNA repair and cell cycle progression, and their absence or modification by mutation result in loss of cell cycle control which can favor progression toward cell transformation.

Fidelity of DNA replication

The DNA replication fidelity measured in model systems shows that errors occur at 10^{-10} per base incorporated. This extraordinary high fidelity of replication can be attributed to different types of enzyme activity that exist in cells. DNA polymerases which replicate DNA by incorporation of the correct base by the Watson-Crick pairing rule, also possess proofreading activity with a fidelity of 10^{-6} ensuring that the correct base has been incorporated. Any errors that remain are detected by enzymes that recognize mismatches which after repair give a replication fidelity level of 10^{-10}. Mismatch repair, therefore, allows for the correction of errors not seen by the DNA polymerases and enables the integrity of the genetic information in the parental cell to be maintained. Bacteria deficient in these mismatch enzymes have been found to have 100- to 1,000-fold higher spontaneous mutation frequencies. In fact, mismatch repair and the genes involved is this repair pathway (Fig. 2) have been very well characterized in bacteria [3].

Four highly evolutionary conserved genes (from yeast to man) are essential for mismatch repair, mut S, mut L, mut U and mut H. The human hMSH2 gene (a homologue of mut S) codes for a protein which recognizes and binds mismatches. The human homologue to bacterial Mut L, hMLHI, codes for a protein which triggers the mismatch-repair process.

Genetic instability in hereditary colon cancers

Recent studies have demonstrated novel alterations of microsatellite DNA in tumor tissue and the instability of these highly polymorphic, short tandem repeats is due to errors in mismatch repair. In fact, these repetitions of di-, tri- or tetra-nucleotide motifs are difficult to replicate and are hotspots for replication errors as the DNA polymerase tends to "slip or slide" over these sequences either adding or deleting some of the repeat elements. Mismatch repair enzymes normally correct such errors and a defect in these enzymes results in microsatellite alterations. Indeed, the relationship between DNA microsatellite instability and mismatch repair defect was demonstrated clearly during genetic linkage analysis of hereditary nonpolyposis colon carcinoma (HNPCC) families. The HNPCC tumor cells are deficient in repair due to germ line mutations of hMSH2 [4] or hMLHI [5]. Two similar genes carrying mutations have also been isolated from some HNPCC patients. A genetic transmission

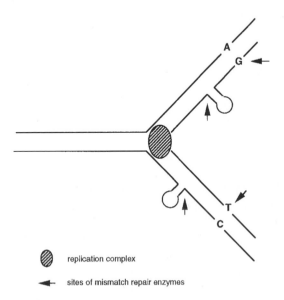

replication complex

sites of mismatch repair enzymes

Fig. 2. The role of mismatch repair enzymes in eliminating errors made by the DNA replication complex. After replication, errors left by the proofreading activity of the DNA polymerases can still exist. The mismatch repair complex is able to eliminate the mistakes (at sites of arrows) and gives rise to the normal genetic message.

of the mutated repair gene, followed by mutation of the second allele, gives rise to the colon cancers and a higher frequency of endometrial, stomach and urinary tract cancers [6,7].

Colon carcinoma cells in culture have mutation frequencies 500- to 1,000-fold higher than normal in certain target cells [8]. Hence, these tumor cells present a mutator phenotype which leads to the accumulation of mutations in the cell genome and in particular result in modifications of oncogenes and tumor suppressor genes.

At least 20 genes have been implicated in the regulation of spontaneous mutation levels in bacteria. So far only four human genes have been isolated, but one can easily predict that many more genes must be necessary for this regulation in mammalian cells. Modification in the expression of these genes can also initiate carcinogenesis (Fig. 1) as the gene product may be involved in any one of the regulatory pathways of the cell: DNA replication or repair, control of chromatin and chromosome structure integrity, control of gene copy number, regulation of recombination or transposition, etc.

Effects of genotoxic agents

All living cells are continuously submitted to DNA damage inflicted by a variety of genotoxic agents either endogenous (metabolically created free radicals, unstable nucleotide bases) or exogenous (UV or ionizing irradiation, chemical carcinogens, antitumor drugs). The existence of a number of repair systems protects the cells from the harmful effects of these agents by efficient removal of the lesions. Nucleotide excision repair (NER) is one of the highly conserved and most important and efficient pathways for eliminating the majority of DNA lesions [9,10]. Lesions produced by ultraviolet light (UV), the majority of chemical carcinogens (Aflatoxin B_1, polycyclic hydrocarbons, aromatic amines) or by certain drugs (mitomycin C, cisplatine, UVA psoralen/DNA cross-links) are all efficiently removed by NER (Fig. 3). Other repair mechanisms (base excision repair) can occur under specific conditions where alkylated bases or apurinic sites are repaired by specific DNA glycosylases.

It is evident that in the absence of efficient repair irreversible modifications of crucial genes can lead to tumor induction and/or progression [9,10]. This view is strengthened by the existence of highly cancer-prone human repair deficient syndromes which are particularly sensitive to specific genotoxic agents. Table 1 presents some of the more important syndromes including those hypersensitive to UV light, ionizing irradiation or cross-linking agents.

Spontaneous or induced chromosome instability

Spontaneous chromosome instability is found in three of the hereditary syndromes (see Table 1). Ataxia telangiectasia (AT) presents a particularly good correlation between genetic instability and cancer induction. Ataxia telangiectasia is an autosomal recessive disorder characterized by a particularly high sensitivity to ionizing irradiation. The incidence of AT in the population is 1 in 40,000 which gives rise to

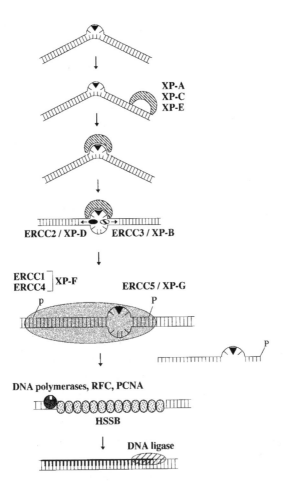

Fig. 3. Repair of UV-induced DNA lesions by the nucleotide excision repair pathway. After UV irradiation, DNA lesions such as cyclobutane pyrimidine dimer (CPD) and pyrimidine (6-4) pyrimidone (6-4) are produced (▲). The DNA repair pathway eliminates these lesions using various enzymes deficient in xeroderma pigmentosum patients (XPA to XPG). XPA, XPC and XPE proteins are part of a multicomplex pathway able to recognize DNA lesion. The separation of the two strands is obtained through the two helicase activities of XPB (ERCC3) and XPD (ERCC2) enzymes. Two endonucleases cut the damaged strand (XPF on the 5′ side and XPG on the 3′). After the removal of the damaged oligonucleotide, DNA polymerases and accessory proteins are able to fill in the gap which is then ligated to parental DNA.

1% AT heterozygotes in the general population [11]. Clinical symptoms are manifested at an early age by a progressive cerebellar ataxia together with neurological deterioration, skin disorders and a partial immunodeficiency. Patients who do not succumb to infectious diseases develop cancers, particularly B and T cell lymphomas and leukemias, as well as some solid tumors before the age of 20. The heterozygote parents of AT patients are also more susceptible to developing lymphomas and breast

Table 1. Main hereditary diseases linked to genetic instability.

Syndrome	Clinical characteristics	Tumor appearance	Biochemical and cellular characteristics
Xeroderma pigmentosum	– sun hypersensitivity – epithelioma on sun-exposed skin – neurological disorders	++++	– UV-hypermutability and hypersensitivity – excision repair deficiency – 8 genes
Cockayne's syndrome	– sun sensitivity – growth retardation – neurological disorders	–	– UV-hypersensitivity and hypermutability – deficient in preferential repair – 5 genes
Trichothiodystrophy	– growth and mental retardation – brittle hair – sun sensitivity	–	– UV-hypersensitivity and hypermutability – excision repair deficiency – low cystine level in hair protein – 4 genes
Ataxia telangiectasia	– progressive ataxia – neurological disorders – partial immunodeficiency – sensitive to ionizing radiations – lymphoma	++++	– hypersensitivity to ionizing radiations – chromosomal aberrations – abnormality in p53 induction – 1 gene
Fanconi's anemia	– anemia – growth retardation – leukemia	++	– hypersensitivity and crosslinking genotoxics – chromosomal aberrations – 4 genes
Bloom's syndrome	– sun hypersensitivity – growth retardation – all types of cancers	++++	– chromosomal aberrations – sister chromatid exchange increase – spontaneous recombinogenic activity – 1 gene

cancers are more common in young AT heterozygote women [12]. In fact, 5% of all cancers in the general populations appearing before the age of 45 are supposed to be related to the AT phenotype [11].

The high level of spontaneous chromosome aberrations found in AT patients together with their sensitivity to ionizing irradiation leads to a significant increase in chromosome rearrangements following radiation treatment. These anomalies concern in particular chromosomes 2, 7, 14 and 22 in AT patients and recent evidence has shown that the immunoglobulin genes or lymphocyte T receptors are implicated in these chromosome rearrangements [11].

AT is genetically heterogeneous, with four complementation groups suspected to represent different genes. Recently, the ATM gene, with a 12 kb transcript has been found to be mutated in AT patients from all complementation groups indicating it is probably the sole gene responsible for the disorder [13]. The ATM gene codes for a putative phosphatidylinositol-3' kinase active in mitogenic signal transduction, meiotic recombination and cell cycle control. Chromosome instability and the acute ionizing irradiation sensitivity shown by AT patients are not due to a known DNA repair defect. Irradiated ataxia telangiectasia cells present a peculiar characteristic in that they fail to show cell cycle arrest despite the presence of DNA lesions. In fact, the delay or absence of induction of the p53 protein and the gadd 45 gene can account for the cell cycle checkpoint failure in AT cells [14]. Without induction of p53, the G1/S checkpoint in the cell cycle is abolished and replication of DNA containing lesions results in the accumulation of genetic alterations (Fig. 1).

Hypersensibility to UV light and genetic instability

Several gravely afflicting human syndromes are characterized by UV hypersensitivity due to a defect in nucleotide excision repair (see Table 1). Among these rare, recessively transmitted hereditary syndromes, xeroderma pigmentosum, "XP", patients display an extraordinarily high frequency of skin cancers [9,10,15–17].

The severely photosensitive "XP" patients are characterized by an incidence of skin cancers on exposed parts of the body 1,000- to 4,000-fold higher than that found in the "normal" population [15,16]. In the most severe cases, "XP" patients start developing numerous cutaneous cancers on the face, hands and forearms from the age of 4 years onwards. Twenty to thirty percent of the "XP" patients present severe neurological disorders and symptoms vary greatly among "XP" patients indicating genetic heterogeneity. Indeed, "XP" presents the best model to date of a direct correlation between unrepaired DNA lesions and the early onset of cancers on sun-exposed skin. The analysis of cell lines established from the UV-sensitive patients has allowed the characterization and isolation of six human genes involved in nucleotide excision repair [17].

It is clear that in the absence of efficient repair, cells accumulate mutations following genotoxic insult. The direct relationship between such mutations and unrepaired DNA lesions is demonstrated by the specific mutation spectra observed in the ras oncogenes and p53 tumor suppressor gene of skin tumors from xeroderma pigmentosum patients [18–20]. Moreover, these spectra are identical to those found on target genes using in vitro model systems irradiated with UVB or C as the mutagenic agent. These results clearly indicate that the persistence of UV-induced DNA lesions in repair-deficient cells give rise to the UV-specific point mutations found in "XP" skin tumors [19,20].

Indeed, in "XP" tumors the presence of UV-specific point mutations results in a high level of gene modifications including amplification of several oncogenes. Therefore, "XP" represents a particularly important model in man of the effect of DNA repair defects which lead to a genetic instability of cells that can be directly associated to a high cancer incidence.

Multistep carcinogenesis

It is clear that human cancers develop by a complex multistep process that involves many genetic modifications. Major aberrations include chromosome gain or loss, rearrangements, as well as the more discrete, but nevertheless important, point mutations in the genome. It is clear that mutations accumulate with age and this can account for the long latent periods generally observed in the development of human cancers in general. Hence, one can hypothesize that the continued induction of mutations in cells leads to the formation of genetically modified target cells which after clonal selection evolve towards the establishment of a malignant phenotype. Therefore, during the aging process, more and more cells are able to gradually evolve towards a transformed phenotype or acquire metastatic properties (Fig. 4). Recessive germ line mutations of critical genes are a major characteristic of tumors found in families with a predisposition to cancer. Thus, in these familial cancer-prone syndromes, point mutations in a tumor suppressor gene (p53, Wt 1, retinoblastoma) result in very rapid formation of specific tumors. Hence, many of the steps necessary

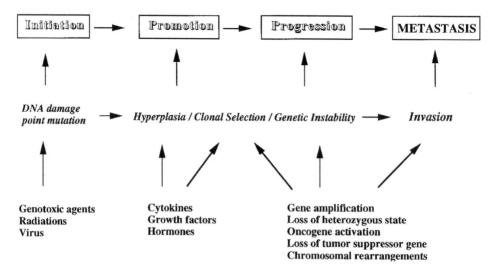

Fig. 4. Schematic overview of the main steps of the carcinogenesis mechanism.

in normal carcinogenesis progression are short circuited and cancer development is greatly accelerated. For example, mutation of the p53 gene results in a genetically unstable cell phenotype because the p53 protein cannot function normally as the "guardian of the genome" monitoring cells for DNA damage [21]. Wild-type p53 usually blocks the cell cycle following DNA damage in order to allow repair to take place before cell division. In the absence of this regulation, replication errors occur due to the presence of unrepaired lesions on the DNA, resulting in chromosome modifications of daughter cells rending them pretumoral.

Finally, the importance of the genes regulating DNA replication fidelity has come to light by the finding that the somatic or germline mutations in these genes result in a mutator phenotype. These cells undergo massive genetic modifications and mutations which result in an outbreak of tumoral cell clones (Fig. 4).

Conclusions

We have shown here that genetic instability can be due to a wide variety of factors and that the biological consequences may be very dramatic. Serious genetic aberrations can result in cell death or progression towards a transformed phenotype and other modifications can give rise to gravely afflicting illnesses. However, to a certain extent genetic instability is necessary to provide variation during evolution of the species. The ease with which some viruses can survive today by constant modification of their genomes has highlighted the importance of understanding the role of the regulatory mechanisms which exist for maintaining the integrity of the genome as this is crucial for mankind's future.

References

1. Chu EHY, Boehnke M, Hanash SM, Kuick RD, Lamb BJ, Neel JV, Niezgoda W, Pivirotto S, Sundling G. Estimation of mutation rates based on the analysis of polypeptide constituents of cultured human lymphoblastoid cell. Genetics 1988;119:693–703.
2. Loeb LA. Mutator phenotype may be required for multistage carcinogenesis. Cancer Res 1991;51: 3075–3079.
3. Radman M, Taddei F, Halliday J. Correction des erreurs dans l'ADN: de la génétique bactérienne aux mécanismes de prédisposition héréditaire aux cancers chez l'homme. Médecine/Sciences 1994; 10:1024–1030.
4. Peltomaki P, Aaltonen LA, Sistonen P et al. Genetic mapping of a locus predisposing to human colorectal cancer. Science (Washington DC) 1993;260:810–819.
5. Bronner CE, Baker SM, Morrison PT et al. Mutation in the DNA mismatch repair gene homologue hMLH1 is associated with hereditary nonpolyposis colon cancer. Nature (Lond) 1994;368:258–261.
6. Honchel R, Halling KC, Schaid DJ, Pittelkow M, Thibodeau SN. Microsatellite instability in Muir-Torre syndrome. Cancer Res 1994;54:1159–1163.
7. Thibodeau SN, Bren G, Schaid D. Microsatellite instability in cancer of the proximal colon. Science (Washington DC) 1993;260:816–819.
8. Bhattacharyya NP, Skandalis A, Ganesh A, Groden J, Meuth M. Mutator phenotypes in human colorectal carcinoma cell lines. Proc Natl Acad Sci USA 1994;91:6319–6323.
9. Hanawalt PC, Sarasin A. Cancer-prone hereditary diseases with DNA processing abnormalities. Trends Genet 1986;2:124–129.
10. Sarasin A. The paradox of DNA repair-deficient diseases. Cancer J 1991;4:233–237.

11. Aurias A. Ataxia-télangiectasie: aspects cliniques, épidémiologiques et génétiques. Médecine/Sciences 1994;10:957–961.
12. Swift M, Morrel D, Massey RB, Chase CL. Incidence of cancer in 161 families affected by ataxia-telangiectasia. N Engl J Med 1991;325:1831–1836.
13. Savitsky K, Bar-Shira A, Gilad S, Rotman G, Ziv Y, Vanagaite L, Tagle DA, Smith S, Uziel T, Sfez S et al. A single ataxia telangiectasia gene with a product similar to PI-3 kinase. Science 1995;268: 1749–1753.
14. Kastan MB, Zhan Q, El-Deiry W et al. A mammalian cell cycle checkpoint pathway utilizing p53 and GADD45 is defective in ataxiatelangiectasia. Cell 1992;71:587–597.
15. Cleaver JE. Defective repair replication of DNA in xeroderma pigmentosum. Nature 1968;218: 652–656.
16. Kraemer KH, Lee MM, Scotto J. Xeroderma pigmentosum. Cutaneous, ocular, and neurologic abnormalities in 830 published cases. Arch Dermatol 1987;123:241–250.
17. Stary A, Sarasin A. The genetic basis of xeroderma pigmentosum and trichothiodystrophy syndromes. Canc Surv 1996;26:(In Press).
18. Dumaz N, Drougard C, Sarasin A, Daya-Grosjean L. Specific UV-induced mutation spectrum in the P53 gene of skin tumors from DNA repair deficient xeroderma pigmentosum patients. Proc Natl Acad Sci USA 1993;90:10529–10533.
19. Dumaz N, Stary A, Soussi T, Daya-Grosjean L, Sarasin A. Can we predict solar ultraviolet radiation as a causal event in human tumors by analysing the mutation spectra of the p53 gene? Mutat Res 1994;307:375–386.
20. Daya-Grosjean L, Robert C, Drougard C, Suarez HG, Sarasin A. High mutation frequency in ras genes of skin tumors isolated from DNA repair deficient xeroderma pigmentosum patients. Cancer Res 1993;53:1625–1629.
21. Lu X, Lane DP. Differential induction of transcriptionally active p53 following UV or ionizing radiation: defects in chromosome instability syndromes? Cell 1993;75:765–768.

Genetic instability and cancer

Claes Ramel

Department of Genetic and Cellular Toxicology, Stockholm University, S-106 91 Stockholm, Sweden

Abstract. Since the 1970s, genetic instability and the dynamics of DNA have been the center of attention in genetic and molecular biology. An important source of this instability is provided by repeated DNA sequences, i.e., associated with many transposable elements. A major part of the noncoding DNA is organized as tandem repeats with units of different lengths, constituting mini- and microsatellites. This satellite DNA often exhibits an extreme variability and mutability. During the last few years it has been shown that such repeated sequences are responsible for several serious human diseases, including cancer. Mutations causing loss of mismatch repair results in increased instability of satellite DNA and increase of cancer, in particular colon cancer. The repeated DNA sequences of the ends of the chromosomes, constituting the telomeres, seem to play an important role in immortalization of cancer cells. While shortening of the chromosome ends cause a programmed cell death of normal somatic cells, the chromosomes of cancer cells are maintained intact by activation of the enzyme telomerase.

Key words: microsatellite, minisatellite, mismatch repair, telomere, transposition.

Introduction

When Watson and Crick presented their double-helix model of DNA, they provided a logical explanation of the high accuracy that the transfer of genetic information requires between cell generations. It was also soon demonstrated through in vitro experiments by Kornberg and others, that DNA replication did proceed with an extremely low frequency of errors. The precision of the replication process was only interrupted by the rare occurrence of spontaneous or induced mutations. The stability of DNA and the fidelity of the genetic system was almost a self-evident foundation in genetic research. The rigidity and exactness of the genetic system was manifested by the formulation of the central dogma, that the flow of information in the cells proceeded from DNA to RNA and from RNA to protein.

In the 1970s this concept of the stability of DNA and the genetic system was rather abruptly changed. DNA turned out to be far more dynamic than one had been able to foresee. The central dogma turned out to be not invariably true. The detection of reversed transcriptase showed that RNA could be transcribed to DNA and that had important consequences for the understanding of many processes such as insertion mutations, the foundation of pseudogenes from mRNA and retrovirus replication.

During the last few years, much debated reports by Cairns [1] and Hall [2] have even indicated the possibility that the substrate may influence the mutation direction of DNA in bacteria, which would hint at an influence from the opposite end of the genetic system.

In the early 1970s other signs of DNA dynamics became apparent such as restriction enzymes, reversible methylation of cytosine and the recognition of the significance of mobile DNA elements first recognized by McClintock almost 50 years ago.

It is tempting to make the general statement that genetic research concentrated on the stability of the genetic system before 1970 and on genetic instability since then. It, nevertheless, is a fact that the dynamics of DNA and the genetic system has played a crucial role in modern biological and medical research. In the last few years much data has been presented, which indicate the importance of genetic instability in cancer induction as well as several other diseases.

Genetic instability and the dynamics of DNA involve many diverse phenomena and no attempt will be made to cover all these aspects. The present survey will focus particularly on genetic instability associated with repeated DNA sequences.

Transpositions

The first accounts and analyses of genetic instability were provided by Barbara McClintock with the observation of genomic stress in maize, which led to her discovery of the transposition of mobile elements Ac (Activator) and Ds (Dissociation) almost 50 years ago (for an overview see [3]). In spite of McClintock's high reputation as a geneticist, the importance of her findings was not fully recognized until the 1970s when the same phenomenon was reported in *Drosophila* bacteria and subsequently in a wide variety of organisms. When McClintock received the Nobel prize in 1980, it was clear that unstable and mobile DNA elements occur throughout the organism world from bacteria to humans. As a matter of concern it can be mentioned that the wrinkled, recessive mutant of peas that Mendel used in his original experiment, in fact, constituted an insertion of a mobile DNA element, and the same is true for the first mutant analyzed by Morgan in *Drosophila*, i.e., white eyes.

The transposable elements are characterized by their ability to "jump" and settle down elsewhere in the genome, often causing mutational alterations. Although transposable elements have a wide distribution in all kinds of organisms, their contribution to mutagenesis varies between organisms. In *Drosophila* about 50% of all spontaneous mutations arc associated with transpositions of mobile elements. In man the contribution of transpositions seem to be far less; Kazazian [4] has estimated the frequency to about 1 out of 500 mutations.

Of evolutionary interest is the fact that a transfer of mobile elements from one species to another has been indicated in later years. One illustrative example of such a probable horizontal transfer of genetic material is provided by Robertson on a mobile element named mariner, which was first described in a species of *Drosophila* from Mauritius [5]. It turned out that the mariner transposon occurs in a wide variety of arthropods. By comparing the DNA sequence in different species one could build-up an evolutionary tree, indicating that the transposon had evolved about 200 million years ago. The development of the mariner transposon was in accordance with other phyllogenetic data, except on one point. Earwigs and bees had almost identical mariner sequence, in spite of the fact that they had separated about 150 million years ago. It indicated that the element must have been incorporated by horizontal transfer between the species. Interestingly, mariner transposons have also been found lately in humans and the data also indicate the occurrence of horizontal transfer [6].

The transposing elements are built-up according to a limited number of basic types. Two major groups can be identified — one that jumps from one place to another by means of RNA and reverse transcriptase, and one that jumps as DNA. The transposition of RNA to DNA requires a specific enzyme, transposase, which can be provided by the transposon itself or elsewhere in the genome.

Humans have a large number of potentially mobile elements, such as short interspersed elements (SINE) and long interspersed elements (LINE). SINE occur in 50,000 to 300,000 copies, LINE in about 100,000 copies. Both these elements move as RNA and get inserted by means of reverse transcriptase [7]. This enzyme is only coded by some LINE elements and they provide the enzyme machinery for the reverse transcription of other mobile elements lacking reverse transcriptase, such as the specific human Alu sequence. Beside these mobile elements HIV can also be considered a human retroviral transposon.

Transpositions of these mobile elements can evidently cause mutations and there are, for instance, cases of hemophilia which have been caused by the insertion of L1LINE retrotransposon. In one such case the origin of LINE could be established to chromosome 22. Seven L1 insertions and four Alu insertions causing diseases have been observed (one in a tumor suppressor gene, three in Duchenne/Becker muscular dystrophy) [4].

It is of interest in this context that stress situations can cause transpositions in experimental organisms. One example is what McClintock called "genomic stress" (see [3] for an overview). Experiments with maize, [8] and presumably, also in *Drosophila* [9], indicate that transposing elements can be mobilized by viral infections. Data by Biemond et al. [10] furthermore indicate that inbreeding also could cause mobilization of retrotransposons.

The occurrence, behavior and mutagenesis of mobile elements makes it highly probable that these elements are involved in carcinogenesis. The genetic instability at the later stages of carcinogenesis can be assumed to cause transpositions and mutations. It may also be of relevance with the observation in maize that mobile elements are inserted primarily at demethylated sites [11]. This is of interest because of the observation of hypomethylation of DNA in neoplastic cells [12]. However, the direct evidence of an association between transpositions and carcinogenicity is limited as yet. Integration of retrotransposons such as LINE in tumors have been recorded in the oncogenes c-mos [13] and in c-myc [14—16]. Integration of Alu has been observed in a plasmid introduced in human lung carcinoma cells [17]. It can also be mentioned that transformed cells (C3H10 1/2) contain RNA(s) with long terminal repeats, characteristic of retroviral transposons [18].

The fact that transposing elements have such a global occurrence in all kinds of organisms would indicate that these elements either fulfil some function or else behave as efficient parasite DNA, surviving by means of reproduction and transpositions. To my knowledge there is no convincing proof of an evolutionary function of transposable elements — it seems that, if anything, they cause trouble to the carriers. That would mean that the transposable elements would join the large group of DNA for which no adaptive function can be discerned and which has been characterized as "selfish" DNA by Orgel and Crick [19] and others. Other names such as parasite and "junk" DNA reflect the confusion about the function of this mostly noncoding DNA. As a matter of fact, only 3–4% of human DNA is transcribed into proteins. Even if some of the remaining 96 or 97% of DNA can be ascribed to regulatory functions, there is a large amount of DNA which seems to be dispensable. Another indication of this is the fact that some organisms have disproportionately large amounts of DNA. It is, for instance, certainly difficult to see why salamanders would need 20 times more DNA than man [19]. The transposable elements point to the large part of the genome without any obvious function, but which is responsible for a great deal of the instability of DNA. One predominant characteristic of that dynamic DNA is the organization with repeated sequence, which also applies to many of the transposable elements. Such repeat sequences constitute somewhat of a "biological dynamite". In later years this "junk" DNA has been subjected to intense research and although it still is difficult to discern any positive function of that DNA, it has been shown to be associated with several serious human diseases, including cancer.

"Extra" DNA

The 96–97% of the nuclear genome which does not contribute directly to genes transcribed into proteins, constitute DNA of different organizations. In order not to mark all this DNA as useless, a better name than "junk" or "selfish" DNA would be the more neutral expression of "extra" DNA. As a matter of fact, this "extra" DNA comprises of functional sequences for gene control as targets for transcription factors. There seems to be at least five regulatory sequences for each transcribed gene. The "extra" DNA can also count the introns of eukarote genes, which are spliced off at transcription.

Much of the "extra" DNA is organized as repeated sequences without any obvious function. It should be emphasized that amplification of DNA is not restricted to the "extra" DNA, but also many coding genes are amplified or can be induced to go through such a process. In many cases, an amplification of coding genes is an adaptive reaction towards an external influence, for instance, as a defence mechanism for detoxication of toxic agents such as amplification of metallothionein genes against heavy metals [20], and the amplification of the dehydrofolate gene giving resistance to methotrexate [21]. Another adaptive amplification occurs in *Drosophila* with the proximal heterochromatin coding for ribosomal DNA. In case of deletion of a part of that heterochromatin, the optimal number of genes is gradually restored [22]. Of particular importance in the present context is the amplification of nuclear oncogenes such as c-myc which results in an increase of their expression, which contributes to the induction of cancer.

The repeated DNA sequences of the "extra" DNA, mostly not transcribed, have been classified in:

— minisatellites: up to 100 bp, but mostly 9—30 bp;
— microsatellites: mostly 2—4 bp; and
— telomeres, telomerlike sequences, and centromeres.

Mini- and microsatellites often constitute highly unstable genetic systems with a high rate of length mutations — "dynamic mutations" — and sometimes also nucleotide mutations. The research concerning the distribution, properties and genetic alterations of these repeated sequences is only at the beginning, and therefore, the full consequences of such alterations, for example, concerning cancer induction, must be regarded as fragmentary at this point. But even so, the rapidly increasing number of cases, when alterations of the repeated sequences are associated with serious human diseases including cancer, suggests that further research will provide many additional examples of pathological effects of these repeated sequences, including induction of neoplasm.

Minisatellites

Minisatellites are noncoding repeats of up to 100 bp [23,24]. The number of minisatellite loci in the human genome has been estimated to 1,500/haploid genome [25,26]. Many of the minisatellite loci show an extreme polymorphism due to variation in the number of repeats, Variable Number of Tandem Repeats (VNTR). The genetic variability is due to a length mutation rate that can exceed 10% per gamete [27]. By means of DNA probes, which are able to simultaneously detect large numbers of hypervariable minisatellites, a pattern of fragments can be discerned in electrophoresis, which is unique for unrelated individuals. These properties provide the background for the "DNA fingerprinting" [28] which has obtained several important applications, such as a powerful tool in forensic medicine, as markers for linkage studies in genetic analyses, and for establishing paternity and kinship between individuals, both in human epidemiology and in animal biology populations.

In accordance with most other repeated sequences of the "extra" DNA, no obvious evolutionary advantage or function of the minisatellites can be established. On the other hand, there are some cases of pathogenic minisatellites. The best known case is the connection between cancer induction and minisatellite connected with the Ha-ras proto-oncogene locus, HRAS1 VNTR. That minisatellite is located 1,000 bp downstream of the polyadenylation signal [29]. The minisatellite is built-up by 28 bp, giving rise to about 30 alleles. Those alleles emanate from four alleles, comprising 94% of all existing alleles [30]. It was found that the rare alleles are three times more common in cancer patients than in controls, and those alleles are associated with multiple forms of cancer. Krontiris [31] has estimated that not less than one out of 11 cancer cases are associated with this minisatellite. The odds ratios for the association between the rare HRAS1 minisatellite alleles and cancer, according to Krontiris et al. [32], are shown in Table 1.

The mechanism behind this association between the HRAS1 minisatellite and cancer is not known, but two possibilities have been discussed [32,31]. It could be

Table 1.

Cancer	Odds ratio	p-value
Bladder	2.30	<0.001
Breast	1.68	0.001
Colorectal	2.21	0.002
Leukemia	2.29	0.001
Lung	1.55	0.051
Melanoma	1.56	0.091

the question of a linkage between the rare alleles and a potential disease locus. The minisatellite alleles would then only function as a marker for the disease locus and the risk of cancer. Considering the fact that the high-risk alleles derive from all four common alleles and presumably from many ancestral chromosomes, this hypothesis is not likely. An alternative hypothesis is based on the finding that the HRAS1 minisatellite binds to the rel NF-kB family of transcriptional regulatory factors [33,34]. It is suggested that the pathogenic minisatellite may disrupt nonpathogenic interactions with rel proteins.

It can be added that a somewhat similar pathogenic situation has been indicated for minisatellite mutations linked with the insulin gene (INS). The presence of one class of minisatellite alleles is associated with a doubling of the relative risk for type 1 diabetes mellitus [31]. Likewise, a minisatellite upstream of the human immuno-globulin heavy-chain gene IGH enhancer may have a suppression effect on immuno-globulin gene expression by a similar transcriptional control as HRAS1 [35].

Microsatellites

Microsatellite DNA, built-up of short-repeat units, have a wide distribution in multicellular organisms. Tandem repetitions of these short sequences can be formed as an error during DNA replication, and further amplification through strand slippage can take place at successive DNA replication. The evolution of microsatellites varies from a high stability with conserved sequences for millions of years, to an exceedingly high instability, when every cell has a different length of the microsatellite. The high instability is associated with GC-rich trinucleotides and CA dinucleotides, which can exhibit mutation frequency orders of magnitudes higher than other tandem repeats [36].

As with other repeated "extra" DNA sequences, hardly anything but disadvantages can be discerned with the microsatellites. The accumulation of simple repeat sequences can be expected to imply an increased risk of homologous recombination between different chromosomal segments, resulting in translocations, deletions and inversions. Fungi-like *Neurospora* does not seem to tolerate the accumulation of these DNA sequences, and they have developed a specific system to get rid of excessive "extra" DNA of that kind — Repeat Induced Point Mutations (RIP) [37]. RIP recognizes amplified sequences and induces GC to AT mutations, probably through methylation of cytosine and deamination of 5-methylcytosin. This kind of "genome cleaning" apparently functions as a defence mechanism not only against "extra" DNA but also against viruses and transposons. Although vertebrates have a higher tolerance level for this kind of "extra" DNA, Kricker et al. [38] have pointed out that also the accumulation of repeated sequences would imply a "genetic time bomb" because of illegitimate recombination. Therefore, also in vertebrates, a strategy based on methylation and deamination of CpG has been developed. These data indicate that at least most microsatellites lack any biological function and they constitute true "parasite" DNA.

It should be added that there are connections between the different "extra" DNA sequences in vertebrates. It is, thus, likely that minisatellites have evolved from microsatellite sequences and in that process transpositions may have been involved. In a "transposition model" Jeffreys et al. [23] have proposed that related core sequences which can be observed between minisatellites are the result of transpositions, mediated by sequences flanking the minisatellites. In support of that hypothesis it has been observed that some minisatellites have dispersed repetitive sequences such as the human Alu and other transposonlike sequences. The involvement of microsatellites in the formation of minisatellites is also indicated by the occurrence of microsatellite sequences in close association or with minisatellite VNTR(s) [39].

Microsatellites and human diseases

During the last few years, microsatellites have been the subject of much scientific attention because of the direct connection between microsatellites and several human neurological disorders. Although no such causative association has been established between microsatellites and cancer induction as mentioned above, we are probably only in the beginning of perceiving pathological effects of microsatellites, and it seems likely that some steps in cancer induction will be shown to be affected by microsatellites.

For this reason it may be justified to give a brief overview of diseases caused by microsatellite mutations. The main neurological diseases that have been associated with an expansion of CG rich trinucleotides [40] are shown in Table 2. These microsatellites are linked to coding genes which are inactivated by an expansion of

Table 2.

Disease	Reiterated Trinucleotide	Normal range of reiteration	Disease range of reiteration
Spinal and muscular atrophy, Kennedy's disease	CAG	11–33	40–62
Huntington's disease	CAG	11–34	42–100
Spinocerebellar ataxia type 1	CAG	<29–36	43–>60
Fragile X	CGG	6–54	250–4.000
Myotonic dystrophy	CTG	5–30	>50

the microsatellite sequence above a certain number, usually about 35 tandem copies. The diseases represent two classes of microsatellite interactions. In Fragile X and Myotonic dystrophy the microsatellite is not included in the coding part of the genes, while in Huntington's disease, Kennedy's disease and Spinocerebellar ataxia, the microsatellite is located within the coding part of the gene, giving rise to polyglutamine. Above a critical number of repeats the system becomes unstable and more sequences are added, eventually resulting in symptoms. Another characteristic of these diseases is the fact that the symptoms tend to be more severe and appear in younger age in subsequent generations. This is due to an expansion of the trinucleotide sequence during gametogenesis or in the zygote, a process which has been named genetic anticipation. The molecular background of this effect by microsatellite expansion is not clear, although some possible hypothesis have been proposed, based on an interaction with the secondary structure of DNA [41,42] and interactions with nucleosomes [43,44].

Microsatellites and mismatch repair

There is another reason for bringing up microsatellites in the present context with cancer induction. The loss of the mismatch repair function in humans has been shown to lead to a genetic instability and the induction of cancer. This genetic instability causes a burst of mutations in microsatellites in which length mutations are dependent on mismatch repair. Such a genetic instability of microsatellites has been observed in colorectal and several other cancer forms. Microsatellites and microsatellite instability have, therefore, become markers for cancer.

The genetic background of hereditary nonpolyposis colon cancer, HNPCC, which is responsible for 15% of colorectal cancers, was shown, by two research groups with DelaChapelle and Vogelstein [45,46], to be associated with a gene in chromosome 2. In tumors of HNPCC patients a pronounced instability of microsatellites could be observed. The similarity of this phenomenon with a deficiency of mismatch repair in coli bacteria and yeast, *Saccharomyces cerevisiae*, [47] lead to the discovery that HNPCC cases depended on the loss of functional mismatch repair genes, closely homologous to corresponding bacterial and yeast mismatch repair genes.

Further research has revealed and identified three more human mismatch repair genes. The genes linked to HNPCC are shown in Table 3 [48].

The induction of colon cancer is caused by a loss of heterozygosity for the wildtype allele and consequently loss of mismatch repair function. Up to 1/200 have been

Table 3. Mismatch repair genes

E. coli	S. cerevisiae	Homo	% HNPCC
MutS	MSH2	hMSH2	50
MutL	MLH1	hMLH1	30
MutL	PMS1	hPMS1	5
MutL		HPMS2	5

estimated to carry mutant alleles of these genes. The induction of colon cancer is caused by a loss of heterozygosity for the wild-type allele and consequently, loss of mismatch repair function. Up to 1/200 have been estimated to carry mutant alleles of these genes. The induction of cancer is caused by the large increase of mutations by deficiency of the mismatch repair function. The situation is, however, more complicated. Parsons et al. [48] have reported that a subset of HNPCC patients have a high frequency of microsatellite mutations not only in the tumors but also in nonneoplastic cells. Nevertheless, these patients had very few tumors. Loss of mismatch repair and the accompanying mutations can evidently be compatible with normal development and is not sufficient for tumor development. This data has caused Bridges [49] to raise the question whether mutation induction constitutes a rate-limited step in carcinogenesis.

Telomeres

The DNA polymerase cannot replicate both DNA strands to the end and in order not to lose any coding sequence the chromosomes have ends with repeated nucleotide sequences of 5–8 bp, which constitute the telomeres. The shortening of the telomeres at each cell division is counteracted by an enzyme synthesizing new telomere sequences, telomerase. The telomerase has an unusual organization with a protein and a stretch of RNA. The repeated DNA of the telomere is replaced by means of reverse transcription of the RNA part of the enzyme [50,51]. The composition of the telomere repeats varies considerably between organisms. *Drosophila* has an exceptional telomere with elements like LINE mobile elements, and the replacement of the telomeres does not occur by means of telomerase, but through transposition of the telomere sequence to the chromosome ends [52].

It has been shown that somatic cells lose their telomerase activity and consequently the chromosomes shorten at each cell division, ending with the death of the cell. It has been hypothesized that this system constitutes a biological clock, resulting in a programmed cell death after a certain number of cell divisions [53]. Of importance in the present context is the observation that while the telomerase activity was repressed in normal somatic cells, the telomerase activity was reactivated in immortal cancer cells [54]. The immortalization of the cells is an important property of neoplastic transformation. The connection between telomerase activity and immortalization opens the possibility of using the telomere and telomerase as a target for cancer therapy.

Telomere repeats in mammalian cells (TTAGGG) also occur interstitially. Such telomerelike repeats (TLR) show an elevated frequency of chromosome breaks and chromosome aberrations. There are also indications of an increased amplification, and, at least in Paramecium, illegitimate recombination. The high frequency of chromosome aberrations with TLR can probably be linked to the tendency of G-rich DNA to get involved in non-Watson-Crick pairing, notably G-quartets. This property of G-rich DNA is also manifested in the formation of the bouquet stage in the beginning of meiosis, when the chromosome ends pair.

Genetic instability and multistage carcinogenesis

The development of cancer is a multistep process involving both genetic and non-genetic alterations. On the basis of skin-painting experiment on mice, the sequence of events has been classified into initiation, promotion and progression [55]. As shown by Vogelstien and his group [56] the induction of colorectal cancer involves a series of up to eight mutations of oncogenes and suppressor genes. The accumulation of such a series of mutations in one and the same cell cannot occur as a random process, but must be the result of selection and/or a genetic instability, increasing the mutation frequency drastically. Clonal expansion of mutated oncogenes and suppressor genes have been postulated and observed [57,58] and it is a well-known fact that the later stages of tumor induction, the progression, is often characterized by a high degree of genetic instability, giving rise to a cascade of chromosome aberrations, aneuploidy and other genetic alterations. There are several possible mechanisms for this genetic instability. An obvious one is the loss of DNA repair capacity, such as the loss of mismatch repair function, as mentioned before. Another similar kind of mutator phenotype can be brought about by eliminating the control of the cell cycle. The tumor-suppressor gene p53 functions as a checkpoint of the cell cycle at least at two points. Thus, p53 stops the cell division at G1 if DNA is damaged. Such damaged cells will be subjected to programmed cell death (apoptosis) or possibly temporary arrest until the DNA damage is repaired. A loss of this check point will evidently result in a mutator phenotype with an increase of mutations. Another checkpoint by p53 has been identified before mitosis, arresting the cells in case of spindle fiber disturbance, thus preventing the formation of polyploid or aneuploid cells [59].

Inactivation of p53 also might lead to other genomic instability. Human and mouse fibroblasts, which lack functional p53, show higher frequency of gene amplification than cells with wild-type p53 [60,61].

References

1. Cairns J, Overbaugh J, Miller S. The origin of mutants. Nature 1988;335:142–145.
2. Hall BG. Adaptive evolution that requires multiple spontaneous mutations. I. Mutatins involving insertion sequence. Genetics 1988;120:887.
3. McClintock B. The significance of response of the genome to change. Science 1984;226:792–801.
4. Plasterk RHA. Molecular mechanisms of transposition and its control. Cell 1993;74:781–786.
5. Robertson HM. The mariner transposable element is widespread in insects. Nature 1993;362: 241–245.
6. Oousumi T, Belknap WR. Mariner transposon in humans. Nature 1995;378:672.
7. McDonald JF. Evolution and consequences of transposable element. Curr Opin Genet Devel 1993; 3:855–864.
8. Johns MA, Mottinger J, Freeling M. A low copy number, copia-like transposons in maize. EMBO J 1985;4:1093–1101.
9. Gershenson SM. Viruses as mutagenic factors. Mutat Res 1986;167:203–213.
10. Biémond C, Aouar A, Arnault C. Genome reshuffling of the copia element of an inbred line of *Drosophila melanogaster*. Nature 1987;329:742–744.
11. Wessler SR. Phenotypic diversity mediated by the maize transposable element Ac and Spm. Science

1988;242:399—405.

12. Feinberg AP, Vogelstein B. Hypomethylation distinguishes genes of some human cancers from their normal counterpart. Nature 1983;301:89—92.

13. Rechavi G, Givol D, Canaani E. Activation of cellular oncogene by DNA rearrangement: possible involvement of an IS-like element. Nature 1982;300:607—611.

14. Katzir N, Rechavi G, Cohen JB, Unger T, Simoni R, Cohen D, Givol D. "Retroposon" insertion into the cellular oncogene c-myc in canine transmissible venerial tumor. Proc Nat Acad Sci 1985;82:1054—1058.

15. Pear WS, Wahlström G, Nelson SF, Axelson H, Szeler A, Wiener F, Bazin H, Klein G, Sümegi J. 6,7 chromosomal translocation in spontaneously arising rat immunocytomas; evidence for c-myc breakpoint clearing and correlation between isotypic expression and the c-myc target. Molec Cell Biol 1988;8:441—451.

16. Morse B, Rothberg PG, South VJ, Spandorfer JM, Astrin SM. Insertional mutagenesis of the myc locus by a LINE-1 sequence in a human breast carcinoma. Nature 1988;333:87—90.

17. Lin CS, Goldtwait DA, Samols D. Identification of Alu transposition in human lung carcinoma cells. Cell 1988;54:153—159.

18. Kirschmeyer P, Gattonicelli D, Dina D, Weinstein IB. Carcinogen-transformed and radiation-transformed CH3 10 1/2 cells contain RNAs homologous to the long terminal repeat sequence of a murine leukemia virus. Proc Nat Acad Sci 1982;74:2773.

19. Orgel LE, Crick FHC. Selfish DNA: The ultimate parasite. Nature 1980;284:604—607.

20. Hamer DH. Metallothionein. Ann Rev Biochem 1986;55:913—951.

21. Schimke RT. Gene amplification, drug resistance and cancer. Cancer Res 1984;44:1735—1742.

22. Ritossa FM. Unstable redundancy of genes for ribosomal RNA. Proc Nat Acad Sci USA 1968;600:509—516.

23. Jeffreys AJ, Wilson V, Thein SL. Hypervariable minisatellite region in human DNA. Nature 1985a;314:67—73.

24. Nakamura Y, Leppert M, O'Connell P et al. Variable number of tandem repeat (VNTR) markers for human mapping. Science 1987;235:1616—1622.

25. Braman J, Barker D, Schumm J, Knowlton R, Donis-Keller H. Characterization of very high polymorphic RFLP probes. Cytogenet Cell Genet 1985;40:589.

26. Jeffreys AJ. 23rd Colworth medal lecture: Highly variable minisatellites and DNA fingerprint. Biochem Soc Trans 1987;15:309.

27. Jeffreys AJ, Royle NJ, Wilson V, Wong Z. Spontaneous mutation rates to new length alleles at tandem repetitive hypervariable loci in human DNA. Nature 1988;332:278—281.

28. Jeffreys AJ, Wilson V, Thein SL. Individual-specific "fingerprints" of human DNA. Nature 1985b;314:76—79.

29. Capon DJ, Chen EY, Levinson AD, Seeburg PH, Goedder DV. Complete nucleotide sequence of the T24 human bladder carcinoma oncogene and its normal homologue. Nature 1983;302:33—37.

30. Kasperszyk A, DiMartino NA, Krontiris TG. Minisatellite allele diversification: the origin of rare alleles of the HRAS1 locus. Am J Human Genet 1990;47:854—859.

31. Krontiris TG. Minisatellites and human disease. Science 1995;269:1682—1683.

32. Krontiris TG, Derlin B, Karp DD, Robert NJ, Risch N. An association between the risk of cancer and mutations in the HRAS1 minisatellite locus. N Engl J Med 1993;329:517—523.

33. Trepicchio WL, Krontiris TG. Members of the rel/NF-kB family of transcriptional regulatory factors bind the HRAS1 minisatellite DNA sequence. Nuc Acid Res 1992;20:2427—2434.

34. Green M, Krontiris TG. Allelic variation in reporter gene activation by the HRAS1 minisatellite. Genomics 1993;345:429—434.

35. Trepicchio WL. IGH minisatellite suppression of USF-binding site and Em-mediated transcriptional activation of the adenovirus major late promoter. Nuc Acid Res 1993;21:977—985.

36. Kuhl DPA, Caskey CT. Trinucleotide repeats and genome variation. Curr Opin Genet Devel 1993;3:404—407.

37. Selker EU. Premeiotic instability of reperated sequences in Neurospora crassa. Ann Rev Genet

24:579—613.
38. Kricker MC, Drake, JW, Radman M. Duplication-targeted DNA methylation and mutagenesis in the evolution of eukaryotic chromosomes. Proc Nat Acad Sci 1992;89:1075—1079.
39. Wright JM. Are minisatellites the evolutionary progeny of microsatellites? Genome 37:335—346.
40. Green H. Human genetic diseases due to codon reiteration: relationship to an evolutionary mechanism. Cell 1993;74:955—956.
41. Yano-Yanagisawa H, Li Y, Wang H, Kohwi Y. Single-stranded DNA binding proteins isolated from mouse brain recognize specific trinucleotide repeat sequences in vitro. Nuc Acid Res 1995;23: 2654—2660.
42. Gacy AM, Goellner G, Juranic N, Macura S, McMurray CT. Trinucleotide repeats that expand in human disease form hairpin structures in vitro. Cell 1995;81:533—540.
43. Wang Y-H, Amirhaeri S, Kang S, Wells RD, Griffith JD. Preferential nucleosome assembly at DNA triplet repeats from Myotonus Dystrophy gene. Science 1994;265:669—671.
44. Aaltonen LA, Peltomäki P. Leach FS et al. Clues to the pathogenesis of familial colorectal cancer. Science 1993;260:812—816.
45. Peltomäki P, Aaltonen LA, Sistonen P et al. Genetic mapping of a locus predisposing to human colorectal cancer. Science 1993;260:810—812.
46. Strand M, Prolla TA, Liskay RM, Petes T. Destabilization of tracts of simple repetititve DNA in yeats by mutations affecting DNA mismatch repair. Nature 1993;365:274—276.
47. Modrich P. Mismatch repair, genetic stability, and cancer. Science 1994;266:1959—1960.
48. Parsons R, Li G-M, Longley M et al. Mismatch repair deficiency in phenotypically normal human cells. Science 1995;268:738—740.
49. Bridges B. Mutations not sufficient for carcinogenesis? Science 1995;269:898.
50. Zakian VA. Telomeres; Beginning to understand the end. Science 1995;270:1601—1607.
51. Lingner J, Cooper JP, Cech TR. Telomerase and DNA end replication; No longer a lagging strand problem? Science 1995;269:1533—1534.
52. Mason JM, Biessmann H. The unusual telomeres of Drosophila. Trends Genet 1995;11:58—62.
53. Harley CB, Futcher AB, Greider CW. Telomeres shorten during ageing of human fibroblasts. Nature 1990;345:458—460.
54. Kim NW, Piatyszek MA, Prowse KR et al. Specific association of human telomerase activity with immortal cells and cancer. Science 1994;266:2011—2015.
55. Berenblum I. The mechanism of carcinogenesis. Cancer Res 1941;1:807.
56. Fearon ER, Vogelstein B. A genetic model for colorectal tumorigenesis. Cell 1990;61:759—767.
57. Nowell P. The clonal evolution of tumor cell populations. Science 1976;194:23—28.
58. Sidransky D, Mikkelsen T, Schwechheimer K, Rosenblum ML, Cavanee W, Vogelstein B. Clonal expansion of p53 mutant cells is associated with brain tumor progression. Nature 1992;355:846—847.
59. Cross SM, Sanchez CA, Morgan CA, Schimke MK, Ramel S, Iczerda RL, Raskind WH, Reid BJ. A p53-dependent mouse spindle checkpoint. Science 1995;267:1353—1356.
60. Livingstone LR, White A, Sprouse J, Livanos E, Jacke T, Tlsty TD. Altered cell cycle arrest and gene amplification potential accompany loss of wild-type p53. Cell 1992;70:923—935.
61. Yin Y, Tainsky MA, Bischoff FZ, Strong LC, Wahl GM. Wild-type p53 restores cell cycle control and inhibits gene amplification in cells with mutant p53 alleles. Cell 1992;70:937—948.

The Scientific Bases of Cancer Chemoprevention.
C. Maltoni, M. Soffritti and W. Davis, editors.

Disturbances in cell cycle control as targets for cancer chemoprevention: the cyclin D1 paradigm

Alessandro Sgambato[*], Ping Zhou, Nadir Arber, Wei Jiang[**] and I. Bernard Weinstein

Columbia-Presbyterian Comprehensive Cancer Center, Columbia University, College of Physicians and Surgeons, New York, USA

Abstract. A characteristic feature of the carcinogenic process is the long-latency period. In humans this time interval is usually decades. At the mechanistic level the basis for the latency period most likely reflects the time required for the successive acquisition of numerous mutations in DNA, repetitive cycles of clonal expansion and cell selection, and epigenetic changes in gene expression, in the evolving tumor.

An optimistic aspect of the latency period and the multistage nature of the carcinogenic process is that it offers numerous opportunities for intervention before fully malignant tumors develop, using various approaches including chemoprevention. At the same time, a rationale scientific approach to cancer chemoprevention and the development of more clinically effective agents requires a better understanding of the cellular and molecular events involved in the various stages of the carcinogenic process. A large number of so-called oncogenes and tumor-suppressor genes have been implicated in the multistage carcinogenic process. Functionally, they can be divided into two categories: 1) those that control intracellular circuitry and signal transduction pathways which ultimately influence gene expression, and 2) those that play a direct role in cell surface and extracellular functions.

Recent studies indicate that the function of genes that control the cell cycle, particularly cyclin D1, are also disturbed during the carcinogenic process and that these changes perturb both cell proliferation and genomic instability, thus enhancing the process of tumor progression. Therefore, cyclin D1 and related proteins might be useful biomarkers and also targets for cancer chemoprevention.

Key words: cancer, cell cycle, chemoprevention, cyclins, cyclin-dependent kinases.

Introduction

Chemoprevention is rapidly evolving as a new strategy for cancer control based on pharmacological or nutritional interventions to prevent, block or reverse the process of tumor formation before fully malignant tumors develop.

Carcinogenesis is a multistep process in which several events are required to produce cancer. An understanding of these different steps at the cellular and molecular level is required for a rationale scientific approach to cancer chemoprevention and the development of more clinically effective agents.

Several models have been proposed to explain the process of tumor development.

Address for correspondence: Bernard Weinstein, Columbia-Presbyterian Cancer Center, 701W 168th Street Room 1509, New York, NY 10032, USA. Tel.: +1-212-305-6921. Fax: +1-212-305-6889.
*Current address: Centro di Ricerche Oncologiche "Giovanni XXIII", Catholic University, Largo Francesco Vito 1, 00168 Rome, Italy.
**Current address: The Salk Institute, La Jolla, CA 92037, USA.

Table 1. Cellular and molecular events in cancer development

1. Successive acquisition of numerous mutations in various cellular genes.
2. Repetitive cycles of clonal expansion and cell selection.
3. Epigenetic changes in gene expression.
4. Progressive acquisition of genome instability.

One of these is the model of clonal evolution, first proposed by Nowell in 1976 [1]. In this model, the accumulation of multiple mutations in the progeny of cells derived from a single cell, which originally acquires a cancer predisposing mutation, is responsible for the development of a fully malignant tumor. Subsequent research has elucidated that several types of events are required for this process (Table 1). Thus, the occurrence of multiple mutations is associated with repetitive cycles of cell selection and clonal expansion. Genomic instability plays an important role by facilitating the formation of mutant cells in the expanding tumor population. Mutations which confer a selective growth advantage over the surrounding cells will be retained and will contribute to the formation of sublines that are increasingly abnormal and genetically unstable. Epigenetic (i.e., nonmutational) changes probably also contribute to this process by altering gene expression, although this aspect requires more intensive studies.

The complexity of these events is responsible for a characteristic feature of the carcinogenic process, observed both in experimental models and in humans, which is the long period of latency between the first exposure to carcinogenic factors and the development of a fully malignant tumor. Several types of evidence confirm the existence of the latent period (Table 2) and different factors may affect, both positively and negatively, its length (Table 3).

An optimistic aspect of the latency period is that it offers numerous opportunities for intervention before fully malignant tumors develop. Chemoprevention strategies are possible at different levels. Thus, chemopreventive agents include substances that reduce absorption of carcinogens, such as dietary fibers; substances that reduce the synthesis of carcinogens in the body, such as vitamin C which inhibits the formation of nitrosamines in the stomach; chemicals that inhibit the metabolic activation of carcinogens or enhance their detoxification and/or excretion such as benzyl isothiocyanate, which is present in cruciferous vegetables, selenium, β-carotene and other antioxidants; chemicals that trap ultimate carcinogens preventing their

Table 2. Evidence for the latent period in cancer development

1. Experimental studies.
2. In humans - can be years or decades:
   a. radiation exposure;
   b. cigarette smoking;
   c. occupational carcinogenesis; and
   d. chemotherapy.
3. Can be "transplacental".

Table 3. Factors that influence the latent period

1. Carcinogenic dose.
2. Tissue site.
3. Presence of tumor promoters or other factors.
4. Anticarcinogens.

interaction with DNA, such as elagic acid or flavonoids, present in fruits and vegetables. The latter category of compounds is referred to as carcinogen-blocking agents. Other compounds, referred to as promotion-suppressing agents, prevent the evolution of the carcinogenic process in initiated cells. They include retinoids, β-carotene and α-tocopherol, which are present in fruit and vegetables, and other chemicals such as aspirin and other nonsteroidal anti-inflammatory drugs. Experimental and epidemiological studies suggest that other substances, such as organosulfur compounds in garlic and onion, curcumin in tumeric/curry, polyphenols in green tea and various protease inhibitors might also be useful in preventing tumor formation. However, their mechanisms of action are still unknown.

Within the past few decades great advances have been made in understanding the genetic and molecular mechanisms which underlie the process of tumor development. As mentioned above, the major feature of this process is the progressive acquisition of mutations in a variety of cellular genes which eventually leads to the appearance of a fully malignant phenotype. The identification of these genes and the specific mechanisms by which they contribute to this process is essential for developing effective chemopreventive agents. In fact, alterations in these genes might help to identify individuals at risk to develop cancer, provide useful targets for chemoprevention, or provide biological markers to be used as intermediate end points for assessing the efficacy of chemoprevention agents in clinical trials.

The genes involved in the carcinogenic process have been classically subdivided into two major groups [2,3]: 1) oncogenes, which are dominant-acting genes that normally mediate agonist-induced signal transduction pathways and whose increased activity contributes to tumor development; and 2) antioncogenes (or tumor-suppressor genes), which are recessive-acting genes whose functional loss contributes to the progression of cells towards the neoplastic state.

This classification, however, does not indicate the biochemical function of these genes, nor at what level they act to contribute to cancer formation. Therefore, we suggest a new classification scheme for these genes (Table 4). According to this

Table 4. Categories of genes involved in carcinogenesis

1. Intracellular circuitry.
   a. agonist-induced signal transduction;
   b. cell-cycle control and apoptosis;
   c. DNA replication and repair; and
   d. differentiation.
2. Cell surface/extracellular functions:
   adhesion, proteases, angiogenesis, etc.

scheme, the genes mutated in cancer cells can be functionally divided into two major categories: 1) those that control intracellular regulatory circuitry, and 2) those that influence cell surface and extracellular functions. The latter category refers to genes involved in the interactions between tumor cells and the surrounding host environment. They are especially relevant to tumor cell invasion and metastasis and include genes encoding various cell surface proteins, cell adhesion molecules, extracellular matrix proteases and other proteins, and angiogenesis factors.

The first category can be further divided into four subcategories. The genes in the first subcategory are involved in the responses of cells to external regulatory signals. These genes encode growth factors, membrane receptors and all of the coupling proteins which transduce the message through the cytosol to the nucleus to activate or inactivate the transcription of specific genes. Most of the classical oncogenes fit into this subcategory. The second subcategory includes genes involved in the regulation of cell proliferation and programmed cell death (or apoptosis). This category is rapidly expanding due to the increased understanding of the molecular mechanisms regulating the cell cycle machinery. The two major tumor-suppressor genes, Rb and p53, fit into this subcategory. We will discuss this category in greater detail later. The third subcategory includes genes involved in DNA replication, repair and recombination. Mutations in these genes (for example in DNA mismatch repair genes) can lead to genomic instability. Finally, the fourth subcategory refers to genes, such as MyoD, which normally regulate cell differentiation but, if altered, might also contribute to tumor development.

This classification clearly suggests how multiple pathways involved in cell proliferation, cell differentiation and cell death can all contribute to the multistep process of tumor formation, through complex and intricate interactions, many of which are still unknown. From this point of view, the neoplastic phenotype might be considered as a condition in which the normal balance between these diverse cellular processes is altered so as to impair cellular differentiation and enhance cell proliferation.

Cell cycle control and cancer

During the past decade rapid advances have been made in our understanding of the normal cell cycle machinery and there is accumulating evidence that disruption of the normal cell cycle is one of the most important alterations involved in cancer development (for review see [4,5]).

A central role in the control of the eukaryotic cell cycle is played by a family of cyclin-dependent kinases (CDKs) which are regulated by positive regulatory subunits called cyclins. Cyclins control the timing of activation and the substrate specificity of a series of CDKs, which are sequentially activated during specific phases of the cell cycle.

G1 cyclins regulate the progression of cells through the G1 phase and drive entry into the S-phase. Three D-type cyclins, D1, D2 and D3, act at mid-G1 by complexing with either CDK4 or CDK6. Cyclin E acts in late G1 by complexing with CDK2 [5] (Fig. 1).

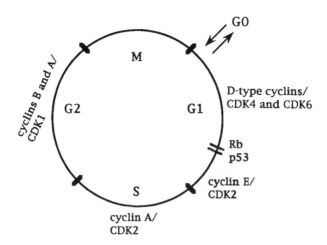

Fig. 1. A schematic diagram of the mammalian cell cycle indicating the GO phase of nondividing cells, the G1 phase when cells enter the cell cycle and prepare for the S-phase, the S-phase in which DNA synthesis occurs, and the G2/M phase in which cells prepare for and undergo mitosis. Also shown are the major cyclins and CDKs which regulate the transitions through these specific phases of the cell cycle; and the Rb and p53 tumor suppressor genes which can act at the G1/S checkpoint (also called restriction point) to inhibit cell cycle progression.

Cyclin accumulation and CDK binding are not the only level of regulation of CDK activity. Both positive and negative phosphorylation events, as well as the association with specific inhibitory proteins also play a critical role in regulating CDK activity. The CDK inhibitors (CDI) identified in mammalian cells are classified into two major categories: 1) p15, p16 and p18 mainly inhibit CDK4 and CDK6 by binding to the CDK subunit itself; and 2) p21, p27, p28 and p57 inhibit a broader range of CDKs by binding to several cyclin/CDK complexes [6,7]. A schematic representation of the multiple mechanisms regulating the activity of the cyclin D1/CDK4 complex is shown in Fig. 2. The same scheme also shows one of the major targets of this complex, the Rb protein, a product of the Rb tumor-suppressor gene. Rb is an inhibitor of cell proliferation and mainly acts in early mid-G1 by binding to E2F, a transcription factor whose activity is required for the G1 to S transition. E2F cannot activate S-phase genes when it is bound to Rb. The binding of Rb to E2F can be prevented by phosphorylation of Rb, which occurs in midlate G1. The cyclin D1/CDK4 complex plays the major role in phosphorylating the Rb protein, thus inhibiting its function: when Rb is phosphorylated, free E2F is released, which then activates the transcription of genes required for progression through the S-phase.

Since the major regulatory events leading to mammalian cell proliferation and differentiation occur in the G1 phase of the cell cycle, deregulated expression of the G1 cyclins and CDKs might cause a loss of cell cycle control and thus enhance oncogenesis.

40

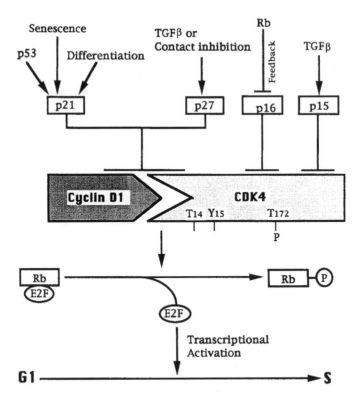

Fig. 2. Schematic representation of the multiple levels of regulation of cyclin/CDK activity. The cyclin D1/CDK4 complex is shown but similar mechanisms also regulate the activity of other cyclin/CDK complexes. The binding of cyclin D1 to CDK4 is essential to activate the kinase activity. However, phosphorylation of specific sites (tyrosine 172) and dephosphorylation of others (tyrosine 15 and threonine 14) is also necessary for kinase activity. Specific kinases and phosphatase regulate the phosphorylation and dephosphorylation of these sites during the cell cycle. Finally, a group of inhibitory proteins, which are in turn regulated by several external factors, also contribute to regulate the final activity of cyclin/CDK complexes. Also shown is the product of the Rb tumor suppressor gene, a major target of cyclinD1/CDK4 complex, which can inhibit cell cycle progression by binding to and blocking the activity of the E2F transcription factor, whose activity is essential for S-phase progression. Phosphorylation by cyclin D1/CDK4 (and by cyclin E-A/CDK2 complexes) prevents Rb from binding to E2F, thus allowing the G1 to S progression.

Cyclin D1 plays multiple roles in cancer development and is a useful target for cancer chemoprevention

Several types of evidence have been obtained which implicate cyclin D1 in the process of neoplastic transformation. Thus, Rat-6 fibroblasts engineered to stably overexpress cyclin D1 displayed a decrease in the duration of G1, increased growth, decreased cell size; and they induced tumors when injected into nude mice [8]. Furthermore, cyclin D1 was shown to cooperate in vitro with other oncogenes to induce cell transformation [9,10], and overexpression of a MMTV-cyclin D1 construct in mammary cells in transgenic mice was associated with an increase in mammary hyperplasia and mammary carcinomas [11]. Taken together, these results provide direct evidence that overexpression of cyclin D1 can cause disturbances in cell cycle control and enhance tumorigenesis both in vitro and in vivo.

The chromosome 11q13 region is amplified in a variety of human tumors, including esophageal tumors. Indeed, about 20–50% of esophageal carcinomas display amplification of the hst1 and int2 genes which are located on chromosome 11q13. However, little or no expression of these two genes is detectable in the corresponding cells. Thus, when it was found that cyclin D1 mapped to the chromosome 11q13 locus, it was of interest to examine the status of the cyclin D1 gene in esophageal carcinomas. Our laboratory discovered that there was a 3- to 10-fold amplification of the cyclin D1 gene in about 30% of squamous esophageal tumors and several esophageal carcinomas cell lines. We also demonstrated by western blot analysis and immunostaining that cyclin D1 protein expression level was increased in both the cell lines and primary tumors [12].

We further observed that all of the tumors that showed amplification and overexpression of cyclin D1 were positive by immunostaining for Rb expression (group 1). In the remaining tumors, in which cyclin D1 was not overexpressed, some had undetectable Rb protein expression (group 2) but the remainders were Rb-positive (group 3), although we did not exclude the possibility that in some of the Rb-positive cases a mutant protein was expressed [13]. This reciprocal relationship between overexpression of cyclin D1 and loss of expression of the Rb protein was statistically significant and suggested a model in which, during the multistep evolution of esophageal tumors, the normal inhibitory role of the Rb protein was abrogated by various mechanisms including: 1) loss of expression of the Rb protein (group 2); and 2) increased expression of cyclin D1 (group 1); or other, at that time unknown, mechanisms (group 3).

This model has been subsequently confirmed and extended to other types of tumors. Alternative mechanisms for Rb inactivation later became apparent in the group 3 tumors. These include loss of inhibitory proteins (such as p16) or amplification and overexpression of CDK4, which have the same final effects on this important pathway of cell-growth regulation.

This example provides a paradigm which demonstrates that the analysis of entire pathways of cell-growth regulation is more informative than simply the study of single genes in understanding tumor cell biology. In fact, tumors that are heterogeneous with respect to mutations of specific genes might actually display deregulation in a common regulatory pathway, and thus have similar biological properties.

Cyclin D1 has also been found to be amplified and/or overexpressed in a variety of human tumors, including breast cancers [14]. As mentioned above, to develop more effective strategies for cancer prevention and treatment we need a better understanding of all of the stages of the carcinogenic process, including the initiating events. These events cannot be readily studied in humans. An experimental model is needed that mimics the human disease and allows one to elucidate the first phases of the tumorigenic process, and whether it can be manipulated by treatment of the host. Thus, it was of interest to determine whether carcinogen-induced rat mammary tumors, which represent a widely used experimental model for mammary tumorigenesis, also display abnormalities in the expression of cyclin D1. Indeed, we found that primary rat mammary carcinomas induced by the carcinogen N-methyl-N-nitrosourea (NMU) frequently show deregulated expression of cyclin D1 and other cell cycle-related genes [15], thus confirming the utility of this model for studies on mammary tumorigenesis.

Since cyclin D1 is part of a very large amplicon, which includes several genes; its amplification and overexpression in tumor cells does not exclude the possibility that genes in this amplicon, other than cyclin D1, play an important role in oncogenesis. To address this question, we introduced an antisense cyclin D1 cDNA construct into a human esophageal cell line which has cyclin D1 amplification and overexpression, and then analyzed possible effects on the growth and tumorigenicity of these cells. We found that the reduction in expression of cyclin D1 in these derivatives was associated with a marked inhibition of both anchorage-dependent and -independent growth in vitro and a complete loss of tumorigenicity when these cells were injected into nude mice [16]. These results provided direct evidence that overexpression of cyclin D1 in these tumor cells plays a critical role in maintaining their abnormal growth and tumorigenicity.

Studies on the cell cycle have shown that normal cells have checkpoint controls at the G1/S and G2/M transition which delay further cell cycle progression to permit repair of damaged DNA. A defect in these cell cycle checkpoints due to loss of the p53 tumor suppressor gene has been associated with genomic instability. Deregulated expression of cyclin D1 can also disrupt normal cell cycle control, and therefore, it might also enhance genomic instability. To test this hypothesis we overexpressed cyclin D1 in a rat liver epithelial cell line which has a normal p53 gene, and using a specific cell selection system, we evaluated the occurrence of gene amplification which is a good marker of genomic instability. We observed that while the occurrence of gene amplification was virtually absent in the parental cell line, the cyclin D1 overexpressing derivatives showed a very high frequency of gene amplification [17]. This finding suggests that overexpression of cyclin D1 can disrupt genomic integrity and thereby accelerate the process of tumor progression.

Thus, all of the above studies provide evidence for multiple roles of cyclin D1 overexpression in tumorigenesis, since overexpression of this gene could promote tumor progression by enhancing genomic instability, and also play a role in maintaining the transformed phenotype in certain types of tumor cells.

To extend the relevance of these findings to the development of human tumors in vivo, we have analyzed the expression of cyclin D1 in a variety of human tumors including esophageal, gastric, colon and breast cancers, by using a simple immuno-staining procedure. Cyclin D1 overexpression was observed in all of these types of tumors, and ranged between 30–60% of the samples analyzed. An interesting finding was that cyclin D1 overexpression can be an early event in the multistep process of carcinogenesis, since cyclin D1 overexpression was detected in adenomatous polyps in the colon, in Barrett's esophagus and in situ carcinomas of the breast ([18,19] and unpublished data).

These findings, together with the above-mentioned results, and findings by other investigators, emphasize the importance of increased expression of cyclin D1 in the development of human tumors. They also suggest that cyclin D1 or cyclin D1/CDK4 activity might be useful targets for cancer chemoprevention, since this abnormality is a fairly early event in the process of tumor development and may directly contribute to tumor progression.

Conclusion

In the last few decades, enormous advances have been made in our understanding of cancer causation and formation. There is now compelling evidence that cancer arises via a multistep process and that at a molecular level this process includes the progressive accumulation of genetic changes in a variety of cellular genes. The identification of these genes and the profound insights obtained into the biochemistry and molecular biology of cancer cells have shifted the focus of cancer research to the molecular level. Thus, we have entered the era of "molecular oncology" which should provide a link between basic research and cancer prevention and treatment.

The studies on cyclin D1 provide a paradigm of how advances in the genetics, molecular biology and biochemistry of cancer cells can contribute to the development of new agents for cancer chemoprevention and chemotherapy. The identification of other molecular markers which can alone, or in combination with cyclin D1, contribute to the process of tumor formation is expected to have a major impact on the development of more effective strategies for reducing both cancer incidence and mortality.

Acknowledgements

This research was supported in part by Grant No. DAMRD17-94-J-4101, AIBS, 2584 from the US Army Medical Research Acquisition Activity and NCI Grant no. Ro1 63467 (to IBW). AS is supported by a fellowship from the Italian Association for Cancer Research (AIRC). The authors are indebted to numerous other investigators in this laboratory for their valuable contributions to these studies.

References

1. Nowell PC. The clonal evolution of tumor cell populations. Science 1976;194;23.
2. Bishop JM. Molecular themes in oncogenesis. Cell 1991;64:235—248.
3. Weinberg RA. Tumor suppressor genes. Science 1991;254:1138—1145.
4. Hunter T, Pines J. Cyclins and cancer II: cyclin D and CDK inhibitors come of age. Cell 1994;79:573—582.
5. Sherr CJ. G1 phase progression: cycling on cue. Cell 1994;79:551—555.
6. Morgan DO. Principles of CDK regulation. Nature 1995;374:131—134.
7. Peter M, Herskowitz I. Joining the complex: cyclin-dependent kinase inhibitory proteins and the cell cycle. Cell 1994;79:181—184.

8. Jiang W, Kahn SM, Zhou P, Zhang YJ, Cacace AM, Infante AS, Doi S, Santella RM, Weinstein IB. Overexpression of cyclin D1 in rat fibroblasts causes abnormalities in growth control, cell cycle progression and gene expression. Oncogene 1993;8(12):3447–3457.

9. Lovec H, Grzeschiczek A, Kowalski MB, Moroy T. Cyclin D1/bcl-1 cooperates with myc genes in the generation of B-cell lymphoma in transgenic mice. EMBO J 1994;13(15):3487–3495.

10. Lovec H, Sewing A, Lucibello FC, Muller R, Moroy T. Oncogenic activity of cyclin D1 revealed through cooperation with Ha-ras: link between cell cycle control and malignant transformation. Oncogene 1994;9:323–326.

11. Wang TC, Cardiff RD, Zukerberg L, Lees E, Arnold A, Schmidt EV. Mammary hyperplasia and carcinoma in MMTV-cyclin D1 transgenic mice. Nature 1994;369:669–671.

12. Jiang W, Kahn SM, Tomita N, Zhang Y-J, Lu S-H, Weinstein IB. Amplification and expression of human cyclin D gene in esophageal cancer. Cancer Res 1992;52:2980–2983.

13. Jiang W, Zhang Y-J, Kahn SM, Hollestein MC, Santella RM, Lu SH, Harris CC, Montesano R, Weinstein IB. Altered expression of the cyclin D1 and retinoblastoma genes in human esophageal cancer. Proc Natl Acad Sci USA 1993;90:9026–9030.

14. Bartkova J, Lukas J, Strauss M, Bartek J. Cyclin D1 oncoprotein aberrantly accumulates in malignancies of diverse histogenesis. Oncogene 1995;10(4):775–778.

15. Sgambato A, Han EK-H, Zhang Y-J, Moon RC, Santella RM, Weinstein IB. Deregulated expression of cyclin D1 and other cell-cycle-related genes in carcinogen-induced rat mammary tumors. Carcinogenesis 1995;16:2193–2198.

16. Zhou P, Jiang W, Zhang Y, Kahn SM, Schieren I, Santella RM, Weinstein IB. Antisense to cyclin D1 inhibits growth and reverses the transformed phenotype of human esophageal cancer cells. Oncogene 1995;11:571–580.

17. Zhou P, Jiang W, Weghorst CM, Weinstein IB. Overexpression of cyclin D1 enhances gene amplification. Cancer Res 1995.

18. Arber N, Lightdale C, Rotterdam H, Han EK-H, Sgambato A, Yap E, Ahsan H, Finegold J, Stevens PD, Green PHR, Hibshoosh H, Neugut AI, Holt PR, Weinstein IB. Increased expression of the cyclin D1 gene in Barrett's esophagus. Cancer Epidem Biomarker Prev 1996;(In press).

19. Arber N, Hibshoosh H, Moss SF, Sutter T, Zhang Y, Begg M, Wang S, Weinstein IB, Holt PR. Increased expressiss of cyclin D1 is an early event in multistage colorectal carcinogenesiss. Gastroenterology 1996;110:669–674.

1996 Elsevier Science B.V.
The Scientific Bases of Cancer Chemoprevention.
C. Maltoni, M. Soffritti and W. Davis, editors.

The contribution of rodent liver and lung carcinogenesis models to our knowledge of the cancer latent period

Theodora R. Devereux[1], David E. Malarkey[2] and Robert R. Maronpot[2]

[1]*Laboratory of Molecular Toxicology; and* [2]*Laboratory of Experimental Pathology, National Institute of Environmental Health Sciences, Research Triangle Park, North Carolina, USA*

Abstract. Historically, scientists have conducted rodent bioassays to identify potentially hazardous substances by determining whether the agent in question increases the incidence of various types of neoplasms. These studies have contributed to our knowledge of the cancer latent period, broadly defined here as the time between carcinogen exposure and appearance of malignant neoplasia. Thus, this interval includes the promutagenic event (initiation), fixation of the mutation (cell proliferation), clonal expansion (promotion) and progression. Various rodent models have been utilized for these studies, but we have concentrated on liver and lung carcinogenesis in this chapter.

Many approaches have been used to elucidate the events occurring during latency. Originally, studies examined mainly the tumor endpoints, the quantitation of preneoplastic lesions and benign and malignant tumor incidence and multiplicity. From these studies we learned that there is a large tissue-specific difference in susceptibility of strains of mice to both spontaneous and chemically induced lung or liver carcinogenesis. Strain differences in susceptibility to carcinogenesis, in part, appear to involve differences in growth rates of cells, thus directly affecting latency periods. Both genetics and the chemical carcinogen are driving forces in determining tumor development and latency. More recently, studies of oncogene activation and tumor suppressor gene inactivation, alterations in growth-related gene expression, DNA adduct formation and repair, and DNA methylation have been utilized to gain a better understanding of cancer latency. Many of these processes, which directly or indirectly affect the balance of cell proliferation and apoptosis, are altered during latency and thus, play critical roles in carcinogenesis. Understanding of the changes that occur in these processes during latency will ultimately provide clues for developing cancer chemoprevention strategies.

Key words: cancer latency, experimental carcinogenesis, rodent carcinogenesis models.

Introduction

For decades scientists have known that the cancer process in humans usually involves a long latency. During this period, a series of genetic and epigenetic changes accumulates in the tissue until signs or symptoms of these changes are detected. Animal models have been developed that allow us to study some of these changes and the nature of the latent period.

Scientists at our institute and elsewhere have conducted rodent bioassays to identify potentially hazardous substances by determining whether the agent in question increases the age-specific incidence of various types of neoplasms. One of

Address for correspondence: Theodora R. Devereux, Laboratory of Molecular Toxicology, National Institute of Environmental Health Sciences, Research Triangle Park, NC 27709, USA.

the criteria used in these studies to determine if the chemical in question is a carcinogen is reduced latency. Rodent bioassays have contributed to our knowledge of cancer latency by identifying some of the factors that appear to influence the duration of this period. The genetic background is the most influential factor and may play the greatest role in determining the length of latency periods [1—3]. Also, sex of the experimental animals [4,5], the dose of the carcinogen administered [6,7], the age at administration of the carcinogen [8—11], and the presence of promoters [8,12—14] or anticarcinogens [15—17] all appear to influence cancer latency. In this review we will examine some of the rodent liver and lung carcinogenesis models and experiments that have identified some of these conditions and factors.

Diverse approaches have been utilized to explore events of the cancer latent period in animal models. Besides studies that have concentrated on the cancer endpoint, studies on the role of cell proliferation, especially in rodent liver carcinogenesis models, have added to our knowledge of latency. Recent reports have demonstrated that some chemicals may act as carcinogens by inhibiting apoptosis rather than or in addition to stimulating cell proliferation [18,19]. Studies on ras proto-oncogene mutation in mouse lung and liver carcinogenesis have also added to our knowledge of cancer latency and will be discussed. Additionally, studies that are identifying tumor susceptibility genes will be considered.

Genetic background of experimental animals

Cancer latency is influenced to a great extent by the genetic background of the experimental animals, especially with reference to strain differences in tumor susceptibility. Inbred mouse strains vary considerably in their susceptibility to the development of both spontaneous and chemically induced lung and liver tumors [2,3,20,21]. Tissue-specific patterns of tumor incidence, multiplicity and latency are observed that may vary by as much as 100-fold in different strains of mice (Fig. 1). For example, A/J mice are among the most lung tumor susceptible strains and yet are resistant to liver tumor formation. In contrast, C3H mice are susceptible to hepatocellular carcinogenesis but resistant to lung tumors. The Balb/c strain has intermediate susceptibility to both hepatocellular and pulmonary carcinogenesis. Hybrid mouse strains, such as the B6C3F1 mouse that is used frequently for toxicity and carcinogenicity studies and is derived from susceptible C3H mice crossed to resistant C57BL/6 mice, often have intermediate susceptibility.

Apparent differences in susceptibility to carcinogenesis may be due to genetic differences in chemical metabolism, promutagenic adduct repair, cell proliferation, or genomic stability. In some rodent hepatocarcinogenesis models the promotion stage appears to be influenced more by the genetic background of the animals than does the initiation stage. For example, Drinkwater and Ginsler [20] found that a single genetic locus was largely responsible for the difference in hepatocarcinogenesis susceptibility between C3H/HeJ and C57BL/6J mouse strains. These authors observed similar numbers of preneoplastic lesions in livers from both mouse strains following diethylnitrosamine treatment, which suggested no difference in the initiation stage of

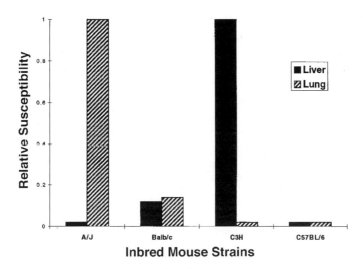

Fig. 1. Strain and tissue specificity in susceptibility of inbred mice to chemically induced liver and lung carcinogenesis. Relative susceptibility is shown with 1.0 representing the most susceptible strain. Lung tumors were induced with urethan (Malkinson 1989) and liver tumors with N-ethyl-N-nitrosourea or N,N-diethylnitrosamine. Modified from Drinkwater and Bennett, 1991.

carcinogenesis. In another study from that laboratory [22], preneoplastic liver lesions in C3H/HeJ mice after treatment with ethylnitrosourea at 12 days of age were shown to have a much greater growth rate relative to those from C57BL/6J mice. Intrinsic hepatocyte growth rates may play a large role in determining susceptibility differences in different inbred mouse strains [2]. Several related studies have provided evidence that mouse strain differences in hepatocarcinogenesis susceptibility are due primarily to differences in the promotional stage of tumor development [1,12,23]. Sometimes differences in hepatocellular tumor latency have been observed between strains, such as for the B6C3F1 and B6D2F1 mice following chronic treatment with chlordane as illustrated in Fig. 2, even though tumor incidence and multiplicity may be similar [24]. Thus, although most studies compare number of tumors in different strains of mice formed by a certain time point, the implication of these studies is that differences in tumor susceptibility affect the length of the cancer latent period. In other words, given enough time, resistant strains may also develop a level of tumor multiplicity similar to that in susceptible strains.

Sex hormonal environment

It has been observed in some studies that male mice have a stronger liver tumor response than females, indicating that the sex hormonal environment of the animals influences liver tumor development. Vesselinovitch [4] demonstrated that the sex hormonal environment of the host altered both the rate of tumor development and the number of tumors formed. The male hormonal environment enhanced liver tumor

48

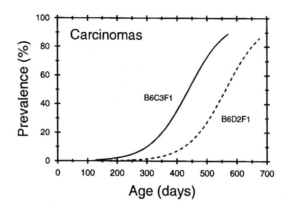

Fig. 2. Prevalence of hepatocellular carcinomas in B6C3F1 and B6D2F1 mice following chronic administration of chlordane shows strain differences in cancer latency. Modified from Malarkey et al., 1995.

formation in B6C3F1 mice, while female hormones appeared to suppress tumor development. The timing of male castration or female ovariectomy in these experiments was critical, suggesting that sex hormones influence both the growth and latency of initiated cells. However, in some rodent carcinogenesis models females were found to be more susceptible than males. A positive role for estrogen has been demonstrated in 2,3,7,8-tetrachlorodibenzo-p-dioxin (TCDD)-induced rat hepatocellular carcinogenesis as evidenced by potent hepatocarcinogenicity in females but not in males [25,26]. Thus, the sex hormonal environment appears to play an important role in carcinogenesis, but its influence is varied depending on the model being studied.

The nature of the carcinogen

Historically, researchers classified carcinogens as initiators, promoters, or complete carcinogens. However, as new information about the carcinogenic process has become available, it has become increasingly difficult to rigidly define a chemical as either an initiator or a promoter. Genotoxic carcinogens or their metabolites damage DNA directly, whereas nongenotoxic carcinogens do not directly interact with DNA. Often, a genotoxic carcinogen will act as an initiator at a low dose and a complete carcinogen at a somewhat higher dose, while latency may be shortened by chronic treatment with another chemical (e.g., promoter) that may not itself cause a strong tumor response. Fixation and replication of the chemically induced DNA damage appear essential for manifestation of mutation induction and contribute to tumor development. Nongenotoxic carcinogens are believed to cause stimulation of cell growth with preferential outgrowth of preneoplastic cells, and increased cell proliferation enhances the clonal expansion of spontaneously initiated cells.

Presence of promoters

The initiation-promotion two-stage paradigm of chemical carcinogenesis has been demonstrated for a variety of tissues [27] and has been studied extensively in rodent liver models [12,28]. According to this model, initiation is an irreversible event, whereas the promotion stage is reversible. In some but not all models chronic treatment with phenobarbital or other promoters has been shown to enhance spontaneously initiated liver tumor development in mouse strains susceptible to hepatocellular carcinogenesis such as the C3H inbred and B6C3F1 hybrid strains [29–31]. In these and other strains, phenobarbital also increased the formation of liver tumors initiated by genotoxic carcinogens [32]. Some studies have demonstrated that the removal of the promoter during the latency period reverses the progression of carcinogenesis [24,33,34].

The tumor-promoting activity of TCDD has been demonstrated in several models [13,19,25]. In a recent study, we compared the liver tumor response in an initiation-promotion protocol-utilizing chronic treatment with TCDD after vinyl carbamate or no initiation in susceptible B6C3F1 mice and resistant C57BL/6 mice [13]. Evidence of cytotoxicity was observed in the livers after TCDD treatment, and TCDD was shown to stimulate DNA synthesis, thereby enhancing cell proliferation in hepatocytes from B6C3F1 mice [35]. Tumor prevalence results, cytotoxicity data, and H-ras mutation spectra provided evidence that TCDD acted in B6C3F1 mice as a promoter of lesions initiated both spontaneously and by vinyl carbamate. The large tumor response in the C57BL/6 mice after TCDD or VC+TCDD suggested that TCDD affects the genes that confer resistance in the C57BL/6 mice, likely genes that are involved in cell proliferation [2].

Role of cell proliferation and apoptosis

The balance of cell proliferation and cell death determines the growth of a tissue, and alterations in that balance can contribute to the formation of tumors. The clonal expansion and growth of initiated cell populations and cancer cells appear to be maintained by increased cell division and/or reduced apoptosis. Chemically induced cell proliferation and apoptosis, especially utilizing rodent liver models, are being intensely investigated [36–38]. The nature of the proliferative response following chemical exposures in the rodent liver often has been classified as either cytotoxic or mitogenic. Cytotoxicants are lethal to cells and lead to a regenerative cell proliferation, while mitogens do not cause cell death. In the rodent liver, mitogenic carcinogens often produce an early transient increase in hepatocyte proliferation and a sustained increase in liver weight for the duration of exposure [36]. Mitogenic agents may provide a selective growth advantage to initiated cells by decreasing apoptosis, inhibiting normal hepatocyte proliferation, or increasing cell proliferation in preneoplastic cell populations.

No simple relationship exists between cell proliferation and carcinogenesis. Although it is widely accepted that cell proliferation is essential for carcinogenesis, it is not sufficient by itself to cause neoplasia. Cell proliferation is an integral part of the process of converting DNA adducts to permanent mutations, required for tumor promotion and growth, and a risk factor for tumor development in both man and animals. Regenerative cell division in response to chronic inflammation, chronic toxicity, partial hepatectomy, and irritants have all been linked to increased cancer risks in humans and animals [39–41]. Cell replication may contribute to an increased error susceptibility rate for the genetic base pairing which contributes to progression of cancer [42]. The role of sustained, enhanced cell proliferation in experimental chemical carcinogenesis is controversial. While there are some examples where induced proliferation correlates with cancer induction, there are many where it does not [43–45]. For carcinogenesis that is unrelated to enhanced cell replication, Ward et al. [46] suggested that mutations may be time dependent rather than replication dependent.

The phenomenon of apoptosis was first defined in the 1970s and has since been recognized to be widespread in multicellular organisms. Apoptosis (or active cell death) is a programmed cell death in which the cell actively participates by providing energy and molecules that are directly or indirectly involved in allowing death to proceed. This "programmed cell death" underlies normal developmental processes such as embryonic organogenesis, tissue homeostasis, and the "editing" of the immune system to remove autoreactive clones. Apoptosis which can be induced by toxic insults, particularly those that damage DNA, is frequently seen in tumors, and may influence the kinetics of tumor growth [47–49]. The study of the molecular basis of apoptosis is in the early stages and recent studies have revealed that there are dominant oncogenes and tumor suppressor genes that can drive apoptosis and/or act to promote cell survival [50]. Some of the pathways leading to cell death can be tied to the same signals that activate proliferation [48–50].

Suppression of programmed cell death during carcinogenesis is thought to play a central role in the development and progression of some cancers. Moreover, the "protective effect" of food restriction or other treatments on tumorigenesis are believed to act, at least in part, by stimulating apoptosis. Marsman and Barrett [47] proposed that some tumor promoters may act by inhibiting apoptosis and that these surviving cells may have more accumulated genetic damage, persist in the tissue, and have a growth advantage over their neighboring cells. Replication of these cells would leave a population of cells susceptible to further mutations and perhaps lead to the clonal expansion of neoplastic cells that grow independent of the tumor promoter. Recently, TCDD used as a promoter in a rat hepatocarcinogenesis model, has been shown to promote focal growth, not only by increasing cell proliferation, but by primarily inhibiting apoptosis [19]. Withdrawal of similar acting agents such as phenobarbital and cyproterone acetate leads to tumor regression by stimulating apoptosis [51]. Food restriction [52] and treatment with monoterpene perillyl alcohol [53] have been shown to prevent preneoplastic growth and liver tumor development by enhancing lesion-specific apoptosis.

Alterations in gene expression and DNA methylation patterns

Upregulation of several growth-related genes has been observed to occur early in rat liver tumor development. Increased expression of H- and K-ras, c-fos, c-myc, and c-raf was detected in preneoplastic foci of rat livers following initiation/promotion protocols [54—56]. Also, a role for the transforming growth factor gene (TGFα) has also been implicated by its increased expression in many types of tumors and transformed cell lines [57—59]. In in vitro experiments, TGFα has been shown to regulate both cell proliferation and differentiation [60]. Transgenic mice, created by using a fusion transgene with the rat TGFα coding sequence and a mouse metal-lothionein-I enhancer/promoter sequence, exhibited an increased incidence of mammary and liver tumors [61].

In addition, alteration of DNA methylation patterns during rat liver tumorigenesis has been demonstrated. DNA methylation appears to regulate gene expression, and evidence is mounting that both global and gene-specific methylation patterns play a role in carcinogenesis. Growth-related genes are both overexpressed and hypomethylated in preneoplastic liver foci [62,63]. Additionally, certain chemical carcinogens inhibit DNA methylation [64], and some hypomethylating agents are promoters of carcinogenesis [65]. In one study feeding of S-adenosyl methionine to rats administered as an initiation/promotion protocol, caused increased DNA methylation and inhibition of both protooncogene expression and growth of altered foci [66]. Recent reports showing hypermethylation of the promoter regions in important tumor-suppressor genes such as p16 in various human cancers suggest that failure of function is due to loss of transcription caused by hypermethylation [67].

Studies on ras protooncogene activation

Activation of the H- and K-ras members of the ras family of protooncogenes appears to be important in the carcinogenesis process in both humans and rodents [68—70]. Profiles of activating mutations in K- and H-ras protooncogenes in carcinogen-induced lung and liver tumors in mice often differ from the pattern identified in spontaneous tumors and appear to be chemical specific (Table 1). In cases involving genotoxic carcinogens, the activating mutation often can be correlated with the DNA adduct produced by the chemical [71—73]. Also, in some studies H-ras mutations have been detected in liver foci (refs). These studies have provided evidence that mutation of ras is an early event in some mouse liver and lung carcinogenesis models [71,74] and suggested association of the ras mutation with initiation. Even for so-called nongenotoxic carcinogens, patterns of ras mutations have provided information that has proved valuable in interpreting tumor endpoint data. For example, exposure of B6C3F1 mice to methylene chloride caused an increase of both liver and lung tumors [75]. Although some in vitro experiments implicated methylene chloride as a genotoxin [76], our data on ras mutation spectra in liver and lung tumors suggested a promotional mechanism [77]. In these tumors, the methylene chloride associated ras mutation profiles were similar to those in the corresponding (liver or lung)

Table 1. H-ras codon 61 mutation patterns in hepatocellular tumors from B6C3F1 mice following different chemical treatment regimens

Treatment	H-ras activation at codon 61	Codon 61 (n = CAA)		
		AAA	CGA	CTA
Control	183/333 (56%)[a]	106	50	21
TCDD	23/45 (51%)[b]	16	4	3
Vinyl carbamate	27/38 (71%)[b]	5	5	17
VC+TCDD	52/67 (78%)[b]	6	8	39
Chlordane	0/30 (0%)[c]	0	0	0

[a]Maronpot et al. Toxicology 1995;101:125—156; [b]Watson et al. Carcinogenesis 1995;16:1705—1710; [c]Malarkey et al. Carcinogenesis 1995;16:2617—2625.

spontaneous tumors. These studies, in which a large proportion of tumors lacked activated ras oncogenes, suggested that at least two populations of cells, those with ras mutations and those without, give rise to hepatocellular tumors. Thus, methylene chloride appeared to promote both ras-activated and non-ras-activated lesions.

Based on H-ras mutation patterns, some nongenotoxic compounds appear to promote hepatocellular lesions preferentially by a pathway independent of ras mutation (Table 1) [24,78,79]. For example, the frequency of H-ras mutations detected in liver tumors from B6C3F1 mice treated with phenobarbital, ciprofibrate or chloroform was significantly less than in spontaneous tumors [78]. In a recent study from our laboratory, chronic treatment with chlordane enhanced liver tumor formation in both B6C3F1 and B6D2F1 mice [24]. None of the tumors examined from the treated mice had H-ras mutations, suggesting a preferential promotion of the cells without ras activation. Some of the benign and malignant tumors regressed when the chlordane treatment was discontinued, providing evidence that chlordane was acting as a promoter and that the promotion stage was reversible.

Studies on the carcinogenic effects of oxazepam and diethylnitrosamine (DEN) in B6C3F1 mice, in which more than one dose of carcinogen was examined, showed that the proportion of liver tumors with H-ras mutations decreased with increasing dose of carcinogen [7,79]. Furthermore, the study on liver tumor induction by DEN and lung tumor formation by 4-(nitrosamino)-1-(3-pyridyl)-1-butanone (NNK) indicated that different mechanisms of tumor induction may occur at high and low doses [7]. For chemicals such as DEN or NNK, which require metabolism before exerting their genotoxicity, different metabolic pathways may be active at different concentrations of the carcinogen, yielding altered proportions of adducts with distinct mutagenic potentials. Alternatively, high concentrations of certain carcinogens may cause cytotoxicity and cell proliferation, thus influencing/altering the pathways to carcinogenesis.

Tumor development in mouse lung models

Besides rodent hepatocarcinogenesis studies, reports on lung tumorigenesis in animal models have provided additional information to our knowledge of cancer latency as well as reinforcing some principles defined in other models. For example, in one study from our laboratory [74], we examined the proliferation of lesions in lung tumor susceptible A/J mice after treatment with the tobacco-specific nitrosamine, NNK. Histological evidence at 14 weeks after a single dose of NNK indicated that the proliferating cells within the hyperplastic lesions in the lungs resembled alveolar type II cells, suggesting cell specificity in proliferation. At later time points, histological evidence of progression of the lesions demonstrated adenomas arising within hyperplasias and carcinomas within adenomas. Furthermore, lesion quantitation data indicated that the number of hyperplasias decreased with time after 14 weeks while the adenoma frequency increased, and was followed at a later time by a rise in carcinomas (Fig. 3). These observations indicate a continuum of progression in this model from cell-specific hyperplasia to adenoma to carcinoma.

In other experiments with these mice after administration of NNK, analysis of O^6MG DNA adducts in isolated lung cells showed higher levels in type II cells and nonciliated bronchiolar epithelial cells than in other cells of lung [74]. In addition, K-ras codon 12 GGT to GAT mutations were identified in 75% of lung hyperplasias examined from these same mice. These results are consistent with the hypothesis that the mutations were an early event and were derived from the O^6MG adduct, and that clonal expansion of a specific cell type was involved in tumor development.

The findings that the H- or K-ras protooncogene is mutated early in mouse lung and liver tumor development, and that chemicals appear to induce specific patterns of mutations, suggests that the ras mutation is an initiating event in many of these

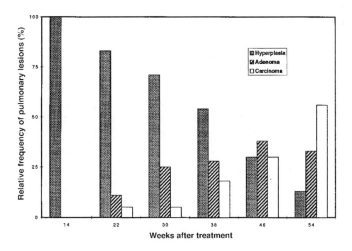

Fig. 3. Progression of lesions in lungs of A/J mice following treatment with the tobacco-specific nitrosamine, NNK. The relative frequency of lesion is shown beginning at 14 weeks after a single-dose administration of NNK. Modified from Belinsky et al., 1992.

models. Additionally, K-ras mutations have been detected in lung tumors from resistant C3H and C57BL/6 mice [80,81], indicating that the K-ras mutation itself does not confer tumor susceptibility. Similar levels of O^{6}MG adducts were also formed and persisted in the lungs of these resistant mice as compared to those of susceptible A/J mice following treatment with NNK [81]. These data suggest that differences in metabolism of NNK by cytochrome P-450s are not likely to be involved in lung tumor susceptibility differences between these strains of mice. Thus, like studies on hepatocarcinogenesis, our studies on a lung carcinogenesis model provide evidence that the initiation stage of carcinogenesis is not strongly influenced by genetic background. Furthermore, K-ras mutation alone in lungs of these mice is not sufficient for a strong tumor response; the tumors in the resistant mice were small and took much longer to develop than in the susceptible strain. Thus, it appears that other events in the susceptible mice, in addition to or in cooperation with activation of K-ras are important for lung tumorigenesis.

In order to identify the events and factors necessary for lung tumor development in mice, our laboratory and others have conducted genetic studies to map and identify loci responsible for differences in lung tumorigenesis between resistant (C3H or C57BL/6) and susceptible (A/J) mouse strains [82–84]. In all these studies, a major susceptibility locus was mapped to distal chromosome 6 in the region of K-ras, and evidence has been obtained from other studies also linking the K-ras gene to mouse lung tumor susceptibility [85,86]. The studies of Festing et al. [84] and Devereux et al. [83] also mapped minor susceptibility loci to chromosomes 9, 17 and 19. These loci appeared to represent modifier or enhancer genes of the major locus. It is proposed that these genes interact with K-ras (or the major gene located near K-ras) to enhance tumor formation in the susceptible A/J strain. Investigations on the identification of these loci are continuing in our laboratory.

Rodent models of chemoprevention

Rodent liver and lung carcinogenesis models have been used to test chemoprevention strategies. A wide variety of agents that inhibit cell proliferation, stimulate apoptosis, or increase DNA methylation have been examined as anticarcinogens. For example, protocols that decrease cell proliferation and increase apoptosis such as food restriction, the natural monterpene perillyl alcohol, or S-adenosyl methionine, all inhibit carcinogenesis in the rat liver two-stage model [52,53,62]. The A/J mouse lung carcinogenesis model following NNK treatment has also been used successfully in tests of chemoprevention [17] as well as chemointervention [87]. Ellagic acid, 2,3-BHA, and the anti-inflammatory agent, sulindac all reduced the multiplicity of adenomas formed when compared to NNK controls [17]. These compounds may work in part by inhibiting the metabolism of NNK. Thus, there are many stages of carcinogenesis that may be slowed down or reversed by chemoprevention.

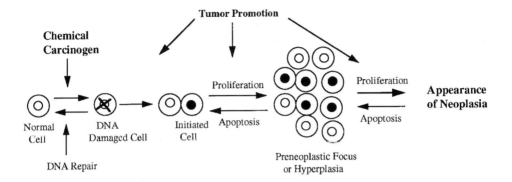

Fig. 4. Experimental model of cancer latency illustrating events that occur between chemical exposure and appearance of neoplasia. Following DNA damage to the cell, the mutation is repaired or becomes fixed in the target cells. Tumor promotion then drives the balance between apoptosis and cell proliferation towards increasing the survival and growth of the initiated target cell population. Increased growth-related gene expression, regulated in part by decreased DNA methylation, and accumulating genetic instability help drive the development of neoplasia. Modified from Goldsworthy et al., 1995.

Conclusions

Although many of the individual changes that occur early in the development of cancer seem "invisible", evidence is accumulating that numerous events take place during cancer latency (Fig. 4). Experimental carcinogenesis models demonstrate that both the genetic background of the animal and the nature of the chemical exposure are major driving forces in determining the carcinogenic response. Protooncogene activation plays a large role in mouse lung and liver carcinogenesis, and in combination with other events provides a growth advantage to some cells in these models. Rodent models have also provided information on the upregulation of growth-regulatory genes that occur during the cancer latent period. Studies on tumor promotion, cell proliferation and apoptosis in the early stages of rodent liver carcinogenesis have given us information important in developing chemopreventive strategies. While we may not be able to control the genetic make-up of an individual that determines susceptibility to carcinogenesis, we may be able to intervene to reverse or slow the progression of preneoplastic or neoplastic lesions.

References

1. Diwan B, Rice J, Ohshima M et al. Interstrain differences in susceptibility to liver carcinogenesis initiated by N-nitrosodiethylamine and its promotion by phenobarbital in C57BL/6NCr, C3H/HeNCrMTV- and DBA/2NCr mice. Carcinogenesis 1986;7:215—220.
2. Drinkwater N, Bennett L. Genetic control of carcinogenesis in experimental animals. In: Sugano NIaH (ed) Modification of Tumor Development in Rodents. Karger: Basel, 1991;1—20.
3. Malkinson A. The genetic basis of susceptibility to lung tumors in mice. Toxicology 1989;54:241—271.
4. Vesselinovitch SD. Certain aspects of hepatocarcinogenesis in the infant mouse model. Toxicol Pathol 1987;15:221—228.

5. Vesselinovitch SD. Perinatal mouse liver carcinogenesis as a sensitive carcinogenesis model and the role of the sex hormonal environment in tumor development. Prog Clin Biol Res 1990;331:53–68.
6. Guess H, Hoel D. The effect of dose on cancer latency period. J Environ Pathol Toxicol 1977;1: 279–286.
7. Chen B, Liu L, Castonguay A et al. Dose-dependent ras mutation spectra in N-nitrosodiethylamine induced mouse liver tumors and 4-(methylnitrosamino)-1-(3-pyridyl)-1-butanone induced mouse lung tumors. Carcinogenesis 1993;14:1603–1608.
8. Ward JM, Diwan BA, Lubet RA et al. Liver tumor promoters and other mouse liver carcinogens. Prog Clin Biol Res 1990;331:85–108.
9. Weghorst CM, Devor DE, Henneman JR et al. Promotion of hepatocellular foci and adenomas by di(2-ethylhexyl) phthalate and phenobarbital in C3H/HeNCr mice following exposure to N-nitrosodiethylamine at 15 days of age. Exp Toxicol Pathol 1994;45:423–431.
10. Beebe LE, Kim YE, Amin S et al. Comparison of transplacental and neonatal initiation of mouse lung and liver tumors by N-nitrosodimethylamine (NDMA) and 4-(methylnitrosamino)-1-(3-pyridyl)-1-butanone (NNK) and promotability by a polychlorinated biphenyls mixture (Aroclor 1254). Carcinogenesis 1993;14:1545–1548.
11. McCullough K, Coleman W, Smith G et al. Age-dependent regulation of the tumorigenic potential of neoplastically transformed rat liver epithelial cells by the liver microenvironment. Cancer Res 1994;54:3668–3671.
12. Diwan BA, Rice JM, Ward JM. Strain-dependent effects of phenobarbital on liver tumor promotion in inbred mice. Prog Clin Biol Res 1990;331:69–83.
13. Watson MA, Devereux TR, Malarkey DE et al. H-ras oncogene mutation spectra in B6C3F1 and C57BL/6 mouse liver tumors provide evidence for TCDD promotion of spontaneous and vinyl carbamate-initiated liver cells. Carcinogenesis 1995;16:1705–1710.
14. Anderson L, Logsdon D, Ruskie S et al. Promotion by polychlorinated biphenyls of lung and liver tumors in mice. Carcinogenesis 1994;15:2245–2248.
15. Klaunig J. Chemopreventive effects of green tea components on hepatic carcinogenesis. Prev Med 1992;21:510–519.
16. Hong JY, Wang ZY, Smith TJ et al. Inhibitory effects of diallyl sulfide on the metabolism and tumorigenicity of the tobacco-specific carcinogen 4-(methylnitrosamino)-1-(3-pyridyl)-1-butanone (NNK) in A/J mouse lung. Carcinogenesis 1992;13:901–904.
17. Castonguay A, Pepin P, Stoner GD. Lung tumorigenicity of NNK given orally to A/J mice: its application to chemopreventive efficacy studies. Exp Lung Res 1991;17:485–499.
18. Schulte-Hermann R, Timmermann-Trosiener I, Barthel G et al. DNA synthesis, apoptosis, and phenotype expression as determinants of growth of altered foci in rat liver during phenobarbital promotion. Cancer Res 1990;50:5127–5135.
19. Stinchcombe S, Buchmann A, Bock K et al. Inhibition of apoptosis during 2,3,7,8-tetrachlorodibenzo-p-dioxin-mediated tumour promotion in rat liver. Carcinogenesis 1995;16:1271–1275.
20. Drinkwater N, Ginsler J. Genetic control of hepatocarcinogenesis in C57BL/6J and C3H/HeJ inbred mice. Carcinogenesis 1986;7:1701–1707.
21. Malkinson A, Nesbitt M, Skamene E. Susceptibility to urethan-induced pulmonary adenomas between A/J and C57BL/6J mice: Use of AxB and BxA recombinant inbred lines indicating a three locus model. J Natl Cancer Inst 1985;75:971–974.
22. Hanigan M, Kemp C, Ginsler J. Rapid growth of preneoplatic lesions in hepatocarcinogen-sensitive C3H/HeJ male mice relative to C57BL/6J male mice. Carcinogenesis 1988;9:885–890.
23. Della-Porta G, Dragani TA, Manenti G. Two-stage liver carcinogenesis in the mouse. Toxicol Pathol 1987;15:229–233.
24. Malarkey D, Devereux T, Dinse G et al. Hepatocarcinogenicity of chlordane in B6C3F1 and B6D2F1 male mice: evidence for regression in B6C3F1 mice and carcinogenesis independent of ras proto-oncogene activation. Carcinogenesis 1995;16:2617–2625.
25. Kociba R, Keyes D, Beyer J. Results of a two year chronic toxicity and oncogenicity study of 2,3,7,8-tetrachlorodibengo-p-dioxin in rats. Toxicol App Pharmacol 1978;46:279–303.

26. Lucier G, Tritscher A, Goldsworthy T et al. Ovarian hormones enhance 2,3,7,8-tetrachlorodibenzo-p-dioxin mediated increases in cell proliferation and preneoplastic foci in a two-stage model for rat hepatocarcinogenesis. Cancer Res 1991;51:1391–1397.

27. Peraino C, Richards W, Stevens F. Multistage Carcinogenesis. In: Slage T (ed) Mechanisms of Tumor Promotion, Vol. 1. Boca Raton, FL: CRC Press, 1983;1–53.

28. Pitot H, Sirica A. The stages of initiation and promotion of hepatocarcinogenesis. Biochem Biophys Acta 1980;605:191–215.

29. Ward JM, Rice JM, Creasia D et al. Dissimilar patterns of promotion by di(2-ethylhexyl)phthalate and phenobarbital of hepatocellular neoplasia initiated by diethylnitrosamine in B6C3F1 mice. Carcinogenesis 1983;4:1021–1029.

30. Dragani TA, Manenti G, Galliani G et al. Promoting effects of 1,4-bis[2-(3,5-dichloropyridyl-oxy)]benzene in mouse hepatocarcinogenesis. Carcinogenesis 1985;6:225–228.

31. Peraino C, Fry R, Staffeldt E. Enhancement of spontaneous hepatic tumorigenesis in C3H mice by dietary phenobarbital. J Natl Cancer Inst 1973;51:1349–1350.

32. Uchida E, Hirono I. Effect of phenobarbital on induction of liver and lung tumors by dimethyl-nitrosamine in newborn mice. Gann 1979;70:639–640.

33. Ito N, Hananouchi M, Sugihara S et al. Reversibility and irreversibility of liver tumors in mice induced by the a isomer of 1,2,3,4,5,6-hexachlorocyclohexane. Cancer Res 1976;36:2227–2234.

34. Marsman D, Popp J. Biological potential of basophilic hepatocellular foci and hepatic adenoma induced by the peroxisome proliferator, Wy-14,643. Carcinogenesis 1994;15:111–117.

35. Busser MT, Lutz WK. Stimulation of DNA synthesis in rat and mouse liver by various tumor promoters. Carcinogenesis 1987;8:1433–1437.

36. Goldsworthy TL, Fransson-Steen R, Maronpot RR. Importance of and approaches to quantification of hepatocyte apoptosis. Toxicol Pathol 1996;24:24–35.

37. Butterworth BE, Goldsworthy TL. The role of cell proliferation in multistage carcinogenesis. Proc Soc Exp Biol Med 1991;198:683–688.

38. Butterworth BE, Popp JA, Connolly RB et al. Chemically induced cell proliferation in carcinogenesis. In: Vainio H et al. (eds) Mechanisms of Carcinogenesis in Risk Identification. Lyon: International Agency for Research on Cancer (IARC), 1992;279–305.

39. Preston-Martin S, Pike MC, Ross RK et al. Epidemiologic evidence for the increased cell proliferation model of carcinogenesis. Environ Health Perspec 1993;101:137–138.

40. Bartsch H, Preat V, Aitio A et al. Partial hepatectomy of rats ten weeks before carcinogen administration can enhance liver carcinogenesis: preliminary observations. Carcinogenesis 1988;9:2315–2317.

41. Ohshima H, Bartsch H. Chronic infections and inflammatory processes as cancer risk factors: possible role of nitric oxide carcinogenesis. Mutat Res 1994;305:253–264.

42. Cohen SM, Ellwein LB. Genetic errors, cell proliferation, and carcinogenesis. Cancer Res 1991;51:6493–6505.

43. Cunningham ML. Role of increased DNA replication in the carcinogenic risk of nonmutagenic chemical carcinogens. Mutat Res 1996;(In press).

44. Melnick RL. Does chemically induced hepatocyte proliferation predict liver carcinogenesis? FASEB 1992;J6:2698–2706.

45. Butterworth BE, Eldridge SR. A decision tree approach for carcinogen risk assessment. In: McClain RM et al. (eds) Growth Factors and Tumor Promotion: Implications for Risk Assessment. New York: Wiley-Liss Inc., 1995;49–70.

46. Ward JM, Uno H, Kurata Y et al. Cell proliferation not associated with carcinogenesis in rodents and humans. Environ Health Perspec 1993;101:125–136.

47. Marsman DS, Barrett JC. Apoptosis and chemical carcinogenesis. J Risk Analysis 1994;14:321–326.

48. Green DR, Bissonnette RP, Cotter TG. Apoptosis and cancer. Prin Prac Oncol 1994;8:1–14.

49. Marx J. Cell death studies yield cancer clues. Science 1993;259:760–761.

50. Harrington EA, Fanidi A, Evan GI. Oncogenes and cell death. Curr Opin Genet Devel 1994;4:120–129.

51. Bursch W, Paffe S, Putz B et al. Determination of the length fo the histologic stages of apoptosis in normal and in altered hepatic foci of rats. Carcinogenesis 1990;11:847–853.

52. Grasl-Kraupp B, Bursch W, Ruttkay-Nedecky B et al. Food restriction eliminates preneoplastci cells through apoptosis and antagonizes carcinogenesis in rat liver. Proc Natl Acad Sci USA 1994;91: 9995–9999.

53. Mills J, Chari R, Boyer I et al. Induction of apoptosis in liver tumors by the monoterpene perillyl alcohol. Cancer Res 1995;55:979–983.

54. Porsch-Hallstrom I, Blank A, Eriksson L et al. Expression of c-myc, c-fos and c-ras protooncogenes during sex-differentiated rat liver carcinogenesis in the resistant hepatocyte model. Carcinogenesis 1989;10:1793–1800.

55. Yaswen P, Goyette M, Shank P et al. Expression of c-Ki-ras, c-Ha-ras and c-myc in specific cell types during hepatocarcinogenesis. Molec Cell Biol 1985;5:780–786.

56. Pascale RM, Simile MM, Feo F. Genomic abnormalities in hepatocarcinogenesis. Implications for a chemopreventive strategy. Anticancer Res 1993;13:1341–1356.

57. Lee L, Raymond V, Tsao M et al. Clonal cosegregation of tumorigenicity with overexpression of c-myc and transforming growth factor alpha genes in chemically transformed rat liver epithelial cells. Cancer Res 1991;51:5238–5244.

58. Liu C, Tsao M, Grisham J. Transforming growth factors produced by normal and neoplastically transformed rat liver epithelial cells in culture. Cancer Res 1988.

59. Raymond V, Lee D, Grisham J et al. Regulation of transforming growth factor alpha messenger RNA expression in a chemically transformed rat hepatic epithelial cell line by phorbol ester and hormones. Cancer Res 1989;49:3608–3612.

60. Luetteke N, Lee D. Transforming growth factor alpha: expression, regulation and biological activion of its integral-membrane precursor. Sem Cancer Biol 1990;1:265–275.

61. Sandgren EP, Luetteke NC, Qiu TH et al. Transforming growth factor alpha dramatically enhances oncogene-induced carcinogenesis in transgenic mouse pancreas and liver. Molec Cell Biol 1993;13: 320–330.

62. Garcea R, Daino L, Pascale R et al. Protooncogene methylation and expression in regenerating liver and preneoplastic liver nodules induced in the rat by diethylnitrosamine: effect of variations of S-adenosylmethionine:S-adenosylhomocysteine ratio. Carcinogenesis 1989;10:1183–1192.

63. Rao PM, Antony A, Rajalakshmi S et al. Studies on hypomethylation of liver DNA during early stages of chemical carcinogenesis in rat liver. Carcinogenesis 1989;10:933–937.

64. Ruchirawat M, Becker F, Lepeyre J. Interaction of DNA methyltransferase with aminofluorene and N-acetylaminofluorene modified poly(dC-dG). Nucl Acid Res 1984;12:3357–3372.

65. Carr B, Reilly J, Smith S et al. The tumorigenesis of 5-azacytidine in male Fisher rats. Carcinogenesis 1984;5:1897–1902.

66. Simile MM, Pascale R, De-Miglio MR et al. Correlation between S-adenosyl-L-methionine content and production of c-myc, c-Ha-ras, and c-Ki-ras mRNA transcripts in the early stages of rat liver carcinogenesis. Cancer Lett 1994;79:9–16.

67. Merlo A, Herman J, Mao L et al. 5′CpG island methylation is associated with transcriptional silencing of the tumour suppressor p16/CDKN2/MTS1 in human cancers. Nature Med 1995;1:686–692.

68. Vogelstein B, Fearon E, Hamilton S et al. Genetic alterations during colrectal-tumor development. N Engl J Med 1988;319:525–532.

69. Rodenhuis S, Slebos R, Boot A et al. Incidence and possible clinical significance of K-ras oncogene activation in adenocarcinoma of the human lung. Cancer Res 1988;48:5738–5741.

70. Zarbl H, Sukumar S, Arthur A et al. Direct mutagenesis of Ha-ras-1 oncogenes by N-nitroso-N-methylurea during initiation of mammary carcinogenesis in rats. Nature 1985;315:382–385.

71. Wiseman R, Stowers S, Miller E et al. Activating mutations of the c-Ha-ras protooncogene in chemically induced hepatomas of the male B6C3F1 mouse. Proc Natl Acad Sci (USA) 1986;83: 5825–5829.

72. You M, Candrian U, Maronpot R et al. Activation of the K-ras protooncogene in spontaneously occurring and chemically induced lung tumors of the strain A mouse. Proc Natl Acad Sci USA 1989;

86:3070—3074.

73. Belinsky S, Devereux T, Maronpot R et al. Relationship between the formation of promutagenic adducts and the activation of the K-ras protooncogene in lung tumors from A/J mice treated with nitrosamines. Cancer Res 1989;49:5305—5311.

74. Belinsky S, Devereux T, Foley J et al. Role of the alveolar type II cell in the development and progression of pulmonary tumors induced by 4-(methylnitrosamino)-1-(3 pyridyl)-1-butanone tumorigenesis in the A/J mouse. Cancer Res 1992;52:3164—3173.

75. Kari F, Foley J, Seilkop S et al. Effect of varying exposure regimens on the tumorigenicity of methylene chloride in female B6C3F1 mice. Carcinogenesis 1993;14:819—826.

76. Green T. The metabolic activation of dichloromethane and chlorofluoromethane in a bacterial mutation assay using Salmonella typhimurium. Mutat Res 1983;118:277—288.

77. Devereux TR, Foley JF, Maronpot RR et al. Ras proto-oncogene activation in liver and lung tumors from B6C3F1 mice exposed chronically to methylene chloride (see comments). Carcinogenesis 1993; 14:795—801.

78. Fox T, Schumann AW, PG, Yano B et al. Mutational analysis of the H-ras oncogene in spontaneous C57BL/6 × C3H/He mouse liver tumors and tumors induced with genotoxic and nongenotoxic hepatocarcinogens. Cancer Res 1990;50:4014—4019.

79. Devereux TR, White CM, Sills RC et al. Low frequency of H-ras mutations in hepatocellular adenomas and carcinomas and in hepatoblastomas from B6C3F1 mice exposed to oxazepam in the diet. Carcinogenesis 1994;15:1083—1087.

80. Devereux T, Anderson M, Belinsky S. Role of ras protooncogene activation in the formation of spontaneous and nitrosamine-induced lung tumors in the resistant C3H mouse. Carcinogenesis 1991.

81. Devereux T, Belinsky S, Maronpot R et al. Comparison of pulmonary O6-methylguanine DNA adduct levels and Ki-ras activation in lung tumors from resistant and susceptible mouse strains. Molec Carcinogen 1993;8:177—185.

82. Gariboldi M, Manenti G, Canzian F et al. A major susceptibility locus to murine lung carcinogenesis maps on chromosome 6. Nature Genetics 1993;3:132—136.

83. Devereux T, Wiseman R, Kaplan N et al. Assignment of a locus for mouse lung tumor susceptibility to proximal chromosome 19. Mamm Genome 1994;5:749—755.

84. Festing M, Yang A, Malkinson A. At least four genes and sex are associated with susceptibility to urethane-induced pulmonary adenomas in mice. Genet Res 1994;64:99—106.

85. Ryan J, Barker P, Nesbitt M et al. KRAS2 as a genetic marker for lung tumor susceptibility in inbred mice. J Natl Cancer Inst 1987;79:1351—1357.

86. You M, Yang Y, Stoner G et al. Parental bias of Ki-ras oncogenes detected in lung tumors from mouse hybrids. Proc Natl Acad Sci USA 1992;89:5804—5808.

87. Belinsky S, Stefanski S, Anderson M. The A/J Mouse Lung as a model for developing new chemointervention strategies. Cancer Res 1993;53:410—416.

88. Goldsworthy TL, Moser GJ, Fransson-Steen RL. Cell proliferation, apoptosis, and hepatocarcinogenesis. Am Coll Veter Pathol Conf Proc 1995:133—164.

Current knowledge of the cancer latent period: chemoprevention strategies during colonic cancer development

Martin Lipkin

Strang Cancer Prevention Center and New York Hospital-Cornell, Medical Center, New York, New York, USA

Abstract. The progressively abnormal development of epithelial cells prior to tumor development has led to different assays of measurement, and to a diversity of approaches to assay the activities of chemopreventive agents. In order to study the influence of inherited and acquired factors during the evolution of tumors, we have developed rodent models in which progressive stages of colonic preneoplasia are expressed. In one model of inherited predisposition to colon cancer, mice carrying a truncated Apc allele with a nonsense mutation in exon 15 have been generated by gene targeting and embryonic stem cell technology (Apc1638 mice). These mice develop multiple gastrointestinal lesions including adenomas and carcinomas, focal areas of high-grade dysplasia (FAD) and polypoid hyperplasias with FADS.

The incidence of inherited colonic neoplasms has now been modulated by a chemopreventive regimen. Colonic lesions significantly increased in Apc1638 mice on a Western-style diet, compared to Apc1638 mice on AIN-76A diet which has lower fat content and higher calcium and vitamin D. These studies have also been carried out in normal mice, and have demonstrated without any chemical carcinogen that a Western-style diet induced colonic tumorigenesis. Modulation of cell proliferation has also been induced by Western-style diets in other organs including mammary gland, pancreas and prostate. These findings are leading to the development of new preclinical models with which to evaluate mutational and epigenetic events leading to neoplasia, and new methods with which to evaluate the efficacy of different classes of chemopreventive agents.

The new preclinical models that we have developed in order to carry out studies of epithelial cells during the evolution of neoplasia are described below.

Gastrointestinal neoplasms in mice carrying a truncated Apc allele

In the past, chemical carcinogens have generally been used in preclinical models to test the possible efficacy of chemopreventive agents. Recently, however, several rodent models have been developed in which neoplastic lesions evolve without chemical carcinogens.

In the first of these rodent models we have studied mice that have a targeted

Address for correspondence: Martin Lipkin MD, Strang Cancer Prevention Center and New York Hospital-Cornell, Medical Center, New York, NY 10021, USA.

mutation in the Apc gene [1]. The adenomatous polyposis coli (APC) gene is important in the development of human gastrointestinal tumors. In our current studies mice carrying a truncated Apc allele with a nonsense mutation in exon 15 were generated by gene targeting and embryonic stem cell technology, and were designated Apc1638 mice.

In an initial study 49 gastrointestinal neoplasms consisting of adenomas and adenocarcinomas developed in 63% of mice carrying the truncated Apc allele. Adenomas and carcinomas were located in stomach, duodenum, jejunum, ileum and colon. Adenomas were tubular, tubulovillous, villous and a majority of adenomas had severe dysplasias. Among the adenocarcinomas most invaded the muscularis mucosa, submucosa or inner layer of propria muscularis. Polypoid hyperplasias with dysplasias were also found in the colons of young mice, and adenomas, focal areas of dysplasias and polypoid hyperplasias were found in older mice. Thus, findings revealed a new rodent model based on a specific Apc gene mutation for the study of tumor development and its prevention in the gastrointestinal tract.

Modulation of colonic lesions induced in Apc1638 mice by a Western-style diet

We recently induced modulation of the colonic lesions in these Apc1638 mice. In young Apc1638 mice colonic polypoid hyperplasias containing dysplasias were significantly increased by feeding the Western-style diet with reduced calcium and vitamin D and increased fat content [2]. Total polypoid hyperplasias in colons of young 18-week-old Apc1638 mice fed a Western-style diet were 10-fold more frequent than in a control AIN-76A diet group. This appears to be the first animal model rapidly producing intestinal and colonic lesions without a chemical carcinogen, and rapidly responding to dietary modulation of developing colonic lesions. In older mice focal areas of dysplasia in the colon were significantly increased by the Western-style diet.

Colonic neoplasms developing in normal mice on a Western-style diet without the use of any chemical carcinogen

Our studies of the evolution of neoplasms in the colons of normal mice have shown that a Western-style diet low in calcium and vitamin D induced hyperproliferation and hyperplasia of colonic epithelial cells.

In normal C57BL/6J mice maintained on a Western-style diet, findings develop similar to those seen in human colon in diseases that increase the risk of colon cancer. In the rodent model they include the early development of increased mitosis, atypical mitosis, increased apoptosis of colonic epithelial cells, and the eventual development of colonic whole-crypt dysplasias — all induced in the rodent model by the Western-style diet without any chemical carcinogen. The development of these findings throughout the entire life span of the rodents has now been quantified [3]. These findings now make it possible to evaluate the ability of numerous chemo-preventive approaches to inhibit colonic neoplasia in the rodent model without a chemical carcinogen, and to utilize this information to further guide comparative measurements carried out on the human colon.

Intermediate endpoints associated with differentiation of colonic epithelial cells following Western-style diets

Previous short-term rodent studies have also identified hyperproliferation in colonic epithelial cells following nutritional diets mimicking a Western-style diet. In a new study [4], two Western-style diets with high fat and phosphate, and low calcium and vitamin D content were now fed to C57BL/6J mice for 12, 24 and 52 weeks. Diet A contained American blend fat, diet B contained corn oil, and diet C control AIN-76A. Chronic feeding of both nutritional stress diets revealed modified colonic epithelial cell differentiation up to 52 weeks of age. Comparisons were made between the Western-style diet and control groups for lectin SBA binding, cytokeratins AE1 and RPN 1160, and acidic mucins including sialo- and sulpho-mucins. In the colonic epithelial cells, lectin SBA binding became significantly increased in the Western-style diet groups compared to controls at all time periods. Significant increases were also found in the expression of cytokeratins AE1 and RPN 1160, and in total acidic mucins at all time periods. These results defined both structural and functional alterations that developed in differentiating colonic epithelial cells under these dietary conditions.

Studies of other organs in addition to colon

The effect of a Western-style diet on early abnormalities associated with breast cancer in the mammary glands of mice

In addition to studies of the colon noted above, we have also begun to study the effects of Western-style diets on other organs, including mammary gland structure and function [5]. In a new study [6], mammary glands of female C57BL/6J mice were analyzed after feeding a Western-style diet or control AIN-76A diet for periods of up to 20 weeks, with mammary glands removed for morphometric and microauto-radiographic measurements. By 14 weeks and 20 weeks of feeding, the number of terminal ducts in the mammary glands of the Western-diet mice significantly increased compared to the control group. This is the area where carcinomas characteristically develop in rodent models and in humans. Moreover, there was a significant increase in the [^{3}H]dThd labeling index of mammary terminal ductal epithelial cells after 14 and 20 weeks of Western-style diet administration. Thus, the Western-style diet induced both increased epithelial cell proliferation and increased numbers of terminal ducts in female mice when fed during young adult growth and development. The findings raise the possibility that in humans the ingestion of a diet containing low calcium and vitamin D content might induce similar changes during the early development of human mammary glands, which is of particular importance in young adolescent women. Studies similar to the above can also be carried out to test the efficacy of chemopreventive agents on mammary gland development in human subjects.

Hyperproliferation in exocrine pancreas and prostate of mice induced by a Western-style diet

We have also begun to study the effects of a Western-style diet with increased fat (corn oil) and low calcium and vitamin D on epithelial cell proliferation in the pancreas, prostate and bladder of C57BL/6J mice [7]. After feeding Western-style diet for periods up to 16 weeks, mice were infused with BrdU for 72 h using subcutaneous Alzet pumps. The findings revealed an unchanged number of pancreatic ducts and acini in the pancreas of mice on Western-style diet or AIN-76A control diets; however, BrdU-labeling indices of epithelial cells lining pancreatic inter- and intralobular ducts, and centroacinar cells significantly increased in Western-style diet compared to control diet groups at all time periods. In prostate BrdU-labeling indices significantly increased in anterior and dorsal but not ventral lobes in Western-style diet compared to control diet groups after feeding Western-style diet for 16 weeks. In bladder epithelial cell BrdU-labeling indices unchanged in Western-style diet and control groups. Findings are thus similar to Western-style diet effects on colon and mammary gland, they also suggest that Western diets play a role in human pancreatic and prostatic carcinogenesis, and chemopreventive strategies that can be considered.

References

1. Fodde R, Edelmann W. Yang K, van Leeuwen C, Carlson C, Renault B, Breukel C, Alt E, Lipkin M, Khan P, Kucherlapati R. A targeted chain-termination mutation in the mouse Apc gene results in multiple intestinal tumors. Proc Natl Acad Sci USA 1994;91:8969–8973.
2. Lipkin M, Yang K, Fan K, Newmark H, Edelmann W, Fodde R, Leung D, Kucherlapati R. Modulation of colonic lesions induced in Apc1638 mice by a Western-style diet. Proc Am Assoc Cancer Res 1995;36:596.
3. Risio M, Lipkin M, Newmark H, Yang K, Steele V, Boone C, Kelloff G. In preparation.
4. Yang K, Fan K, Newmark H, Lipkin M. Intermediate endpoints of colonic epithelial cell differentiation following nutritional stress diets. Proc Am Assoc Cancer Res 1994;35:621.
5. Khan N, Yang K, Newmark H, Wong G, Telang N, Rivlin R, Lipkin M. Mammary ductal epithelial cell hyperproliferation and hyperplasia induced by a nutritional stress diet containing four components of a Western-style diet. Carcinogenesis 1994;15(11):2645–2648.
6. Xue L, Newmark H, Yang K, Lipkin M. Mammary gland hyperproliferation and hyperplasia induced in mice by a Western-style diet. Memorial Sloan-Kettering Cancer Center, New York, NY 10021.
7. Xue L, Newmark H, Yang K, Lipkin M. Hyperproliferation in endocrine pancreas and prostate of mice induced by a Western-style diet. Proc Am Assoc Cancer Res 1996;(In press).

The Scientific Bases of Cancer Chemoprevention.
C. Maltoni, M. Soffritti and W. Davis, editors.

Current knowledge about the cancer latent period: the contribution of epidemiology

John C. Bailar III

University of Chicago, Chicago, Illinois, USA

Abstract. The concept of a latent period for carcinogenesis requires precise definition of each end of the interval between exposure and outcome. These definitions are complex and subject to wide variation from one proposed use to another. The complexities include such things as the difference between individual and population latent period, acute vs. continuing exposure, exposure vs. dose, increase in incidence vs. change in time of appearance, and analogues of the lead time and length bias.

Because many carcinogens, such as dioxin, are stored in body tissues, even a single external exposure may lead to long-term internal exposure. Thus there are few observations about the latent period for acute exposure, and nearly all of those observations are for samples too small to be of use here.

The present analysis considers the time interval between a single, acute exposure to a carcinogen and the clinical detection of cancer. The best information about latency in human cancer is from radiation. Most of the radiation exposure of the atomic bomb survivors was at the time of the blast in August 1945, the exposed populations were relatively large (though not at high doses), and follow-up for neoplasms has been good. However, data have not been reported for the years prior to 1950, so that very short latent periods cannot be documented. Data from 1950 onward are presented. Evidence indicates that the latent period for radiation carcinogenesis varies from one type of cancer to another. Among the common tumors of adults, it is shortest for forms of leukemia.

Key words: cancer, lag, latency, radiation.

Initial considerations

At first, the concept of the latent period for cancer seems simple: it is the time period between exposure to a carcinogenic agent and the occurrence of cancer. On examination, however, this concept requires much elaboration. This is because both ends of the time interval need careful definition and because of other conceptual difficulties.

There is good evidence that many neoplasms go through several steps to reach the point of being independent malignant tumors, and that different agents can alter the timing and extent of these changes. Here I consider a three-step process, but the schema is readily altered for other processes. The first change, initiation, is generally considered to be a point event; the second, promotion, may occur over some period of time; and the third, progression, again seems to depend on a point event. If we are interested in a carcinogenic agent that affects one of these changes, e.g., promotion,

---

Address for correspondence: John C. Bailar III, MD, PhD, University of Chicago, 5841 S. Maryland, MC-2007, Chicago, IL 60637, USA.

the time required for its expression may depend on what other agents the subject has been or will be exposed to. For example, malignant change as a result of exposure to an initiator is likely to take longer if progressors are almost absent than if they are abundant. Similar considerations apply to the study of carcinogens that work at other steps in the development of cancer. Cancer is a multifactorial disease; the factors do not necessarily act independently; and their interrelations may affect the latent period, however, defined.

A second general consideration is that the incidence of every form of cancer changes with age (most, of course, increase monotonically with increasing age), and there may also be other age-related changes, such as sensitivity of hormone-dependent tissues, or the efficacy of repair mechanisms. These, too, can affect the time interval between exposure to a carcinogen and the occurrence of cancer. Thus the study of latent periods may require the study of separate age groups, and appropriate age groups may differ from cancer to cancer. As an example, it appears that many cancers induced by radiation do not appear until the subject reaches an age where the background incidence of that cancer is substantial. For subjects exposed in early childhood, this may be a long wait — 50 years or more — so that the observed latent period depends heavily on age.

Age may enter in another way. An agent can exert a carcinogenic effect only while the subject is alive; the latent period can never exceed the remaining life span of the subject. This means that the possible range of latent periods (and, generally, the probability that an agent will act as a carcinogen) necessarily decreases with age. A person who is first exposed to a carcinogen at age 80 simply cannot express that carcinogenicity over a period of more than, say, 20 years, because competing causes of death leave little likelihood of survival for that long.

A third general concept of latent period is operational. We must estimate the period of latency by using data of the type and quality available. Some events of much interest are simply not observable (e.g., the appearance of the first independent malignant cell at the time of progression). Others may be subject to a range of statistical influences both random and systematic (bias). The clinical detection of a cancer depends on its exact location, rate of growth (rapid change may be alarming to the patient, and lead to early diagnosis), secondary symptoms such as pain or hemorrhage, the acuity of the physician, the use of screening modalities, and many other things. A purely statistical consideration is that carcinogenicity cannot be established, and latency investigated, until the incidence of cancer has risen far enough above the natural or background rate for the change to be demonstrated. The common statement that most cancers have a latent period of at least 10 years may depend critically on our inability to demonstrate small increases in incidence at earlier times. True latent periods may be shorter than we commonly think because of the need for statistical evidence of exposure-related risk.

Fourth, there are almost no earmarks of the cause of a specific malignant neoplasm. The established exceptions are rare cancers with only (or almost only) a single cause, e.g., retinoblastoma and a specific genetic defect; mesothelioma and asbestos; or angiosarcoma of the liver and vinyl chloride. In the future it may be possible to link some other, more common, cancers to specific causes if they leave characteristic changes in DNA, but it seems unlikely that this will ever explain very many cancers.

To illustrate, specific occurrences of leukemias cannot be labeled as to whether the cause was chemical, radiologic, or general background. This raises the more general issue of what is a cause, and whether in a useful and meaningful sense every cancer has a cause, but that matter is beyond the scope of the discussion here. The problem with not knowing which cancers are a result of a specific cause is that any effect must be demonstrated in an entire diluted group of neoplasms. This can have devastating effects on such matter as statistical power to detect an effect, estimation of latent periods, and research on mechanisms of carcinogenesis.

Reasons for interest

One important use for an understanding of latent periods is the identification of carcinogens and an improved understanding of how they work. A second use is in understanding the circumstances of a specific patient for such purposes as determining any familial risk, or perhaps eligibility for workman's compensation. A cancer of, say, the colon that is found 2 years after the subject started work is not likely to be work related, whatever the impact of that work on cancer rates 10 or 20 years later.

A third use, and the one of special interest here, is in defining the time interval where medical intervention may interrupt the sequence of events that leads to cancer, and defining and investigating the appropriate use of chemopreventive agents. For example, a substance that inhibits initiation is not likely to have much effect on observed cancer incidence rates for at least 10 years. Similarly, a highly effective agent that destroys or sterilizes initiated cells must be given at least once during the time interval between initiation and progression (or, possibly, promotion). We may eventually find that effective chemopreventive agents need not be taken every day, or even every month, but the interval must not be so long as to exceed the time window where such agents can be effective.

Specific considerations

Latent period can be defined, in concept, for the individual patient, or it can be defined in terms of the distribution of individual latent periods for members of some population group. In the latter instance, the analyst must decide whether to estimate the average latency (perhaps with its variance), minimum latency, the full distribution, or something else. In my reading of the literature, latency in a population seems to refer most often to the earliest time at which an elevation in cancer rates can be demonstrated, often taken as 10 years, except for leukemia. Hereafter, I will use the term "population latency" in this sense. But the earliest event in a group must occur before the mean time to an event, sometimes very long before, and the largest number of events can occur many years after the increase is demonstrated. Thus, this definition of latency will tend to overstate or understate the rates at which neoplasms develop, and thus to overstate or understate individual risks, unless the analysis includes an appropriate adjustment.

For exposures that occur over some time interval, e.g., exposure to an industrial carcinogen, or to tobacco smoke, the analyst must specify the time point that will be used to determine the start of the latent period. Obvious choices are the onset of exposure, its midpoint, or its end if recent exposures (those within the latent period) are to be excluded in calculating exposure duration or total exposure, so that special attention is needed in deciding just what aspect(s) of the carcinogenic process are to be assessed. (Defining the close of the period of relevant exposure in terms of the latent period involves some recursive difficulties, but these can be solved.)

Special attention must be given also to the difference between exposure and dose, where I use the word exposure to mean the amount or concentration of a carcinogen that reaches or penetrates the "body envelope," and dose to mean the amount or concentration at an internal site such as plasma or intracellular fluid. For agents that are either metabolized rapidly (e.g., formaldehyde) or removed rapidly (e.g., benzene) average dose over a period of months or years may be assumed to be in proportion to exposure, and the analysis can be carried out in terms of exposure alone. For agents retained in the body (e.g., arsenic or dioxin) this is not true because internal dose, and risk, will rise continuously even if exposure remains constant. Thus an adverse event (e.g., initiation) is more likely to have occurred as a result of the more recent, higher dose than from the earlier, lower dose. If exposure is constant and still continues, if dose increases linearly with constant exposure, and if risk is linear in dose, the average time from which latent period should be estimated is not the midpoint of the exposure interval, but its "centroid" at about 70% (actually $1/(\sqrt{2})$) of the way through it. Similarly, if exposure was constant but stopped at some past time, the effective midpoint at which dose began was about 70% of the way through the exposure.

The shape of the dose-response curve for such agents may also be important. Thus if there is a threshold dose for carcinogenesis, the minimum latent period will depend on how long it takes for exposure to generate an internal dose above the threshold. (Dose-response curves may affect latent periods in other ways, too, but those are not discussed here.) Other complexities arise if exposure is intermittent, or if levels fluctuate, but this also is reserved for another time.

Finally, it is not clear how we should estimate latent periods when more than one carcinogen may be at work. But this is almost always true, because almost every form of cancer is found in persons who have multiple (known) exposures, and also in those with no known exposure to a recognized carcinogen. Perhaps we should conclude that life itself is a carcinogen, with an average latent period of about 70 years.

A final comment about age in that we cannot ordinarily tell the difference between an increase in the incidence of some cancers and an advance in the time at which the cancer occurs. I have heard statements that high doses of a carcinogen lead to shorter latent periods, but such a statement needs careful backup to be taken as valid. This may seem true only because the higher risk leads to a demonstrable increase at an earlier time because statistical power at earlier times is increased.

Observations from epidemiology

Laboratory studies can provide great enlightenment about the processes (and control) of cancer, especially when the collection of human data is impossible, not feasible, or unethical. However, animal data cannot answer some critical questions, and here I consider aspects of human data from epidemiologic research.

It is clear that the term "latent period" requires special thought and definition for each use, and that any definition for practical use must attend to the availability of appropriate data. For example, research on industrial carcinogens may properly count exposure (and dose) from the start of employment, if medical care and compensation are tied to the duration of occupational exposure. In contrast, studies of the carcinogenesis process may make the most progress if time is counted from the moment of a single acute exposure, or from the midpoint or centroid (see above) of exposure over a longer time period.

Cancers in children seem to be well detected, with virtually complete reporting that includes accurate statements about age. Such cancers can occur at very early ages, and some have been reported to be present at the time of birth. Latent periods then cannot exceed the length of pregnancy plus attained age. Retinoblastoma, for example, is generally found by 3 years of age. Choriocarcinoma, a malignant tumor of certain cells in the placenta, can also have its origin before birth, and hence a latent period of less than 9 months. I have come to believe, however, that these short latent periods have little to do with the qualities of interest here. Malignant tumors in children are rarely attributable to any external agent. Further, they differ from adult tumors in their types of cell origin, their epidemiology, and their response to treatment. While they are indeed malignant tumors, it seems best for present purposes to regard them as biologic errors in the development of organs or tissues rather than errors in tissue maintenance, repair, or replacement. Thus, I will keep my focus on the more common cancers of adults.

The literature of epidemiology has countless reports about the correlations (sometimes, the lack of correlations) between some exposure and the later development of cancer. However, most of these are of limited value for the present purpose because they do not report individual latent periods in a usable way, exposures were irregular and/or poorly measured, subjects often have concurrent exposure to a variety of other chemical agents, and no adjustment has been made for losses of subjects to competing causes of death. This is not to criticize such studies; in general they were carried out for other purposes (such as the identification of a human carcinogen), and important data items were often not available.

The best population for study of the cancer latent period in humans is the group of Japanese survivors of the atomic bombs that were exploded in Hiroshima and Nagasaki in August, 1945. The sample sizes are quite large in the present context, most of the exposure was instantaneous (despite some delayed exposure from secondary radiation and fallout), doses are rather well estimated, the exposed population was fairly representative of the general Japanese population, follow-up is close to 100%, and the Atomic Bomb Casualty Commission (ABCC) and its successor the Radiation Effects Research Foundation (RERF) have collected and made available large amounts of highly accurate supporting data. Of course, there are problems, too heavy mortality at the time of the bombs and over the following years may have introduced selection biases, generalization of some of the observations to other populations may be less than straightforward, events in the first 5 years after exposure were not recorded and studied in the same way, and findings in radiation carcinogenesis may not apply with full force to chemical carcinogenesis. In addition, times are measured to death rather than to clinical diagnosis. However, the strengths of the data far outweigh these problems.

In summary, the Japanese data show that the relative risk (RR) for death from leukemia (all types combined) was about 12 (i.e., 12 times the rate in an unexposed Japanese control population of the same mix of age and sex) during the years 1950–55 and that it decreased markedly and rather regularly to about 2 (twice normal) in 1971–75, where is has remained. The shape of the RR curve over time, and anecdotal reports of elevated leukemia incidence prior to the start of the ABCC-RERF study, suggest that the latent period for many persons who died of leukemia was shorter than 5 years. I have inquired about data year-by-year for the period 1950–55, but apparently the tabulations and calculations have not yet been carried out using current dose estimates. Such information, when it is available, will add to our understanding about latent period and may be more strongly suggestive of events prior to 1950. Earlier reports, based on less accurate estimates of exposure, suggest that the peak RR for radiation-related leukemia was 6–8 years after exposure. While samples for specific ages and follow-up periods are small, there is a suggestion that the peak in RR was highest, and decayed most rapidly, in children under 10 years of age at the time of exposure. I have not found similar data over time for subtypes of leukemia.

While I have focused here on the course of the RR over time, the background incidence of leukemia in adults rises with age, and there is little evidence that the absolute risk has yet started to decline. In summary, even for leukemia, individual latent periods may be as long as the full human life span.

Of course, radiation can cause many kinds of neoplasms other than leukemia. In the Japanese series, there have been statistically significant excesses of deaths from cancer of the esophagus, stomach, colon, lung, breast, ovary, and urinary bladder, and from multiple myeloma. Elevations in other forms of cancer are suggestive and may yet attain statistical significance. For all cancers excluding leukemia, the relative risk has been low but increasing, especially recently. RRs for all nonleukemia cancers combined were between 1.12 and 1.29 for each 5-year period from 1950 to 1975, but 1.40 and 1.43 for the following two 5-year periods. I do not have more recent data. Because these cancers are much more common than leukemia, most of the excess risk among the atomic bomb survivors is from these long-delayed cancers. Since there is as yet no evidence of a downturn in risk, it is not yet possible to estimate maximum or even average latent periods. Overall, it appears that the population latent period is less than 5 years, but most individual latent periods are measured in decades.

Latent period and cancer chemoprevention

A cancer chemopreventive agent, to be successful, must be applied before the malignant process reaches the stage of progression, but we cannot estimate individual latent periods until after a cancer has appeared (if then). This means that we must use the population incidence curve to estimate latency, and it is likely that specific applications to chemoprevention will require more detailed consideration of single steps in carcinogenesis. Further, to prevent a point change (such as initiation or progression) or to block or retard a continuous process (such as promotion) may well require that the chemopreventive agent act continuously, and this is likely to require that an effective level of the agent itself be present at all times. Exceptions will arise only when the agent reverses some step in the process (as by selective killing of initiated cells). It seems likely that neither this degree of fine-tuning of agents nor the necessary banks of data on timing will be available for many years. At present, strategies for chemoprevention may be substantially illuminated by consideration of the latent period, but the choice of a specific regimen must be based on a much more general appreciation of carcinogenic processes, drug actions, and available data, including results of studies in animals.

The scientific bases of
cancer chemoprevention (2)

The Scientific Bases of Cancer Chemoprevention.
C. Maltoni, M. Soffritti and W. Davis, editors.

The contribution of epidemiology and molecular biology for identifying population groups eligible for cancer chemoprevention

Gary J. Kelloff[1], Charles W. Boone[1], Winfred F. Malone[1], Susan G. Nayfield[1], Ernest T. Hawk[1], James A. Crowell[1], Ronald A. Lubet[1], Vernon E. Steele[1] and Caroline C. Sigman[2]

[1]Chemoprevention Branch, Division of Cancer Prevention and Control, National Cancer Institute, Bethesda, Maryland; and [2]CCS Associates, Mountain View, California, USA

Abstract. Cancer risk factors identified in epidemiological and molecular biological studies demonstrate the need for chemoprevention and define cohorts for chemopreventive intervention. These risk factors can be attributed to both genetic (e.g., familial adenomatous polyposis, BRCA1 mutation, Li-Fraumeni syndrome, genetic polymorphism in carcinogen-metabolizing enzymes) and environmental (e.g., tobacco use, occupational exposure to carcinogens, HPV infection) causes. One aspect of chemoprevention research is identification and validation of early risk biomarkers. Some of these biomarkers measure exposure to carcinogens. Examples are carcinogen-DNA adducts, urinary mutagens/carcinogens, hyperproliferation in mucosal tissue, and nonspecific modifications to DNA and protein indicating oxidative damage. Others are specific, primarily genetic lesions associated with carcinogenesis. Besides germline mutations such as those cited above, these include the presence of activated oncogenes and loss of tumor suppressor function in somatic cells. Also included are measures of genetic susceptibility such as chromosome instability and loss and changes in metabolic phenotype affecting the metabolism of carcinogens. Similarly, histopathological features (e.g., nuclear morphometry) and changes in cell biochemistry associated with carcinogenesis (e.g., G-actin and PSA) are being evaluated as biomarkers of cancer risk.

Besides characterizing cohorts for chemoprevention trials, some of these risk biomarkers can be modulated by chemopreventive agents and, therefore, may be suitable surrogate endpoints for cancer incidence in chemoprevention intervention trials. Risk biomarkers are already being integrated into many chemoprevention intervention trials. Examples are carcinogen-DNA adducts in subjects exposed to aflatoxin B_1, hereditary risk and biomarker abnormalities in a high risk cohort for breast cancer, prostatic intraepithelial neoplasia, oral leukoplakia, bronchial dysplasia, Barrett's esophagus, colorectal adenomas, cervical intraepithelial neoplasia, and breast ductal carcinoma in situ.

Key words: intraepithelial neoplasia, phase II/III clinical trials, risk biomarkers.

Cancer chemoprevention is the use of specific chemical compounds to prevent, inhibit, or reverse carcinogenesis. Many epidemiological and molecular biology studies have identified cancer risk factors ranging from environmental and lifestyle factors [1–3] to familial syndromes [3–7] and specific germline or acquired lesions

---

Address for correspondence: Dr Gary J. Kelloff, Chemoprevention Branch, Division of Cancer Prevention and Control, National Cancer Institute, Executive Plaza North, Suite 201, 6130 Executive Boulevard, Rockville, MD 20852, USA.

[2,8–19]. These well-characterized, quantitative cancer risk factors demonstrate the need for chemoprevention and define cohorts for chemopreventive intervention.

A primary objective of current chemoprevention research is development of strategies for evaluating chemopreventive efficacy in phase II and small phase III clinical trials [20–22]. The discussion following considers the current and potential impact of cancer risk on these chemoprevention strategies. Included are:

1. Definition of risk factors or biomarkers that may be used in selecting cohorts and as endpoints for chemoprevention studies.
2. Criteria for selecting risk biomarkers as endpoints and high risk cohorts for chemoprevention studies.
3. Studies at major target sites that incorporate cancer risk-based measurements in their design.

Cancer risk biomarkers

For chemoprevention, the important cancer risk factors are those that can be measured quantitatively in the subject at risk [23]. These factors can be called "risk" biomarkers and can be used to identify cohorts for chemoprevention. Those that are modulated by chemopreventive agents may also be used as endpoints in chemoprevention studies. Generally, the risk biomarkers fit into categories based on those previously defined by Hulka [24]:

1) carcinogen exposure,
2) carcinogen exposure/effect,
3) genetic predisposition,
4) intermediate biomarkers of cancer, and
5) previous cancers (Table 1).

Carcinogen exposure biomarkers are those measuring the presence of carcinogen in tissue or body fluid. These include chemical mutagens and carcinogens, and viruses such as human papilloma virus (HPV) associated with cervical cancer [25] and hepatitis B virus (HBV) associated with liver cancer [2]. For example, De Flora has described molecular dosimetry methods for detecting urinary mutagen levels, and has used them as an endpoint in chemopreventive intervention studies of N-acetyl-L-cysteine (NAC) in smokers [26]. One result of these studies was that 600–800 mg NAC/day significantly reduced the mutagenicity of smokers' urine extracts in the Ames' Salmonella assay.

Besides detecting the presence of carcinogen, carcinogen exposure/effect biomarkers provide evidence that carcinogen is interacting with tissue, typically at the molecular level, in a way that produces cancer. Such biomarkers are usually the result of very early carcinogen-DNA reactions. For example, Kensler and his colleagues have evaluated the correlation of rat liver tumor induction to urinary DNA adducts with the carcinogen aflatoxin B_1 (AFB_1). As will be described below, AFB_1-DNA adducts are inhibited by the chemopreventive agent oltipraz, and a current phase II clinical chemoprevention trial with oltipraz is using these adducts as an endpoint. Mutational specificity (i.e., the evaluation of mutational spectra and "hotspots") is

Table 1. Risk biomarkers in cancer chemoprevention.

Risk biomarkers in chemoprevention are measures of future cancer potential. This risk is normally quantified as relative risk (RR) once validated studies are done. Included are:

Carcinogen exposure
e.g., Urinary mutagens, HPV or HBV infection, plasma hormone levels.

Carcinogen exposure/effect
e.g., Carcinogen-DNA adducts, hydroxyguanosine residues.

Genetic predisposition
e.g., APC, BRCA1, BRCA2, MLH1. MSH2, Li-Fraumeni syndrome (p53 mutation), ataxia telangiectasia, xeroderma pigmentosum, genetic polymorphism in carcinogen metabolizing enzymes (NAT1, NAT2, CYP45OIAI, GSMT1, GSTP1, SRD5A2), mutagen sensitivity.

Intermediate biomarkers
e.g., intraepithelial neoplasia (histopathology including nuclear/nucleolar morphometry and ploidy in CIN, PIN, DCIS, colorectal adenomas, dysplastic oral leukoplakia, bronchial dysplasia, superficial bladder cancers, actinic keratosis), hyperproliferation, proliferation kinetics, genomic instability, oncogene overexpression/tumor suppressor loss, growth factor and growth factor receptor overexpression (e.g., EFGR), differentiation biomarkers (e.g., G-actin cytokeratins blood group antigens), biochemical changes (PSA levels).

Previous cancers/precancerous lesions
e.g., breast, bladder, colorectal cancers and adenomas, head and neck cancers.
Risk biomarkers can be used to identify clinical cohorts for chemopreventive intervention. In some cases risk biomarkers that are modulatable by chemopreventive agents may be used as endpoints in clinical chemoprevention studies.

Abbreviations: CIN = cervical intraepithelial neoplasia, DCIS = ductal cell carcinoma in situ, EFGR = epidermal growth factor receptor, HBV = hepatitis B virus, HPV = human papilloma virus, LCIS = lobular cell carcinoma in situ, PIN = prostatic intraepithelial neoplasia, PSA = prostate specific antigen.

also highly interesting for evaluating the mechanisms of environmental carcinogenesis. Particularly, a large database is accumulating on human p53 gene mutations and the association of "hotspots" with specific carcinogens (e.g., G→T transversion at codon 249 induced in liver by AFB_1 [27,28] and in lung by radon [29]).

Genetic predisposition includes well-characterized germline mutations, many of which are associated with loss of tumor suppressor functions. Examples are APC (familial adenomatous polyposis leading to colorectal cancer) [8,10], BRCA1 and BRCA2 (breast and ovarian cancers) [6,7,17,19,30,31], and p53 mutation resulting in Li-Fraumeni syndrome (multiple cancers including breast, colorectal, brain and leukemia) [4]. Several cancer-predisposing genes are thought to affect the ability of cells to repair carcinogen-induced damage. Prominent among these are the MLH1 gene on chromosome 3p and the MSH2 gene on chromosome 2p, which have been linked to hereditary nonpolyposis colon cancer (HNPCC) [11,12]. Also, recent cancer epidemiology and pharmacogenetic studies have suggested the importance of genetic polymorphisms affecting the ability to detoxify carcinogens (reviewed in [15,32]), e.g., glutathione S-transferase (GSTM1, GSTM2, GSTP1), N-acetyltransferase (NAT1, NAT2), cytochrome P450IAI, and steroid 5α-reductase type II (SRD5A2). Usually, genetic lesions by themselves do not provide appropriate endpoints for chemoprevention studies, since they are not easily modified by chemopreventive agents and are distal in time and progression from the cancer. However, as will be described below, their presence identifies cohorts for chemopreventive intervention, and in association with other biomarker abnormalities can be useful in defining cohorts for phase II and III clinical chemoprevention trials.

Mutations and changes in expression of tumor suppressors during carcinogenesis are also important. Particularly, Harris and colleagues have reviewed the associations of p53 changes with cancer [9,14]. Similarly, oncogenes and growth factors, which are formed by mutation or are overexpressed during carcinogenesis (e.g., ras, EGFR, c-erbB-2), are significant genetic lesions in cancer (reviewed in [33]). Although it is not likely that any of these lesions will be eradicated by chemopreventive agents, their presence and activity may be decreased by damping the signal transduction pathways in which they participate, thereby selecting against proliferation of cells containing the lesions. Moreover, subjects such as smokers who are at risk for induction of these effects may be good candidates for chemopreventive intervention with antimutagens.

Besides these specific genetic lesions, general indicators of genetic susceptibility have been identified. For example, Spitz [13] has described mutagen sensitivity, as measured by the frequency of bleomycin-induced DNA breaks in lymphocytes in vitro [13]. In lung cancer patients >50% of cases tested had mutagen sensitivity scores >1 break/cell compared with 22% of controls.

Intermediate biomarkers of cancer particularly useful as risk biomarkers are intraepithelial neoplasia (IEN), e.g., prostatic intraepithelial neoplasia (PIN), breast ductal carcinoma in situ (DCIS), colorectal adenomas, and cervical intraepithelial neoplasia (CIN). These lesions are essentially precancers, are directly on the causal pathway to cancer, and their presence puts carriers at high risk for invasive disease [21,22,34–36]. Regression and prevention of recurring IEN are logical endpoints for chemoprevention trials. As will be described below in greater detail, current or previous IEN have already been used to define cohorts for clinical chemoprevention studies.

Other intermediate biomarkers may occur within IEN. Besides the genetic biomarkers described above, biochemical changes associated with carcinogenesis are also being evaluated. For example, Hemstreet has identified G-actin as a differentiation biomarker associated with bladder carcinogenesis [37,38]. Besides genetic damage such as microsatellite instability, Tockman and associates have considered the appearance of p31 antigen in sputum samples from patients with premalignant lung lesions [39]. Coffey has discussed nuclear matrix proteins changes [40] and increasing telomerase activity during prostate carcinogenesis [41].

Previous cancers in many targets such as head and neck, breast and bladder put patients at high risk for recurrence and new primaries. In a trial in head and neck cancer, for instance, the incidence of second primaries was 31% after 4 years follow-up [42,43]. In breast cancer patients, the incidence rate of contralateral breast cancer has been estimated as 0.8%/year [44]. Superficial bladder cancers recur in 60–75% of patients within 2–5 years of treatment [45,46]. Like subjects with precancerous lesions, these patients can be good cohorts for chemoprevention studies. For example, in the head and neck cancer trial just cited, which is Hong's pivotal chemoprevention study, treatment with 13-*cis*-retinoic acid reduced the incidence of second primaries to 14%.

Critical aspects in designing chemoprevention studies with risk biomarkers

Concepts fundamental to evaluating the use of risk biomarkers in chemoprevention studies are:
1. The importance of accumulated risk from one or many factors,
2. The stochastic, multipath mode by which these factors are acquired during carcinogenesis.
3. The long time period required for carcinogenesis [23].

For example, the Gail model [47] defines the contributions to accumulated breast cancer risk from family history, previous breast biopsies, age, parity, and age of menarche. Family history, presumably associated at least partially with genetic predisposition, is the predominant factor. Previous breast biopsies diagnosed as benign suggest the presence and persistence of possible precancerous lesions. One interpretation is that the other factors reflect accumulated estrogen exposure — the relative risk (RR) increasing directly with dose. Similarly, accumulated risk has been demonstrated in epidemiological studies on chronic smokers. In these studies, the RRs for lung cancer repeatedly show a dose-response to number of pack/years of smoking (reviewed in [48]).

Fearon and Vogelstein have described the multipath process of carcinogenesis in colorectal cancer [8]. They have identified the lesions that contribute to cancer risk; namely, germline mutations such as APC, ras mutation and overexpression, hypermethylation, loss of heterozygosity in chromosomes 17p (i.e., loss of p53 function) and 18q. The relevance of their model to this discussion of accumulated risk is that multiple lesions are required for cancer development, not all the lesions are seen in every cancer, and the same lesions are not seen in all cancers.

Carcinogenesis can require 20–40 years [49–54]. Thus, even in very high risk cohorts cancer incidence may be a difficult endpoint to evaluate, requiring very large study populations and long study durations. For example, in the epidemiological studies in smokers cited above, the RRs for lung cancer are as high as 25; however, chronic exposure (for risk accumulation) is critical, and the incidence is still relatively low. It has been estimated that less than 20% of smokers will develop lung cancer in their lifetime [55]. The designs of two lung cancer chemoprevention trials show the impact of these factors on cohort size and study duration. A trial of β-carotene and vitamin E in Finnish male smokers was carried out in 29,000 subjects treated for 5–8 years [56]. The CARET trial of vitamin A and β-carotene planned to accrue

>13,000 chronic smokers for a mean 6 years of treatment [57]. The importance of accumulated risk is shown by another group in this study. With a second risk factor of asbestos exposure added, the number of subjects required dropped to 4,000. However, this cohort is still very large and not feasible for many chemoprevention efficacy studies.

The implications of these concepts for risk biomarkers in chemoprevention clinical trials are summarized in Table 2 (see also [23,36]). The first criterion is that risk biomarkers fit the expected biological mechanism(s) of carcinogenesis in the target tissue. That is, the closer the association of the risk biomarker(s) to the cancer or the higher the accumulated risk associated with the biomarker(s), the higher the likelihood that the biomarker(s) will be useful as endpoints and in selection of cohorts for chemoprevention studies. A corollary is that panels of biomarkers representing the various possible carcinogenicity pathways may be better as endpoints and in defining high risk cohorts. Also, it is desirable that chemoprevention trials be relatively short (e.g., phase II trials are 1 month–3 years in duration; phase III trials may be up to 10 years, but in many cancer targets ≤3 years duration should be feasible). Thus, for risk biomarkers used as endpoints short latency compared with cancer is important, and for risk biomarkers defining cohorts short latency between the appearance of the biomarker and subsequent cancer is wanted.

The second and very important criterion is that the biomarker(s) and assay(s) provide acceptable sensitivity, specificity, and accuracy for evaluating chemopreventive efficacy. These factors ensure that a small trial will produce meaningful results. Many investigators have addressed the important issues in identifying risk biomarkers, particularly those suggesting genetic susceptibility, and have described elegant techniques for assaying them. For example, Sidransky and colleagues have described landmark studies in the detection of clonal genetic alterations that identify tissues at risk for bladder, lung and head and neck cancers [58,59].

Gould has characterized an inherited pattern of allelic imbalance in rats that correlates to susceptibility for mammary gland cancer [60]. This pattern may be a prototype molecular marker of cancer risk. You and colleagues described the use of two-dimensional gel electrophoresis patterns to compare the genomes of CIN and cervical carcinomas with normal cervical tissue [61], and the use of confocal laser scanning microscopy (CLSM) to compare DNA content in normal cervical tissue and CIN III [62]. In the gel electrophoresis study, different patterns were seen in normal and neoplastic tissue, and more changes from normal were seen in the cancers than in the precancerous CIN lesions. Similarly, the DNA index observed by CLSM was significantly higher in CIN than in normal tissue.

Also, Hittelman and his colleagues have delineated the use of chromosome in situ hybridization to detect genetic changes in normal and precancerous tissue adjacent to head and neck cancers [63]. In this study, the degree of genetic change (polysomy) detected correlated to histologic progression of the tissue toward cancer. Very importantly, three of the five patients with premalignant lesions of the oral cavity and high levels of polysomy subsequently developed oral cavity cancers, compared with one of eight patients with less severe genetic changes.

Table 2. Criteria for selecting risk biomarkers in identifying cohorts and as endpoints in cancer chemoprevention trials.

Fits expected biological mechanism
Differentially expressed in normal and high-risk tissue.
On or closely linked to causal pathway for cancer.
Latency is short compared with cancer.

Biomarker and assay provide acceptable sensitivity specificity and accuracy
Assay for biomarker is standardized and validated.
Statistically significant difference between levels in high- and low-risk groups.
Relative risk (RR) has been quantified.

Biomarker is easily measured
Biomarker can be obtained by noninvasive or relatively noninvasive techniques.
Assay for biomarker is not technically difficult.

For risk biomarkers used as endpoints
Modulated by chemopreventive agents.
Biomarker modulation correlates with decreased cancer incidence.
Dose-response effect of the chemopreventive agent is observed.

A very interesting animal model has been identified by Jakoby and his associates [64]. They described the chemopreventive activity of the nonsteroidal anti-inflammatory drug piroxicam on colorectal adenomas and drug effect markers in the Apc^{Min} mouse, which carries a mutation resembling human APC and forms many gastrointestinal dysplasia. As they point out, this and other transgenic strains under development will facilitate the analysis of individual etiological and chemopreventive effects that presumably may be translated to clinical studies.

The third criterion of easy measurement applies to all biomarkers in chemoprevention trials, including those involving risk biomarkers. Biomarkers that can be sampled by noninvasive or relatively noninvasive methods, such as in blood or urine, have higher priority for development than those obtained by biopsy or other surgical procedures. Particularly, this is true for trials in healthier subjects where repeated biopsies would be beyond the limits of accepted medical care. On the other hand, there are high-risk cohorts, such as patients with previous colorectal adenomas or colorectal cancer, where periodic biopsies are an established part of follow-up care. In such cases, biomarkers obtained in biopsy samples are of high priority, because of the opportunity to evaluate the histopathology in the high-risk tissue. Particularly important are measurements of changes in nuclear and nucleolar morphometry that reflect the progression of tissue from preneoplasia through IEN to cancer. We and others have previously described the rationale for these measurements and their quantification [35,36,65–67]. Also, in the study by Hittelman et al. cited above, high levels of genetic changes were seen in tissues distant from the tumor site. Hittelman regarded this result as confirmation of the "field effect" in carcinogenesis [68,69], in that high-risk tissue was detected in a wide area near, but not directly at, the cancer site. Very significantly, this result also suggests that simple biopsies in easily accessed tissues such as oral cavity may provide information for determining cancer risk in nearby but less accessible tissues, such as the other parts of the upper aerodigestive tract.

The special requirement for risk biomarkers used as endpoints in chemoprevention trials is obvious, and is that the expression of the biomarker must be affected by the chemopreventive agent being tested. Further, biomarker modulation should correlate to decreased cancer incidence and show dose-response to the chemopreventive agent. As suggested above, this requirement has important implications for the feasibility of genetic lesions as endpoints. It is not likely that chemopreventive agents will eradicate a genetic lesion per se. However, a genetic lesion can be an endpoint in a chemoprevention trial if: 1) cell populations containing the lesion are diminished by the chemopreventive agent in favor of normal cells, or 2) encoded proteins are modulated by the chemopreventive agent.

Cohorts for chemoprevention trials defined by risk biomarkers

We have recently presented the material in Table 3 and the concepts outlined below for selecting high-risk populations for chemoprevention studies [23]. The first column in Table 3 lists representative cohorts at high-risk for major cancers that are likely to benefit from chemopreventive intervention. The second column lists high-risk cohorts in these same major target sites that would be suitable for phase II and III chemo-prevention trials. As follows from the discussion above, the primary distinction between the two lists is the degree of accumulated risk. The higher the degree of accumulated risk and the closer the association of the risk to cancer, the higher are the feasibility and likely success of a chemoprevention trial in the cohort. The high rates of recurrence and new primaries in patients with previous cancers in targets such as head and neck, bladder, colon and breast suggest that such patients comprise suitable cohorts for chemoprevention trials (reviewed in [21]). The endpoints in these trials would be new lesions or earlier biomarkers of elevated risk. Similarly, patients with previous and current precancerous lesions, particularly IEN, make suitable cohorts for chemopreventive intervention studies. The National Cancer Institute Chemoprevention Branch clinical testing program is currently evaluating chemopre-ventive agents in phase II trials in several groups of patients with precancerous lesions – patients with PIN, DCIS, colorectal adenomas, bronchial dysplasia, superficial bladder lesions (Stage Ta, T1), CIN III, esophageal dysplasia, and dysplastic oral leukoplakia. Table 4 lists these trials. Several of the cohorts for future chemopreventive intervention listed in Table 3 are genetic syndromes. Usually, these cohorts are not good candidates for chemoprevention trials, unless they have histological precancerous lesions, as with many patients bearing APC mutations or hereditary nonpolyposis colorectal carcinoma genes (MSH1, MLH2) who develop early colorectal adenomas. Protocol design and statistical problems of using and evaluating high risk cohorts where a predictive genetic test exists but precancerous lesions do not has been described recently by Schatzkin, Freedman and co-workers

[70,71]. Although they acknowledged that there would be difficulties such as noncompliance of subjects who tested negative for the gene defect and the need for relatively large cohorts, the investigators estimated that there could be savings in size,

Table 3. Representative high-risk cohorts for cancer intervention and clinical trials.

Intervention	Clinical trials
Prostate	
PIN.	PIN.
Family history.	Prostate cancer on biopsy treated by "watchful
PSA >3 ng/ml.	waiting".
Prostatitis.	High PSA.
Genetic polymorphism in testosterone activation (SRD5A2).	Organ-confined prostate cancer, scheduled for prostatectomy (assess PIN and other biomarkers in whole gland).
Breast	
Genetic syndrome (e.g., Li-Fraumeni, BRCA1).	DCIS (intervention in presurgical period).
Family history.	High-risk (family history, precancerous lesion,
Previous breast, endometrial, or ovarian cancer.	previous breast cancer) with multiple biomarker
Precancerous lesion (e.g., atypical hyperplasia, DCIS, LCIS).	abnormalities.
Lung	
Tobacco use (smoking and chewing).	Chronic smoking with previous respiratory tract
Previous respiratory tract cancer.	cancer and bronchial dysplasia.
Bronchial dysplasia.	Chronic smoking or prior respiratory tract cancer.
Genetic polymorphisms in carcinogen-metabolizing enzymes (e.g., CYP45OIAI, GSTM2).	
Occupational exposures (e.g., asbestos, nickel, copper).	
Colon	
Genetic syndrome (e.g., APC, HNPCC).	APC or HNPCC and previous adenomas.
Previous colorectal cancer or adenomas.	Previous colorectal cancer or adenomas.
Family history (colorectal cancer or adenomas).	
Previous breast or endometrial cancer.	
Inflammatory bowel disease.	
Bladder	
Previous superficial bladder cancers (Ta, T1).	Previous superficial bladder cancers (with or
Tobacco smoking.	without TIS)
Occupational exposures (e.g., aromatic amines).	
Genetic polymorphism in carcinogen-metabolizing enzymes (e.g., NAT1, NAT2).	
Cervix	
HPV infection.	CIN II or III.
CIN.	
Tobacco smoking.	

(continued)

Table 3. Continued.

Intervention	Clinical trials
Oral cavity	
Oral leukoplakia.	Dysplastic oral leukoplakia
Tobacco use (smoking or chewing).	
Tobacco with alcohol use.	

Abbreviations: CIN = cervical intraepithelial neoplasia, DCIS - ductal cell carcinoma in situ. HNPCC = hereditary nonpolyposis colorectal cancer, HPV = human papilloma virus, LCIS = lobular cell carcinoma in situ, PIN = prostatic intraepithelial neoplasia, PSA = Prostate specific antigen, TIS = transitional cell carcinoma in situ.

duration and cost for cancer prevention trials using genetic tests. The investigators also touched upon the ethical issues that should be explored in developing clinical study protocols with such cohorts. For instance, two fundamental concerns are the timing of genetic testing and disclosure of the results to the patient. There is concern that positive test results can prematurely limit ability to get health insurance or cause job loss, despite the lack of the more definitive risk of a pathologically evaluated lesion. Similarly, there is concern with falsely worrying the patient with the threat of cancer, where the risks are suspected but not confirmed and no standard of treatment exists. A conservative approach is that such lesions alone are not sufficient to warrant entry into a chemoprevention study, but the possibility of additional risk biomarkers in these patients should be evaluated and could lead to definition of appropriate cohorts for early chemoprevention trials. The design of a trial involving high risk with associated intermediate biomarker abnormalities is described below.

Design of clinical chemoprevention trials based on risk biomarkers

From the discussion above and Table 4, clearly risk biomarkers are already factors in the design of most clinical chemoprevention trials — particularly, in identification of cohorts. However, much additional critical thinking is needed to fully integrate risk factors into chemoprevention studies. Two recent protocols have addressed major issues of risk factors in designing chemoprevention trials.

The first study, designed by Kensler and his colleagues [72], is on the effect of oltipraz against liver carcinogenesis. Both the cohort and the endpoint are based on the risk associated with exposure to the environmental carcinogen AFB_1. Importantly, extensive effort was put into developing the assay for the risk biomarker endpoint and for establishing the correlation of this endpoint to cancer risk. Epidemiologic studies have shown a strong association between estimated aflatoxin intake and primary liver cancer [73]. High levels of aflatoxins, produced by Aspergillus species, have been found in groundnuts and maize in Africa, southeast Asia, and southern China, where these foods are dietary staples. In the chemoprevention study, groups of 80 subjects at high risk for liver cancer from AFB_1 exposure (and also from HBV_1 exposure) in the Qidong region of China were treated with oltipraz at 125 mg qd or 500 mg

Table 4. Current and planned phase II clinical chemoprevention trials in high-risk cohorts.

Target site	Agent(s)	Cohort (Treatment period)	Proposed endpoints
Prostate	DFMO DHEA 4-HPR	Scheduled for prostate cancer surgery (evaluation of biopsy tissue with associated PIN) (2–8 weeks)	Histopathology (PIN grade, nuclear/nucleolar polymorphism, ploidy), proliferation biomarkers (e.g., Lewis^Y antigen) genetic/ regulatory biomarkers (e.g., TGFα, p53, bcl-2, pc-1, chromosome 8p loss)
	CATBN	High grade PIN, no carcinoma (3 years)	Histopathology (PIN grade and incidence, nuclear polymorphism, nucleolar size, ploidy) proliferation biomarkers (e.g., PCNA), genetic/ regulatory biomarkers (e.g., TGFβ, altered oncogene expression), PSA, drug effect markers
Breast	DFMO DHEA Exemestane 4-HPR Tamoxifen 4-HPR + Tamoxifen	Mammographic lesion requiring biopsy (DCIS) (2–4 weeks)	Histopathology (PIN grade and incidence, nuclear polymorphism, nucleolar size, ploidy), proliferation biomarkers (e.g., PCNA, Ki-67, S-phase fraction)
	DFMO DHEA	High risk with ≥2 biomarker abnormalities (p53, EGFR, aneuploidy, ER, c-erbB-2) with or without atypical hyperplasia (6 months)	Histopathology (hyperplasia grade, ploidy), proliferation biomarkers (e.g., PCNA), genetic/regulatory biomarkers (e.g., p53, EGFR, ER, c-erbB-2)
Colon	Aspirin + calcium	Previous colorectal adenomas (6 months)	Proliferation biomarkers (PCNA), PGE$_2$ levels
	Sulindac Calcium Calcitriol Vitamin D$_3$	Previous adenomas (resected within the past 2 years) or colon cancers (6 months)	Histopathology (nuclear polymorphism), proliferation biomarkers (DNA labelling index, crypt proliferation pattern – PCNA), differentiation biomarkers, genetic/regulatory biomarkers (p53 apoptosis)
	Sulindac Sulfone	FAP patients (6 months)	Adenoma size and number, proliferation biomarkers (PCNA), genetic/regulatory biomarkers (apoptosis)
	Aspirin Folic acid Aspirin + folic acid	Previous colorectal adenomas (3 years)	Adenoma size and number

(*continued*)

Table 4. Continued.

Target site	Agents	Cohort (Treatment period)	Proposed endpoints
	Calcium + vitamin D_3	Colorectal adenomas <6mm in diameter (3 years)	Adenoma size and number, histopathology (nuclear/nucleolar polymorphism ploidy), proliferation biomarkers (crypt proliferation pattern — PCNA)
	Sulindac	Colorectal adenomas (left side 5–9 mm diameter) (1 year)	Adenoma size and number. proliferation biomarkers (PCNA)
Lung	4-HPR	Chronic smokers with prior resected head/neck lung or bladder cancer who display bronchial squamous metaplasia (index ≥15%) or dysplasia (6 months)	Histopathology (dysplasia regression, ploidy), proliferation biomarkers (PCNA), genetic/regulatory biomarkers (p53, EGFR), mutagen sensitivity, micronucleated cell frequency
	Oltipraz	Chronic smokers or prior resected carcinoma of respiratory tract (6 months)	Histopathology (nuclear polymorphism, ploidy), proliferation biomarkers (MIB-1), genetic/regulatory biomarkers (p53), agent specific (GSTM phenotype, GST activity in lymphocytes and bronchial cells)
Cervix	DFMO 4-HPR	CIN III (6 months)	Histopathology (CIN grade, nuclear polymorphism, ploidy), proliferation biomarkers (PCNA), differentiation biomarkers (keratins, involucrin, transglutaminase), genetic/regulatory biomarkers (ras, EGFR, TGFα), agent specific (e.g., ODC activity, polyamine levels, RAR)
Bladder	DFMO	Previous superficial bladder cancer (Ta, T1 disease without TIS) (12 months)	Histopathology, proliferation biomarkers (Ki-67), differentiation biomarkers (Lewis^x Antigen), genetic/regulatory biomarkers (EGF, EGFR, p53, PKC isotypes), agent specific (ODC activity, polyamine levels)
	4-HPR	Previous superficial bladder cancer (Ta, T1 disease with TIS treated with BCG) (12 months)	Recurrence, histopathology (ploidy), proliferation biomarkers (Ki-67, DD23, M-344), differentiation biomarkers (G-actin)

(*continued*)

Table 4. Continued.

Target site	Agent	Cohort (Treatment period)	Proposed endpoints
Oral cavity	DFMO 4-HPR 13-cis-Retinoic acid	Dysplastic oral leukoplakia (6 months)	Recurrence, histopathology (dysplasia/leukoplakia grade, nuclear polymorphism, ploidy), native cellular fluorescence, proliferation biomarkers (PCNA, Ki-67, S-Phase fraction), differentiation biomarkers (cytokeratin 19, blood Group antigens), genetic/regulatory biomarkers (TGFβ)
Esophagus	DFMO	Dysplastic/metaplastic Barrett's esophagus (6 months)	Histopathology (nuclear/nucleolar polymorphism, ploidy), proliferation biomarkers (Ki-67), genetic/regulatory biomarkers (p53, TGFα, EGFR, microsatellite instability)
Skin	4-HPR	Actinic keratosis (6 months)	Histopathology (lesion grade), proliferation biomarkers (PCNA), genetic/regulatory biomarkers (EGFR, TGFβ)
Liver	Oltipraz	Aflatoxin exposure (Qidong, China) (2 months)	Urinary aflatoxin-DNA adducts, serum aflatoxin-albumin adducts

Abbreviations: CATBN = chemopreventive agent to-be-named, CIN = cervical intraepithelial neoplasia, DCIS = ductal carcinoma in situ, DFMO = 2-difluoromethylornithine, DHEA = dehydroepiandrosterone, EGF = epidermal growth factor, EGFR = epidermal growth factor receptor, FAP = familial adenomatous polyposis, GST = glutathione-*S*-transferase, 4-HPR = all-trans-*N*-(4-hydroxyphenyl)retinamide, ODC = ornithine decarboxylase, PCNA = proliferating cell nuclear antigen, PG = prostaglandin, PIN = prostatic intraepithelial neoplasia, PKC = protein kinase C, RAR = retinoic acid receptor, TGF = transforming growth factor, TIS = transitional cell carcinoma in situ.

$1\times$/week for 2 months. Treatment was scheduled over the summer months, when AFB_1-exposure is highest. The primary endpoint of the trial is urinary AFB_1-DNA adducts.

Kensler and his colleagues developed the preclinical data supporting the trial design, which is as follows:

1. Oltipraz is a potent inducer of phase II metabolic enzymes such as glutathione (GSH) *S*-transferase (GST), and its chemopreventive activity has been attributed to its ability to enhance these enzymes resulting in conjugation and excretion of carcinogens. In studies with carcinogen-induced animals, lower levels of effective carcinogens are seen in oltipraz-treated animals, as measured, for example, by carcinogen-DNA adducts; particularly, lower levels of AFB_1-DNA adducts have been observed [74,75].

2. Oltipraz suppresses liver adenomas and carcinomas in AFB_1-treated rats [76].
3. Liver tumor inhibition correlates to reduction of liver neoplastic foci, GST enhancement, and reduction of liver AFB_1-DNA adducts [76].
4. Reduction of liver AFB_1-DNA adducts, in turn, correlates to reduction of urinary AFB_1-DNA adducts [77–79].
5. And, weekly and twice weekly oltipraz doses are approximately as effective as daily 500 mg doses in reducing rat liver GST-positive neoplastic foci and increasing rat liver GST [79].

In the second study, Fabian and co-workers have addressed the problem of defining a risk-based cohort that is feasible for a short-term chemoprevention study [80]. In this study, 213 women at high risk for breast cancer were selected based on having first degree relatives with breast cancer (73%), prior biopsy indicating premalignant disease (26%), history of breast cancer (13%) or a combination of these factors (11%). Fine needle aspirates (FNA) from these women and 30 low-risk women were analyzed for abnormalities in cytology and other biomarkers (aneuploidy, epidermal growth factor receptor (EGFR), estrogen receptor (ER), p53 and c-*erb*B-2) and compared. The results suggested that the presence of multiple biomarker abnormalities exclusive of cytology could be used to refine the selection of high-risk subjects. Thirty-one (31%) of the high-risk subjects had two or more biomarker abnormalities, while none of the low-risk group had more than one such abnormality. The presence of multiple biomarker abnormalities increased directly with cytologic atypia, ranging from 16% of subjects with normal cytology to 29% of those with hyperplasia to 60% of those with atypical hyperplasia. No significant differences in the number of biomarker abnormalities or abnormal cytology were seen among the original risk groupings (i.e., first degree relatives, prior positive biopsy, history of breast cancer, or multiple factors). Because of the association of multiple biomarkers to cytological evidence of dysplasia, the investigators have suggested that changes in the pattern of biomarker abnormalities (particularly, p53 and EGFR), as well as atypical hyperplasia, in the FNA could be explored as endpoints in a chemoprevention study in this cohort.

Prospects for risk biomarkers in chemoprevention

Throughout the discussion above, we have cited the challenges associated with using risk biomarkers as a basis for cohort selection and as endpoints in chemoprevention trials. The immediate hurdle is defining risk biomarkers that are highly predictive of cancer incidence, are quantitative, and can be used in short-term clinical trials. We are addressing this challenge conceptually by developing strategies based on accumulated risk — e.g., considering risks from lesions such as IEN which are on the causal pathway and closely resemble cancer, and including multiple-risk factors in defining cohorts and endpoints. Technically sophisticated methods for characterizing risk, such as those based on quantitative analysis of chromosome damage patterns (e.g., electrophoretic genomic scanning, allelic imbalance, mutagen sensitivity, and quantitative measures of nuclear and nucleolar morphometry and cytometry) are also being evaluated. Very importantly, we have begun the process of developing the preclinical and pilot clinical data to support the design of short-term clinical trial protocols based on high-risk cohorts and risk biomarker endpoints.

As we stated above, cancer risk from lifestyle, occupational, environmental, and inherited causes defines the need for and the cohorts who will benefit from chemoprevention. One remarkable achievement in recent years has been the identification of genetic lesions that predispose subjects to cancer — these include both germline and acquired mutations leading to such cancer-promoting events as loss of tumor suppressor function, inability of cells to repair induced damage, overexpression of cellular growth and transcription factors, and inability to detoxify carcinogens. Although subjects with these lesions are not likely to comprise cohorts for phase II and III chemoprevention trials unless they are expressing other lesions associated with carcinogenesis, these lesions suggest types of agents that may be effective and the cohorts to which chemoprevention will ultimately be directed.

References

1. Doll R, Peto R. The causes of cancer. J Natl Cancer Inst 1981;66:1191–1308.
2. Henderson BE, Ross RK, Shibata A, Paganini-Hill A, Yu MC. Environmental carcinogens and anticarcinogens. In: Wattenberg L, Lipkin M, Boone CW, Kelloff GJ (eds) Cancer Chemoprevention. Boca Raton FL: CRC Press, 1992;3–17.
3. Ruddon RW. The epidemiology of human cancer. Cancer Biology. New York: Oxford University Press, 1995;19–60.
4. Li FP. Cancer families: Human models of susceptibility to neoplasia — The Richard and Hinda Rosenthal Foundation Award lecture. Cancer Res 1988;48:5381–5386.
5. Lynch HT, Lynch JF. Familial factors and genetic predisposition to cancer: population studies. Cancer Detect Prev 1991;15:49–57.
6. Easton DF, Bishop DT, Ford D, Crockford GP. Genetic linkage analysis in familial breast and ovarian cancer: results from 214 families. The Breast Cancer Linkage Consortium. Am J Hum Genet 1993;52:678–701.
7. Goldgar DE, Fields P, Lewis CM, Tran TD, Cannon-Albright LA, Ward JH, Swensen J, Skolnick MH. A large kindred with 17q-linked breast and ovarian cancer: Genetic phenotypic and genealogical analysis. J Natl Cancer Inst 1994;86:200–209.
8. Fearon ER, Vogelstein B. A genetic model for colorectal tumorigenesis. Cell 1990;61:759–767.
9. Hollstein M, Sidransky D, Vogelstein B, Harris CC. p53 mutations in human cancers. Science 1991;253:49–53.
10. Goyette MC, Stanbridge EJ. The role of tumor suppressor genes in human colorectal cancer. In: Steele VE, Boone CW, Stoner GD, Kelloff GJ (eds) Cellular and Molecular Targets for Chemoprevention. Boca Raton FL: CRC Press, 1992;133–145.
11. Fishel R, Lescoe MK, Rao MRS, Copeland NG, Jenkins NA, Garber J, Kane M, Kolodner R. The human mutator gene homolog *MSH2* and its association with hereditary nonpolyposis colon cancer. Cell 1993;75:1027–1038.
12. Papadopoulos N, Nicolaides NC, Wei Y-F, Ruben SM, Carter KC, Rosen CA, Haseltine WA, Fleischmann RD, Fraser CM, Adams MD, Venter JC, Hamilton SR, Petersen GM, Watson P, Lynch HT, Peltomäki P, Mecklin J-P, de la Chapelle A, Kinzler KW, Vogelstein B. Mutation of a *mutL* homolog in hereditary colon cancer. Science 1993;263:1625–1629.
13. Spitz MR, Bondy ML. Genetic susceptibility to cancer. Cancer 1993;72:991–995.
14. Greenblatt MS, Bennett WP, Hollstein M, Harris CC. Mutations in the p53 tumor suppressor gene: Clues to cancer etiology and molecular pathogenesis. Cancer Res 1994;54:4855–4878.

15. Inaba T, Nebert DW, Burchell B, Watkins PB, Goldstein JA, Bertilsson L, Tucker GT. Pharmaco-genetics in clinical pharmacology and toxicology. Can J Physiol Pharmacol 1995;73:331—338.

17. Easton DF, Ford D, Bishop DT. Breast and ovarian cancer incidence in BRCA1-mutation carriers. Am J Hum Genet 1995;56:265—271.

19. Collins FS. BRCA — Lots of mutations lots of dilemmas. N Engl J Med 1996;334:186—188.

20. Kelloff GJ, Boone CW, Crowell JA, Steele VE, Lubet R, Sigman CC. Chemopreventive drug development: Perspectives and progress. Cancer Epidemiol Biomarkers Prev 1994;3:85—98.

21. Kelloff GJ, Boone CW, Steele VE, Crowell JA, Lubet R, Sigman CC. Progress in cancer chemoprevention: Perspectives on agent selection and short-term clinical intervention trials. Cancer Res 1994;54:2015S—1024S.

22. Kelloff GJ, Johnson JR, Crowell JA, Boone CW, DeGeorge JJ, Steele VE, Mehta MU, Temeck JW, Schmidt WJ, Burke G, Greenwald P, Temple RJ. Approaches to the development and marketing approval of drugs that prevent cancer. Cancer Epidemiol Biomarkers Prev 1995;4:1—10.

23. Kelloff GJ, Boone CW, Crowell JA, Nayfield SG, Hawk E, Malone WF, Steele VE, Lubet RA, Sigman CC. Risk markers and current strategies for cancer chemoprevention. J Cell Biochem (Suppl 24) (In press).

24. Hulka BS, Wilcosky T. Biological markers in epidemiologic research. Arch Environ Health 1988;43:83—89.

25. Lowy DR, Kirnbauer R, Schiller JT. Genital human papilloma virus infection. Proc Natl Acad Sci USA 1994;91:2436—2440.

26. De Flora S, Cesarone CF, Balansky RM, Albini A, D'Agostini F, Bennicelli C, Bagnasco M, Camoirano A, Scatolini L, Rovida A, Izzotti A. Chemopreventive properties and mechanisms of N-acetylcysteine. The experimental background. J Cell Biochem 1995;22:33—41.

27. Puisieux A, Lim S, Groopman J, Ozturk M. Selective targeting of p53 gene mutational hotspots in human cancer by etiologically defined carcinogens. Cancer Res 1991;51:6185—6189.

28. Cerutti P, Hussain P, Pourzand C, Aguilar F. Mutagenesis of the H-*ras* protooncogene and the p53 tumor suppressor gene. Cancer Res 1994;54:1934S—1938S.

29. Taylor JA, Watson MA, Devereux TR, Michels RY, Saccomanno G, Anderson M. p53 mutation hotspot in radon-associated lung cancer. Lancet 1994;343:86—87.

30. King M-C. Breast cancer genes: How many, where, and who are they? Nat Genet 1992;2:89—90.

31. Smith SA, Easton DF, Evans DGR, Ponder BAJ. Allele losses in the region 17q12—21 in familial breast and ovarian cancer involve the wild-type chromosome. Nat Genet 1992;2:128—131.

32. Hayes JD, Pulford DJ. The glutathione *S*-transferase supergene family: Regulation of GST and the contribution of the isoenzymes to cancer chemoprotection and drug resistance. Crit Rev Biochem Molec Biol 1995;30:445—600.

33. Cooper GM. Oncogenes, 2nd edn. Boston: Jones and Bartlett, 1995.

34. Boone CW, Kelloff GJ, Steele VE. Natural history of intraepithelial neoplasia in humans with implications for cancer chemoprevention strategy. Cancer Res 1992;52:1651—1659.

35. Boone CW, Kelloff GJ, Freedman LS. Intraepithelial and postinvasive neoplasia as a stochastic continuum of clonal evolution and its relationship to mechanisms of chemopreventive drug action. J Cell Biochem 1993;17G:14—25.

36. Kelloff GJ, Boone CW, Crowell JA, Steele VE, Lubet R, Doody LA. Surrogate endpoint biomarkers for Phase II cancer chemoprevention trials. J Cell Biochem 1994;19:1—9.

37. Rao JY, Hemstreet GP III, Hurst RE, Bonner RB, Min KW, Jones PL. Cellular F-actin levels as a marker for cellular transformation: Correlation with bladder cancer risk. Cancer Res 1991;51:2762—2767.

38. Hemstreet GP III, Rao JY, Hurst RE, Bonner RB, Jones PL, Vaidya AM, Fradet Y, Moon RC, Kelloff GJ. Intermediate endpoint biomarkers for chemoprevention. J Cell Biochem 1992;16I:93—110.

39. Tockman MS, Erozan YS, Gupta P, Piantadosi S, Mulshine JL, Ruckdeschel JC. The early detection of second primary lung cancers by sputum immunostaining. LCEWDG Investigators. Lung Cancer Early Detection Group. Chest 1994;106:385S—390S.

40. Partin AW, Getzenberg RH, CarMichael MJ, Vindivich D, Yoo J, Epstein JI, Coffey DS. Nuclear

matrix protein patterns in human benign prostatic hyperplasia and prostate cancer. Cancer Res 1993;53:744–746.

41. Sommerfeld H-J, Meeker AK, Piatyszek MA, Bova GS, Shay JW, Coffey DS. Telomerase activity: A prevalent marker of malignant human prostate tissue. Cancer Res 1996;56:218–222.

42. Hong WK, Lippman SM, Itri LM, Karp DD, Lee JS, Byers RM, Schantz SP, Kramer AM, Lotan R, Peters LJ, Dimery IW, Brown BW, Goepfert H. Prevention of second primary tumors with isotretinoin in squamous-cell carcinoma of the head and neck. N Engl J Med 1990;323:795–801.

43. Lippman SM, Benner SE, Hong WK. Chemoprevention. Strategies for the control of cancer. Cancer 1993;72:984–990.

44. Veronesi U, De Palo G, Costa A, Del Vecchio M, Marubini E, de Yoldi GFC, Attili A, Mascotti G, Moglia D, Magni A, Cerrotta A, Delle Grottaglie M, Crippa A, Palvarini M, Maltoni C, Del Turco MR, Saccani G, Boccardo F. Controlled clinical trials with fenretinide in the prevention of contralateral breast cancer. Rationale design methodological approach and accrual. Serono Symp Pub Raven Press 1992;79:243–259.

45. Harris AL, Neal DE. Bladder cancer – field versus clonal origin. N Engl J Med 1992;326:759–761.

46. Herr HW, Jakse G, Sheinfeld J. The T1 bladder tumor. Sem Urol 1990;8:254–261.

47. Gail MH, Brinton LA, Byar DP, Corle DK, Green SB, Schairer C, Mulvihill JJ. Projecting individualized probabilities of developing breast cancer for white females who are being examined annually. J Natl Cancer Inst 1989;81:1879–1886.

48. Shopland DR, Eyre HJ, Pechacek TF. Smoking-attributable cancer mortality in 1991: Is lung cancer now the leading cause of death among smokers in the United States? J Natl Cancer Inst 1991;83: 1142–1148.

49. Frykberg ER, Bland KI. In situ breast carcinoma. Adv Surg 1993;26:29–72.

50. Chanen W. The CIN saga – The biological and clinical significance of cervical intraepithelial neoplasia. Austr NZ J Obstet Gynaecol 1990;30:18–23.

51. Day DW, Morson BC. The adenoma-carcinoma sequence In: Bennington JL (ed) The Pathogenesis of Colorectal Cancer. Philadelphia PA: WB Saunders Co., 1978;58–71.

52. Page DL, Dupont WD, Rogers LW, Rados MS. Atypical hyperplastic lesions of the female breast. A long-term follow-up study. Cancer 1985;55:2698–2708.

53. Bostwick DG. Prostatic intraepithelial neoplasia (PIN): Current concepts. J Cell Biochem 1992;16H:10–19.

54. Bruzzi P, Bonelli L, Costantini M, Sciallero S, Boni L, Aste H, Gatteschi B, Naldoni C, Bucchi L, Casetti T, Bertinelli E, Lanzanova G, Onofri P, Parri R, Rinaldi P, Castiglione G, Mantellini P, Giannini A. A Multicenter Study of Colorectal Adenomas – Rationale, objectives, methods and characteristics of the study cohort. Tumori 1995;81:157–163.

55. Villeneuve PJ, Mao Y. Lifetime probability of developing lung cancer by smoking status, Canada. Can J Pub Health 1993;85:385–388.

56. The Alpha-Tocopherol Beta Carotene Cancer Prevention Group. The effect of vitamin E and β-carotene on the incidence of lung cancer and other cancers in male smokers. N Engl J Med 1994;330:1029–1035.

57. Omenn GS, Goodman G, Thornquist M, Grizzle J, Rosenstock L, Barnhart S, Balmes J, Cherniack MG, Cullen MR, Glass A, Keogh J, Meyskens F Jr, Valanis B, Williams J Jr. The β-carotene and retinol efficacy trial (CARET) for chemoprevention of lung cancer in high risk populations: Smokers and asbestos-exposed workers. Cancer Res 1994;54:2038S–2043S.

58. Mao L, Lee DJ, Tockman MS, Erozan YS, Askin F, Sidransky D. Microsatellite alterations as clonal markers for the detection of human cancer. Proc Natl Acad Sci USA 1994;91:9871–9875.

59. Sidransky D. Molecular markers in cancer diagnosis. J Natl Cancer Inst Monogr 1995;17:27–29.

60. Gould MN, Lubet RA, Kelloff GJ, Haag JD. Inherited susceptibility and acquired allelic imbalance in rat mammary carcinogenesis. J Cell Biochem (Suppl 24) (In press).

61. Liu J, Wang Y, Gu P, Patrick J, Crist KA, Sabourin C, Stoner GD, Mitchell MF, Fanning JD, Kim K, Goldblatt PJ, Kelloff GJ, Boone CW, You M. Detection of genomic alterations in human cervical cancer by two-dimensional gel electrophoresis. J Cell Biochem (Suppl 24) (In press).

92

62. Crist KA, Kim K, Goldblatt PJ, Boone CW, Kelloff GJ, You M. DNA quantitation in cervical intraepithelial neoplasia thick tissue sections by confocal laser scanning microscopy. J Cell Biochem (Suppl 24) (In press).

63. Hittelman WN, Varavud N, Shin DM, Lee JS, Ro JY, Hong WK. Early genetic changes during upper aerodigestive tract tumorigenesis. J Cell Biochem 1993;17(Suppl F):233–236.

64. Jacoby RF, Marshall DJ, Newton MA, Novakovic K, Tutsch K, Cole CE, Lubet RA, Kelloff GJ, Verma A, Moser AR, Dove WF. Chemoprevention of spontaneous intestinal adenomas in the Apc^{Min} mouse model by the nonsteroidal anti-inflammatory drug piroxicam. Cancer Res 1996;56:710–714.

65. Palcic B. Nuclear texture: Can it be used as a surrogate endpoint biomarker? J Cell Biochem 1994;19:40–46.

66. van Diest PJ, Baak JPA. Biomarkers of breast hyperplasias and in situ carcinomas: An overview. J Cell Biochem 1994;19:99–104.

67. Bacus JW, Bacus JV. Quality control in image cytometry: DNA ploidy. J Cell Biochem 1994;19: 153–164.

68. Slaughter DP, Southwick HW, Smejkel W. "Field cancerization" in oral stratified squamous epithelium: Clinical implications of multicentric origin. Cancer 1953;6:963–968.

69. Benner SE, Lippman SM, Hong WK. Chemoprevention strategies for lung and upper aerodigestive tract cancer. Cancer Res 1992;52:2758S–2763S.

70. Schatzkin A, Goldstein A, Freedman LS. What does it mean to be a cancer gene carrier? Problems in establishing causality from the molecular genetics of cancer. J Natl Cancer Inst 1995;87:1126–1130.

71. Baker SG, Freedman LS. Potential impact of genetic testing on cancer prevention trials using breast cancer as an example. J Natl Cancer Inst 1995;87:1137–1144.

72. Kensler TW, Helzlsouer KJ. Oltipraz: Clinical opportunities for cancer chemoprevention. J Cell Biochem 1995;22:101–107.

73. Vainio H, Heseltine E, Wilbourn J. Report on an IARC Working Group meeting on some naturally occurring substances. Int J Cancer 1993;53:535–537.

74. Kensler TW, Egner PA, Trush MA, Bueding E, Groopman JD. Modification of aflatoxin B$_1$ binding to DNA in vivo in rats fed phenolic antioxidants ethoxyquin and a dithiolthione. Carcinogenesis 1985;6:759–763.

75. Kensler TW, Egner PA, Dolan PM, Groopman JD, Roebuck BD. Mechanism of protection against aflatoxin tumorigenicity in rats fed 5-(2-pyrazinyl)-4-methyl-12-dithiol-3-thione (oltipraz) and related 12-dithiol-3-thiones and 12-dithiol-3-ones. Cancer Res 1987;47:4271–4277.

76. Roebuck BD, Liu Y-L, Rogers AE, Groopman JD, Kensler TW. Protection against aflatoxin B$_1$-induced hepatocarcinogenesis in F344 rats by 5-(2-pyrazinyl)-4-methyl-12-dithiole-3-thione (oltipraz): Predictive role for short-term molecular dosimetry. Cancer Res 1991;51:5501–5506.

77. Groopman JD, Jiaqi Z, Donahue PR, Pikul Λ, Lishheng Z, Jun-shi C, Wogan GN. Molecular dosimetry of urinary aflatoxin-DNA adducts in people living in Guangxi Autonomous Region People's Republic of China. Cancer Res 1992;52:45–52.

78. Groopman JD, DeMatos P, Egner PA, Love-Hunt A, Kensler TW. Molecular dosimetry of urinary aflatoxin-N7-guanine and serum aflatoxin-albumin adducts predicts chemoprotection by 12-dithiole-3-thione in rats. Carcinogenesis 1992;13:101–106.

79. Primiano T, Egner PA, Sutter TR, Kelloff GJ, Roebuck BD, Kensler TW. Intermittent dosing with oltipraz: Relationship between chemoprevention of aflatoxin-induced tumorigenesis and induction of glutathione S-transferases. Cancer Res 1995;55:4319–4324.

80. Fabian CJ, Zalles C, Kamel S, McKittrick R, Moore WP, Zeiger S, Simon C, Kimler B, Cramer A, Garcia F, Jewell W. Biomarkers and cytologic abnormalities in women at high and low risk for breast cancer. J Cell Biochem 1993;17G:153–160.

Genetic predisposition of susceptible groups to cancers

H. John Evans

MRC Human Genetics Unit, Western General Hospital, Edinburgh, UK

Key words: ataxia telangiectasia, breast cancer genes, colon cancer genes, genetic polymorphisms, polyposis coli, replication errors, skin cancer.

Many human cancers can be shown to be associated with exposure to specific environmental agents as a result of lifestyle, diet, occupation, etc., but cancers are, in reality, genetic diseases. They result from a continued abnormal proliferation of cells at the wrong time and in the wrong place, following a failure on the part of these cells to undergo a normal process of differentiation or cell death (apoptosis). Each of these cellular processes is governed by a series of specific genes which in normal circumstances, and in nonmutant forms, control the processes of proliferation, differentiation and apoptosis.

It has long been recognized that the development to a metastatic neoplasm is a multistep process and progressive phases such as initiation, promotion and progression are well documented. Moreover, it is now clear that the development of a malignant tumour requires qualitative or quantitative alterations in the functions of a number of genes, many of which have now been identified, and that exposure to certain environmental factors results in structural and functional changes in these genes.

With the exception of smoking-related cancers, it would be true to say that a family history of the disease, particularly early disease, is the single most important risk for all of the common cancers. This familial predisposition is the consequence of the inheritance of a mutated form of one or other of a number of genes, so that one of the steps towards neoplasia is constitutionally present from birth, and is reflected by the early development of cancer in the affected individual. The other, acquired, mutational changes are somatic events that result from the actions of exogenous or endogenous mutagens, or mutagenic processes, and the induction of these somatic changes by environmental factors is itself under the influence of our genes.

A variety of our genes code for proteins that are, in one way or another, responsible for influencing the effects of potential carcinogens in damaging our DNAs and over the past decade much effort has been expended in studies into the

Address for correspondence: H. John Evans, MRC Human Genetics Unit, Western General Hospital, Edinburgh EH4 2XU, UK.

relation between cancer susceptibility and polymorphic genetic loci coding for proteins that activate procarcinogens, or alternatively, inactivate carcinogens [1]. There are many examples, including of course various forms of the large family of p450 isozymes (e.g., CYP 1A1), glutathione-S-transferase (e.g., GST-mu) and N-acetyltransferase-2, which confer either susceptibility, or resistance, to various environmental, including occupational, exposures. For instance, a number of studies on cohorts of cancer patients have noted an excess of individuals homozygous for a deletion of the GST M1 gene, and, hence, having no GST mu activity, but an excess of a variety of cancers including lung, colon and bladder, and such studies certainly define genetically susceptible groups [2–4]. However, the influence of genetics is more dramatic, and more readily evident, in studies on families with cancer, particularly since virtually all types of cancer may exist in familial forms. Early work on the molecular genetics of familial cancers was largely confined to studies on relatively rare childhood cancers, and hence rare families [5]. Others were concerned with rare autosomal recessive syndromes associated with defective repair of damaged DNA and an increased cancer risk, e.g., Bloom's syndrome [6]. In the last few years, however, dramatic advances have been made in our understanding of the genetic predispositions to many common cancers and I would like to discuss these in the context of some of the commonest of these cancers, namely those of skin, breast and colon.

Skin cancer

Skin cancers, including basal and squamous cell carcinomas and melanomas, are the most common forms of cancer in the Western world and their frequencies are rapidly increasing at a rate of around 10% per annum. I am going to confine myself to by far the commonest of these, namely basal cell carcinomas.

The classical inherited condition that predisposes to skin carcinomas is of course the recessive syndrome of xeroderma pigmentosum (Xp). Xp is rare and is a consequence of homozygosity of one of seven different genes whose products are involved in transcription and, in particular, the excision repair of damaged DNA [7]. Another relatively rare skin cancer syndrome is the naevoid basal cell carcinoma syndrome (NBCCS) of Gorlin in which heterozygote carriers of the mutated gene are characterised by the presence of large numbers of naevi. This condition afflicts some one in 57,000 individuals in the population, but is seen in one in five of those patients presenting with basal cell carcinomas below the age of 19 years [8]. NBCCS is an autosomal dominant condition and the responsible gene is localised to chromosome 9q22.3 [9,10]. One allele of this gene is missing, or defective, in patients with the disease and the normal allele is lost in the tumours that arise in these individuals; the gene, therefore, acts as a typical tumour suppressor gene. Moreover, the chromosome region containing this gene shows loss of heterozygosity in sporadic basal cell carcinomas arising in apparently normal individuals [11]. The major carcinogenic agent resulting in skin cancer in these and in normal individuals is the UV-light from the sun's rays. UV-light produces specific changes in DNA, particularly cyclobutane dimers, and genetic analysis of actinic keratoses and basal cell carcinomas shows that virtually all of these have the footprint of specific UV-induced damage in their mutated p53 genes [12,13].

Now the sensitivity of our skins to the induction of erythema by sunlight is under genetic control and some recent studies by Valverde et al. [14] have disclosed some interesting findings. Our skins are protected from the damaging rays of the sun by melanin pigmentation. The melanin exists in two forms, red phaeomelanin and black cumelanin, and people with red hair and fair skins have a predominance of red phaeomelanin in their hair and skins and a reduced ability to produce eumelanin. The relative proportions of these two melanins are regulated by the melanocyte-stimulating hormone (MSH) which acts on its receptor (MC1R) in melanocytes to increase the synthesis of eumelanin.

Valverde and colleagues sequenced the MC1R gene from blood and mucosa cell DNA's from 60 unrelated individuals, 30 with black/brown hair and a good tanning response to the suns rays, and 30 with various shades of red hair with a poor tanning response. They found that the majority of those with red hair (21 of 30, Table 1) exhibited one or more of a series of variants in the sequence of their MC1R gene, whereas no such variants were found in the dark-haired group. In a further study of 135 individuals, classified according to skin type, over 80% of those who tanned poorly, but less than 4% of those who showed a good response to tanning, had variant MC1R gene sequences. Some of these variants may have little effect on the function of the receptor protein, so that the presence of variants in a very small proportion of those who tan well may not be surprising. I mention this work because there is a strong association between the prevalence of skin carcinoma and skin sensitivity to sunlight. Whether the inherited genetic changes in the MC1R gene are also associated with a predisposition to UV-induced skin cancers is not yet established, but it may well be that mutated MC1R genes may define a large and susceptible group.

Breast cancer

The age standardised incidence of breast cancer varies by at least 10-fold throughout the world. The highest incidence occurs in the Western world where up to one in 10 women eventually develop breast cancer. Studies on populations migrating from low-

Table 1. Relationship between hair colour and genetic variants of the melanocyte receptor gene (after [14]).

Hair colour	Light red	Deep red	Auburn	Dark brown/black
No. unrelated individuals	8	16	6	30
No. with MC1R variants	7	13	1	0

to high-risk regions show that these migrants eventually take on the risk characteristic of their new environment, so that environmental factors, including lifestyle, are important. It has been known for a long time, however, that breast cancers "run in families" and that this is a consequence of a genetic predisposition and not merely the sharing of a common environment. Estimates suggest that from 5—10% of breast cancer is predisposed to by the inheritance of a single, dominantly acting, mutated gene (Table 2). Families possessing such a mutation not only have an increased risk of breast cancer, but have early, and not infrequently, bilateral cancers. The first major breast cancer gene, BRCA1, on chromosome 17q21, was isolated in 1994 [15] and the isolation of the second major gene, BRCA2, followed in December of last year [16]. Mutations in one or other of these two genes are responsible for the bulk of breast cancers that are predisposed to by the inheritance of a single dominant mutation.

Women with a constitutional mutation in the BRCA1 gene have an 80—90% lifetime risk of breast cancer and a 40—50% risk for ovarian cancer [17]. The degree of penetrance of the mutated gene is known to be modified by other genes, e.g., HRAS [18], and mutations in BRCA1 alone account for 10—13% of all breast cancers in women <30—35 years of age [19,20], so that germ line mutations in BRCA1 also occur in young women who do not belong to families with multiple-affected members. The gene is large (22 exons encoding 5,529 nucleotides and spanning some 100 kb of genomic DNA) and codes for a calcium-binding protein (a granin) located within secretory vesicles within the cytoplasm [21]. Almost 100 different kinds of mutation have been reported within BRCA1, so that testing for mutations in possible carriers may not be all that straightforward. However, "founder effects" have been noted, for example, 1% of Ashkenazi Jews carry a single specific mutation in BRCA1 which accounts for 16% of breast cancers and 40% of ovarian cancers in women <50 years of age [22]. Despite the fact that the product of BRCA1 is a secretory protein, early studies on loss of heterozygosity involving the wild-type gene at the 17q21 locus had already indicated that the gene acts as a typical tumour-suppressor gene. Recent studies have, indeed, shown that the introduction of a normal gene, by

Table 2. Constitutional mutations in major genes that predispose to familial breast cancer.

Gene (location)	Principal cancers	% cases <35 years	% of total breast cancer
BRCA1 17q21	breast, ovary	~10—13	~3
BRCA2 13q12	breast, male breast	~8	~3 (?)
ATM 11q22	various, breast	(?)	~7 (?)
TP53 17p13	sarcomas, breast, various	~1	<1

transfection, into breast carcinoma cells inhibits their growth, whereas the introduction of this gene into fibroblasts, lung or colon carcinoma cells is without effect [23].

Since the BRCA2 gene has only recently been identified, we know less about its function or indeed its true frequency. It does, however, share some common motifs, and inherited mutations in the gene are considered to be equally as frequent as mutations in BRCA1. The BRCA2 gene is even larger than BRCA1 (around 10 kb of coding sequence) and may have the same enhanced risk for breast cancer, but in contrast to BRCA1 it does not increase the risk for ovarian cancer, but does markedly increase the risk for breast cancer in males.

Although constitutional mutations in BRCA1 and 2 account for most of the obviously familial breast cancer cases, other genes, recessive or of lower penetrance, also contribute to inherited predispositions to breast cancer. The two genes of particular interest are the p53 gene on chromosome 17p, responsible for the Li-Fraumeni syndrome (Li-F), and the ATM gene, on chromosome 11q, responsible for the ataxia telangiectasia syndrome (A-T). Heterozygote carriers of a mutated p53 gene in Li-F families have a much increased risk of cancer, in particular sarcomas and breast cancers [24,25]. The syndrome is rare, it is the result of a single mutation in a gene that is involved in controlling cellular proliferation and apoptosis, and it effectively acts as a tumour-suppressor gene. The principal feature of the syndrome is the very high cancer risk, but the rarity of the condition suggests that it contributes less than 1% to the total of breast cancers in females. A-T, in contrast, is an autosomal recessive condition associated with a variety of major congenital abnormalities, as well as a very high cancer incidence. Affected (homozygous) individuals are also rare, the condition affecting around one in 40,000–100,000 of the population. However, heterozygotes, having but one mutated ATM allele, are very common, they are physically indistinguishable from the normal and it is estimated that they comprise around 1–4% of the population. Such heterozygotes have long been known to be unduly sensitive to ionising radiations, probably as a consequence of a defect in repairing damaged DNA, and the gene responsible, on chromosome 11q22, has recently been cloned [26]: although no linkage has been observed between this locus and familial breast cancer [27]. The protein gene product is similar to known mammalian PI-3 kinases that are involved in cellular growth control and also, and perhaps more importantly, to a group of proteins involved in the repair of damaged DNA [28,29].

Following original work by Swift and colleagues [30,31], which has been supported by others (e.g., [32]), there has been much interest in the possibility that A-T heterozygotes may constitute a very significant proportion of individuals that are predisposed to developing breast cancer. In Swift et al.'s [31] study of 1,599 adult blood relatives of A-T patients and 821 of their unrelated spouses, the relative cancer rate in blood relatives, over a 6.4-year period and for a range of cancers, was found to be 3.5–3.8× higher than in comparable controls, and 5.1× higher for breast cancer. From these data it was suggested that A-T heterozygotes may constitute from around 9–18% of all persons with breast cancer in the USA.

The increased in vivo radiosensitivity of A-T heterozygotes can also be

98

demonstrated in blood lymphocytes exposed to X-radiation in vitro. Following some earlier work of Sandford [33], Scott and colleagues [34] examined the sensitivity to X-ray-induction of chromosome damage in G_2 lymphocytes in vitro from 74 controls, 28 obligate A-T heterozygotes and 50 breast cancer patients (Fig. 1). They found that 21 (42%) of the unselected apparently sporadic breast cancer patients treated before therapy, compared with seven (9%) of the controls, had a chromosomal sensitivity comparable with that found for the hypersensitive A-T heterozygotes. A proportion of the cancer patients may well have been A-T heterozygotes, but the results raise the possibility that other genes of low penetrance, and which are involved in processing DNA damage, may also predispose to breast cancer. This possibility can now be more readily pursued now that the ATM gene has been cloned.

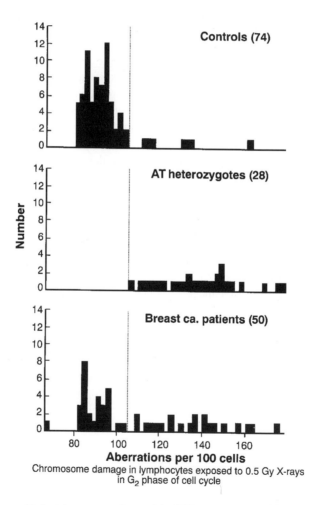

Fig. 1. Radiation sensitivity (chromosome damage) in AT heterozygotes and breast cancer patients (see [34]).

Colon cancer

Familial adenomatous polyposis coli (APC) is the rare, but well-known, syndrome associated with a predisposition to colon cancers. It is an autosomal disease of high penetrance so that 50% of the offspring of an affected parent will themselves be affected. A principal feature of the disease is the development of carpets of many hundreds or thousands of adenomatous polyps lining the lower GI tract, some of which inevitably develop into frank carcinomas in those young people who are heterozygous carriers of a mutation in the gene. The APC gene, on chromosome 5q2.1, has been cloned and characterised and in tumours of these patients the wild-type APC gene is lost, or mutated, so that the normal gene acts as a tumour-suppressor gene. Mutations of the APC gene are also involved in the development of apparently sporadic colon cancers and the introduction of a normal chromosome 5 into neoplastic colorectal cells reverses their neoplasticity [35].

Colorectal cancer is one of the commonest forms of cancer, but the inheritance of a mutated APC gene is a rare event, observed in around one in 10,000 individuals, so that this predisposition can only contribute to less than 1% of the total cases of colon cancer in the population. However, it has long been known that colon cancer may be familial and this is certainly due in part to the sharing of a common diet, but, as Lynch and colleagues have shown [36], it is also quite substantially contributed to by the inheritance of a single predisposing gene or genes. This predisposed colon cancer is referred to as hereditary nonpolyposis colon cancer, or HNPCC [37], and it would appear that it contributes to at least 10–15% of all colorectal cancers.

During 1993/4, and following the assignment by linkage of two different genes, on chromosome 2p [38] and 3p [39], to HNPCC, two further HNPCC genes were identified, on chromosome 2q [40] and 7q [41], and the gene products characterised. More recently a fifth gene, the GTBP gene, has been identified [42]. It transpires that all of these genes are homologous to the mutL and mutS genes of bacteria and yeasts that are involved in long patch excision repair of DNA and, when defective, they result in a mutator phenotype. They code for proteins that recognize mismatched DNA base pairs and excise and replace them with the correct nucleotides [41,43–45]. HNPCC individuals are, therefore, constitutional heterozygotes for a defective DNA repair gene.

Tumours in HNPCC individuals have a replication error, or RER+ phenotype [46], revealed by microsatellite marker probes detecting considerable variation in the size patterns of various repeated DNA sequences as compared with parental patterns. These cancers have acquired a second, somatic, mutation in the corresponding normal allele, so that the cells are homozygous for a defective mismatch DNA repair gene. The consequence of this anomaly is a genetic instability, as a result of polymerase slippage during replication, resulting in insertions and deletions. Some of the microsatellite sequences that show such mutational changes are located within the promotors and coding regions of functional genes, e.g., the p53 and HPRT genes [47]. A significant observation is that of Markowitz and colleagues [48]. They found that the gene coding for the R11 receptor of the growth inhibiting factor TGFβ is

Table 3. Genetic alterations in HNPCC kindreds (see [51]).

Genetic alterations	Kindreds studied	Alterations identified	% alterations
RER+	74	68	92
hMSH2	48	15	31
hMLH1	48	16	33
hPMS1	48	1	2
hPMS2	48	2	4
GTBP	48	0	0
Total[a]	48	34	>69%

[a]Lymphoblasts available from only 48 of the 74 families.

mutated in RER+ colon cancer cells, the mutations occurring in a sequence containing 10 contiguous adenines — exactly what one might predict for a mismatch repair defect. TGFβ is a potent inhibitor of epithelial cell growth and RER+ colon cancer cells deficient for the R11 receptor lose their tumour-forming capacity in nude mice if the cells are transfected with the wild-type R11 gene.

The RER+ phenotype is evident in virtually all tumours seen in HNPCC individuals and it is also seen in around 15% of colon tumours that are of sporadic origin, in a wide variety of other sporadic tumour types [49], and indeed in nontumour cells of HNPCC individuals. Somatically arising mutations in DNA repair genes that result in genetic instabilities would not be unexpected in tumours, but if they are present constitutionally then they clearly predispose the individual to the development of cancers. In the case of HNPCC, a number of current studies are aimed at defining the spectra of mutations in these mismatch genes and in attempting to relate them to the clinical patterns of colorectal disease. Nystrom-Lahti and colleagues [50] have reported that a significant fraction of Scandinavian cases of HNPCC are caused by a small number of mutations within the hMLH1 gene that have spread through the population by a founder effect. In contrast, Liu et al. [51] have found a range of mutations in RER+ patients from North America, Europe and New Zealand. Of interest in their study is that of the mutS homologues, hMSH2 and GTBP, which form a heterodimer complex that binds to mismatched base pairs, only hMSH2 is altered in the germline. Similarly, of the mutL homologues, hMLH2 and hPMS2, which also form heterodimers, only hMLH1 is commonly mutated (Table 3). The relationship between these different mutations and the clinical manifestation of disease is yet to be established, although preliminary findings suggest that colon cancers that are RER+ may have a somewhat better prognosis than those that are RER−.

Concluding comments

In the time available to talk about "susceptible groups", I have attempted to illustrate the importance of genetic predisposition to cancer by reference to mutations in single

Table 4. Approximate number of new cases per year of some common cancers in the UK population (57 × 10⁶ people), and estimates of the proportion genetically predisposed.

Cancers	No. of cases/year[a]	% genetically predisposed
Lung	40000	?
Skin (excl. melanoma)	36000	?
Breast/ovary	30000	7–10%
Colorectal	28000	10–20%
Prostate	14000	5–10%
Bladder	13000	?
Testis	3000	33%
Melanoma	3000	10%

[a]Data derived from UK Cancer Research Campaign Fact Sheets.

genes that strongly predispose to the commonest of cancers; for the greatest risk factors for cancer in the population at large are probably those resulting in evident familial predispositions.

All cancers are, to a greater or lesser extent, predisposed to by an individual's genetic heritage, with genetic factors being paramount for instance in most solid cancers of childhood, but less evident, but by no means absent, for example in smoking-related lung cancer. All cancers also involve the induction of a series of somatic mutations along the road from the initiating events, and genetic factors clearly play a role in modifying the sensitivity of an individual to such changes. Although environmental factors are obvious major determinants, the contribution of our inherited genetic constitutions is vast (Table 4). The fact that we are now in a position to identify various groups of individuals at high risk of contracting specific common cancers is a major advance, and one which we must utilise to the full in the prospective prevention of cancers and in improving their treatment.

References

1. Idle JR. Is environmental carcinogenesis modulated by host polymorphism? Mutat Res 1991;247: 259–266.
2. Bell DA, Taylor JA, Paulson DF, Robertson CN, Mohler JL, Lucier GW. Genetic risk and carcinogenic exposure: a common inherited defect of the carcinogen-metabolism gene glutathione s-transferase M1 (GSTM1) that increases susceptibility to bladder cancer. J Natl Cancer Inst 1993;85:1159–1164.
3. Hirvonen A, Husgafvel-Pursiainen K, Antilla S, Vainio H. The GSTM1 null genotype as a potential risk modifier for squamous carcinoma of the lung. Carcinogenesis 1993;14:1479–1481.
4. Nakachi K, Ianu K, Hayashi SI, Kawajiri K. Polymorphism of the CYP1A1 and glutathione S transferase genes associated with susceptibility to lung cancer in a relation to cigarette dose in a Japanese population. Cancer Res 1993;P53:2994–2999.
5. Evans HJ. Molecular genetic aspects of human cancers: the 1993 Frank Rose Lacture. Br J Cancer 1993;68:1051–1060.
6. Ellis NA, Groden J, Ye T-Z, Straughen J, Lennon DJ, Ciocci S, Proycheva M, German J. The Bloom's syndrome gene product is homologous to RecQ Helicases. Cell 1995;83:655–666.
7. Bootsma D, Hoeijmakers JHJ. Engagement with transcription. Nature (Lond) 1993;363:114–115.

8. Farndon PA, DelMastro RG, Evans DGR, Kilpatrick MW. Location of gene for Gorlin syndrome. Lancet 1992;339:581–582.

9. Farndon PA, Morris DJ, Hardy C, McConville CM, Weissenbach J, Kilpatrick MW, Reis A. Analysis of 133 meiosis places the genes for Nevoid Basal Cell Carcinoma (Gorlins) Syndrome and Fanconi's Anaemia Group C in a 2.6-cm interval and contributes to the fine map of 9q22.3. Genomics 1994;23:486–489.

10. Wicking C, Berkman J, Wainwright B, Chevenix-Trench G. Fine genetic mapping of the gene for Nevoid Basal Cell Carcinoma Syndrome. Genomics 1994;22:505–511.

11. Bonifas JM, Bare JW, Kerschmann RL, Master SP, Epstein EH. Parental origin of chromosome 9q22.3-q31 lost in basal cell carcinomas from basal cell nevus syndrome patients. Hum Molec Genet 1994:3:447–448.

12. Zeigler A, Leffell DJ, Kunala S, Sharma HW, Gailani M, Simon JA, Halperin AJ, Baden HP, Shapiro PE, Bale AE, Brash DE. Mutation hotspots due to sunlight in the p53 gene of non-melanoma skin cancer. Proc Natl Acad Sci USA 1993;90:4216–4220.

13. Zeigler A, Jonasson AS, Leffell DJ, Simon JA, Sharma HW, Kimmelman J, Remington L, Jacks T, Brash DE. Sunburn and p53 in the onset of skin cancer. Nature (Lond) 1994;372:773–776.

14. Valverde P, Healy E, Jackson I, Rees JL, Thoday AJ. Variants of the melanocyte-stimulating hormone receptor gene are associated with red hair and fair skin in humans. Nature Genet 1995;11:328–330.

15. Miki Y, Swensen J, Shattuck-Eidens D, Futreal PA, Harshman K, Tavtigian S, Liu Q, Cochran C, Bennett LM, Ding W, Bell R, Rosenthal J, Hussey C, Tran T, McClure M, Frye C, Hattier T, Phelps R, Haugen-Strano A, Katcher H, Yakumo K, Gholami Z, Shaffer D, Stone G, Bayer S, Wray C, Bogden R, Dayanath P, Ward J, Tonin P, Narod S, Bristow PK, Norris FH, Helvering L, Morrison P, Rosteck P, Lai M, Barrett JC, Lewis C, Neuhausen S, Cannon-Albright L, Goldgar D, Wiseman R, Kamb A, Skolnick MH. A strong candidate for the breast and ovarian cancer susceptibility gene BRCA1. Science 1994;266:66–71.

16. Wooster R, Bignell G, Lancaster J, Swift S, Seal S, Mangion J, Collins N, Gregory S, Gumbs C, Micklem G, Barfoot R, Hamoudi R, Patel S, Rice C, Biggs P, Hashim Y, Smith A, Connor F, Arason A, Gudmundsson J, Ficenec D, Kelsell D, Ford D, Tonon P, Bishop DT, Spurr NK, Ponder BAJ, Eeles R, Peto J, Devilee P, Cornelisse C, Lynch HT, Narod S, Lenoir G, Eglisson V, Barkadottir RB, Easton DF, Bentley DR, Futreal PA, Ashworth A, Stratton MR. Identification of the breast cancer susceptibility gene BRCA2. Nature (Lond) 1995;378:789–792.

17. Ford D, Easton DF, Bishop DT, Narod SA, Goldgar DE, the Breast Cancer Consortium. Risks of cancer in BRCA1 mutation carriers. Lancet 1994;343:692–695.

18. Phelan CM, Rebbeck TR, Weber BL, Devilee P, Ruttledge MH, Lynch HT, Lenoir GM, Stratton MR, Easton DF, Ponder BAJ, Cannon-Albright L, Larsson C, Goldgar DE, Narod SA. Ovarian cancer risk in BRCA1 carriers is modified by the HRAS1 variable number of tandem repeat (VNTR) locus. Nature Genet 1996;12:309–311.

19. FitzGerald MG, MacDonald DJ, Krainer M, Hoover I, O'Neil E, Unsal H, Silva-Arrieto S, Finkelstein DM, Beer-Romero P, Englert C, Sgroi DC, Smith BL, Younger JW, Garber JE, Duda RB, Mayzel KA, Isselbacher KJ, Friend SH, Haber DA. Germ-line BRCA1 mutations in jewish and non-jewish women with early-onset breast cancer. N Eng J Med 1996;2334:143–149.

20. Langston AA, Malone KE, Thompson JD, Daling JR, Ostrander E. BRCA1 mutations in a population-based sample of young women with breast cancer. N Eng J Med 1996;334:137–142.

21. Jensen RA, Thompson ME, Jetton TL, Szabo CS, van der Meer R, Helou B, Tronick SR, Page DL, King M-C, Holt JT. BRCA1 is secreted and exhibits properties of a granin. Nature Genet 1996;12:303–308.

22. Streuwing JP, Abeliovich D, Peretz T, Avishai N, Kaback MM, Collins FS, Brody LC. The carrier frequency of the BRCA1 185delAG mutation is approximately 1% in Ashkenazi Jewish individuals. Nature Genet 1995;11:198–200.

23. Holt JT, Thompson ME, Szabo C, Robinson-Bession C, Arteaga CL, King M-C, Jensen RA. Nature Genet 1996;12:298–302.

24. Malkin D, Li FP, Strong FC, Fraumeni JF, Nelson CE, Kim DH, Kassel J, Gryka MA, Bischoff FZ, Tainsky MA, Friend SH. Germ line p53 mutations in a familial syndrome of breast cancer, sarcomas and other neoplasms. Science 1990;250:1233—1238.

25. Srivastava S, Zou Z, Pirollo K, Blattner W, Chang EH. Germ-line transmission of a mutated p53 gene in a cancer-prone family with Li-Fraumeni syndrome. Nature (Lond) 1990;348:747—749.

26. Savitsky K, Bar-Shira A, Gilad S, Rotman G, Ziv Y, Vanagaite L, Tagle DA, Smith S, Uziel T, Sfez S, Ashkenazi M, Pecker I, Frydman M, Harnik R, Patanjali SR, Simmons A, Clines GA, Sartiel A, Gatti RA, Chessa L, Sanal O, Lavin MF, Jaspers NGJ, Taylor MR, Arlett CF, Miki T, Weissman SM, Lovett M, Collins FS, Shiloh Y. A single ataxia telangiectasia gene with a product similar to PI-3 kinase. Science 1995;268:1749—1753.

27. Wooster R, Ford D, Mangion J, Ponder BAJ, Peto J, Easton DR, Stratton MR. Absence of linkage to the ataxia telangiectasia locus in familial breast cancer. Hum Genet 1993;92:91—94.

28. Hartley KO, Gell D, Smith GCM, Zhang H, Divecha N, Conelly MA, Admon A, Lees-Miller SP, Anderson CW, Jackson SP. DNA-dependant protein kinase catalytic subunit: a relative of phosphatidylinositol 3-kinase and the ataxia telangiectasia gene product. Cell 1995;84:849—856.

29. Zakian VA. ATM-related genes: what do they tell us about function of the human gene. Cell 1995;82:685—687.

30. Swift M, Reitnauer PJ, Morell D, Chase L. Breast and other cancers in families with ataxia telangiectasia. N Engl J Med 1987;316:1289—1294.

31. Swift M, Morell D, Massey RB, Chase CL. Incidence of cancer in 161 families affected by ataxia-telangiectasia. N Engl J Med 1991;325:1831—1836.

32. Borresen A-L, Andersen TI, Treti S, Heiberg A, Moller P. Breast cancer and other cancers in Norwegian families with ataxia-telangiectasia. Genes Chromosomes Cancer 1990;2:339—340.

33. Sandford KK, Parshad R. Detection of cancer-prone individuals using cytogenetic response to X-rays. In: Obe G, Natarajan AT (eds) "Chromosomal Aberrations: Basic and Applied Aspects". Berlin: Springer-Verlag, 1990.

34. Scott D, Spreadborough A, Levine E, Roberts SA. Genetic predisposition in breast cancer. Lancet 1994;344:1444.

35. Fearon E, Vogelstein B. A genetic model for colorectal tumorigenesis. Cell 1990;61:759—767.

36. Lynch HT, Rozen P, Schuelke GS. Hereditary non-polyposis colorectal cancer (Lynch syndromes I and II). Cancer 1985;15:934—938.

37. Vasin HF, Mechlin JP, Meera-Khan P, Lynch HT. The international collaborative group on hereditary non-polyposis colorectal cancer (ICG-HNPCC). Dis Colon Rect 1991;34:424—425.

38. Aaltonen LA, Peltomaki P, Leach FS, Sistonen P, Pylkkanen L, Mecklin J-P, Jarvinen H, Powell SM, Jen J, Hamilton SR, Peterson GM, Kinzler KW, Vogelstein B, de la Chapelle A. Clues to the pathogenesis of familial colorectal cancer. Science 1993;260:812—816.

39. Lindblom A, Tannergard P, Werelius B, Nordenskjold M. Genetic mapping of a second locus predisposing to hereditary non-polyposis colon cancer. Nature Genet 1993;5:279—282.

40. Papodopoulis N, Nicolaides NC, Wei Y-F, Rubens SM, Carter KC, Rosen CA, Haseltine WA, Fleischman RD, Fraser CM, Adams MD, Venter JC, Hamilton SR, Petersen JM, Watson P, Lynch HT, Peltomaki P, Mecklin J-P, de la Chapelle A, Kinzler KW, Vogelstein B. Mutation of a MutL homolog in hereditary colon cancer. Science 1994;263:1625—1629.

41. Nicolaides NC, Papadopoulos N, Liu B, Wei Y-F, Carter KC, Ruben SM, Rosen CA, Haseltine WA, Fleischmann RD, Fraser CM, Adams MD, Venter JC, Dunlop MG, Hamilton SR, Peterson GM, de la Chapelle A, Vogelstein B, Kinzler KW. Mutations of two PMS homologues in hereditary nonpolyposis colon cancer. Nature (Lond) 1994;371:75—80.

42. Drummond JT, Li G-M, Longley MJ, Modrich P. Isolation of an hMSH2 p160 heterodimer that restores mismatch repair to tumor cells. Science 268:1909—1912.

43. Fishel R, Lescoe MK, Rao MRS, Copeland NG, Jenkins NA, Garber J, Kane M, Kolodner R. The human mutator gene homolog MSH2 and its association with hereditary nonpolyposis colon cancer. Cell 1993;75:1027—1038.

44. Leach FS, Nicolaides NC, Papadopoulis N, Liu B, Jen J, Parsons R, Peltomaki P, Sistonen P,

Aaltonen LA, Nystrom-Lahti M, Guan X-Y, Zhang J, Meltzer PS, Yu J-W, Kao F-T, Chen DJ, Cerosaletti KM, Fournier REK, Todd S, Lewis T, Leach RJ, Naylor SL, Weissenbach J, Mecklin JP, Jarvinen H, Petersen GM, Hamilton SR, Green J, Jass J, Watson P, Lynch HT, Trent JM, de la Chapelle A, Kinzler KW, Vogelstein B. Mutations of a mutS homolog in hereditary nonpolyposis colorectal cancer. Cell 1993;75:1215–1225.

45. Bronner CE, Baker SM, Morrison PT, Warren G, Smith LG, Lescoe MK, Kane M, Earabino C, Lipford J, Lindblom A, Tannergard P, Bollag RJ, Godwin AR, Ward DC, Nordenskjold M, Fishel R, Kolodner R, Liskay RM. Mutation in the DNA mismatch repair gene homologue hMLH1 is associated with hereditary non-polyposis colon cancer. Nature (Lond) 1994;368:258–261.

46. Parsons R, Li G-M, Longley MJ, Fang W-H, Papadopoulis N, Jen J, de la Chapelle A, Kinzler KW, Vogelstein B, Modrich P. Hypermutability and mismatch repair deficiency in RER+ tumor cells. Cell 1993;75:1227–1236.

47. Bhattacharya NP, Skandalis A, Ganesh A, Groden J, Meuth M. Mutator phenotype in human colorectal carcinoma cell lines. Proc Natl Acad Sci USA 1994;91:6319–6323.

48. Markowitz S, Wang J, Myerhoff L, Parsons R, Sun L, Lutterbaugh J, Fan RS, Zharowska E, Kinzler KW, Vogelstein B, Brattain M, Wilson JV. Inactivation of the type II TGF-β receptor in colon canver cells with microsatellite instability. Science 1995;268:1336–1338.

49. Mao L, Lee DJ, Tockman MS, Erozan YS, Askin F, Sidransky D. Microsatellite alterations as clonal markers for the detection of human cancer. Proc Natl Acad Sci USA 1994;91:9871–9875.

50. Nystrom-Lahti M, Kristo P, Nicolaides NC, Chang S-Y, Aaltonen LA, Moisio A-L, Jarvinem HJ, Mecklin JP, Kinzler KW, Vogelstein B, de la Chapelle A, Peltomaki P. Founding mutations and Alu-mediated recombination in hereditary colon cancer. Nature Med 1995;1:1203–1206.

51. Liu B, Parsons R, Papadopoulos N, Nicolaides NC, Lynch HT, Watson P, Jass JR, Dunlop MG, Wyllie A, Peltomaki P, de la Chapelle A, Hamilton SR, Vogelstein B, Kinzler KW. Analysis of mismatch repair genes in hereditary nonpolyposis colorectal cancer patients. Nature Med 1996;2:169–174.

Fundamental issues in chemoprevention

Jack Cuzick

Imperial Cancer Research Fund, London, UK

Abstract. Chemoprevention can be defined as the use of natural or synthetic agents to arrest, inhibit or reverse the carcinogenic process before the basement membrane has been breached. There are two key aspects to this definition. Firstly, we are talking about the active prescription of beneficial agents, not the proscription or avoidance of agents or exposures, which currently makes up the bulk of cancer prevention strategies. Secondly, we stop at the basement membrane — anything used after that stage is deemed cancer treatment. However, the control of clinically detected precursor lesions is very much a part of this field.

Animal models and in vitro systems have identified a long list of potential chemopreventive agents in man. A more difficult problem is that of prioritising them for evaluation in humans. With some adaptation, the issues which arise are similar to those for evaluating new screening modalities. These include the public health importance of the cancer site; knowledge of the natural history of the disease process; and the efficacy, safety, and acceptability of the agent. These and other issues related to the evaluation of chemopreventive agents in humans are reviewed.

Key words: chemoprevention, drugs, food constituents, methodologic issues.

Fundamental issues in chemoprevention

Chemoprevention can be defined as the use of natural or synthetic agents to inhibit, arrest, or reverse the carcinogenic process before the basement membrane is breached. There are two important limitations in this definition. Firstly we are only considering the active prescription of preventive agents, as opposed to the avoidance of harmful exposures, which is the mainstay of cancer prevention. Secondly to distinguish chemoprevention from cancer therapy, we only consider control of lesions that have not yet become invasive. Chemoprevention can be used when no lesion is observable or when precursor lesions are found, but once the basement membrane is breached, intervention falls into the domain of cancer treatment. However, even in this case, when all detectable signs of the cancer have been removed, chemoprevention may be important in inhibiting the development of secondary primary cancers.

There is still some disagreement as what constitutes a potential chemopreventive agent. Most researchers would include pharmaceutical drugs, any synthetic compound, micronutrients and other food constituents, and hormonally active agents, but there is less agreement on more diverse agents such as vaccines and whole foods (as opposed to extracted food constituents). There is general agreement that "healthy activities" such as exercise programme would lie outside the scope of this field.

Address for correspondence: Dr Jack Cuzick, Department of Mathematics, Statistics and Epidemiology, Imperial Cancer Research Fund, P.O. Box 123, Lincoln's Inn Fields, London WC2A 3PX, UK.

Several strategies have been used to identify potentially useful chemopreventive agents. Epidemiologic studies have identified certain nutrients which appear to protect against cancer, and demonstrated reduced cancer incidence in individual taking various medications. Animal studies have shown inhibitory effects of various compounds in various model systems and in vitro screening assays have also been used to evaluate a large number of naturally occurring plant extracts and synthetically produced or artificially modified agents. Currently, there are several dozen promising agents that have been identified and evaluated by one or more of these methods [1—3] and a difficult problem is to develop a strategy and priority listing for the human evaluation of these agents.

One approach to this problem is to take a public health/epidemiologic point of view and I have adapted the UICC criteria for evaluating new screening modalities [4] to the case of chemoprevention to provide a framework for this activity.

Important health problem

It is a central tenet of public health medicine to focus resources on the most important health problems. This applies as much to chemoprevention as it does to screening or treatment. For cancer the determination of public health importance is based primarily on mortality rates, but morbidity issues should also be considered, as well as more refined measures of mortality such as total number of years of life lost, which gives greater weight to fatal cancers with an early age at onset. In the Western world it is clear that the four major cancers are those of the lung, bowel, breast, and prostate, followed by those of the stomach, pancreas and bladder (Table 1). In parts of Asia and Africa liver cancer also assumes a major prominence, whereas cervix cancer is still a very common cancer in the developing world [5,6].

Natural history known

An understanding of the natural history of the disease process is even more important for chemoprevention than for screening. In most cases chemopreventive measures are

Table 1. Cancer deaths in England and Wales (1992)

All cancers	146000
•Lung	33700
•Bowel	17400
•Breast	13700
•Prostate	8700
Stomach	8200
Pancreas	6000
Bladder	5100
Ovary	3900

Source OPCS Series DHZ No. 19 (1992).

aimed at intervening in the disease process at an earlier stage than for screening, and an understanding of the preinvasive stages of disease development is vital if these interventions are to be evaluated within a reasonable time frame. Even when chemoprevention is to be used on screened detected preinvasive lesions an understanding of their normal progression and regression rates is needed to evaluate the effect of the intervention.

Intermediate or surrogate endpoints are crucial in this field and their validation is an important research priority. Intermediate endpoints are stages or lesions that all (or almost all) cancers must pass through before becoming fully invasive. It is not necessary that every intermediate endpoint progress eventually to cancer although a high progression rate makes the intermediate endpoint more useful. Much more important is the need for all cancers of a particular type to pass through this stage. Full validation of an intermediate endpoint requires confirmation of this sequence and also evidence that agents affecting the incidence of the surrogate also affect cancer outcome in a direct proportional way. This involves large, expensive studies over a long-term period. A shortcut is to demonstrate that the agent influences the intermediate endpoint in one study and in a separate (simultaneous) study that the intermediate endpoint predicts the final disease state. Such an approach is fraught with potential problems since there may be more than one pathway by which the agent affects the disease, and there may be heterogeneity in the behaviour of intermediate lesion such that in some cases progression is likely, whereas in others stability or even regression is more common. The problem is particularly acute when the agent has been designed or chosen specifically on the basis of influencing this intermediate marker. Thus, a detailed understanding of the causal pathway is needed if these endpoints are to be used.

Biomarkers are another type of surrogate, which are often used to measure exposure at the DNA level, but can also be used to examine other influences on the carcinogenic process without being directly on the causal pathway. Usually they attempt to replace or refine external exposures with internal measures of exposure, but factors influencing the subsequent steps in carcinogenesis such as oncogene or growth factor expression, hormone levels, apoptosis or p53 expression can also be useful biomarkers. Examples include DNA or protein adducts, enzyme levels and changes in metabolic pathways and measures of general damage to the DNA such as micronuclei, sister chromatid exchange rates, etc.

No simple avoidance measures available

Chemoprevention is likely to be a far less effective strategy than avoidance of the carcinogenic agent in the first place. Where this is possible, priority should be given to avoidance measures. Thus, the control of lung cancer must focus on smoking cessation, and the role of chemoprevention is best restricted to attempting to inhibit the development of previous damage in ex-smokers. Avoidance strategies are also appropriate for some occupational or environmental agents, but there is a limit to what can be controlled in this context, and in many cases the causative agents are unknown. This is particularly true in the area of diet. Some types of dietary fat may be associated with cancer development but our understanding of this is still very limited and current evidence suggests that emphasis on protective foods such as fresh fruit and vegetables may be more effective. However, again we have little understanding of which of the multitude of potential chemopreventive agents found in foods are likely to be the most important.

Effective agents

Chemopreventive agents can be identified in a number of ways. Epidemiologic studies have identified a number of foods which appear to protect against cancer. They have also attempted to look at specific nutrients, based on food composition tables (Table 2). However, this is a complicated process because individual foods contain a variety of constituents and the foods themselves are not eaten individually, but as part of an overall diet. Animal studies can be used to look at individual compounds isolated from foods, but the extrapolation from effects on induced tumours caused by single agents (NMU, DMBA, etc.) to those occurring in humans is difficult. Mechanistic studies based on in vitro systems may also be helpful, but there is the major difficulty of knowing which mechanisms are relevant. Randomised trials in humans are the ultimate answer, but they are expensive and very slow. The importance and difficulty of choosing an effective agent for such trials is emphasised by this apparent increase in lung cancer associated with β-carotene consumption in the Finnish trial of heavy smokers [7]. This emphasizes the need for reliable intermediate endpoints and a greater understanding of the carcinogenic process.

Epidemiologic studies of pharmaceutical drugs such as oestrogens, progestins, tamoxifen, aspirin, etc., are more likely to be informative than for dietary studies as the compound under test is better defined and exposure is more easily measured (Table 3). Several studies have shown that oral contraceptives reduce the risk of

Table 2. Possible chemopreventive agents found naturally in food.

Vitamin A	(Lung)
Carotinoids	(Lung)
Vitamin C	(Stomach)
Vitamin E	(Colon)
Calcium/vitamin D_3	(Colon)
Monoterpenes (plant oils, citrus) limonene	(Breast)
Polyphenols	
Green tea	
Curcumin (turmeric)	
Ellagic acid (fruits and nuts)	
3-indole-carbonyl	(Breast)
Isothiocyanates	(Lung)
Broccoli	
Watercress	
Genistein	(Breast)

Table 3. Possible chemopreventive agents used pharmaceutically.

Tamoxifen	Breast
Finasteride	Prostate
Progestins	Endometrium
Oltipraz	Liver (especially if aflatoxin exposure)
Difluoromethylornithene (DFMO)	Colon
NSAIDS	Colon
aspirin	
sulindac	
piroxicam	
ibuprofen	
N-acetylcysteine (NAC)	Lung

ovarian cancer by about 40%, that combined oestrogen-progestin hormone replacement therapy reduces the risk of endometrial cancer, aspirin and others NSAIDs have a large protective effect on colon cancer, and tamoxifen reduces the risk of new contralateral tumours in women taking it to prevent the recurrence of breast cancer. However, confounding factors and biases such as surveillance bias may still be operating in some of these studies and in some cases it is difficult to estimate accurately the benefits for a prospective cohort. A more serious concern in the use of these agents is the likelihood of side effects which, to some degree, occur in any pharmaco-active drug.

Most agents currently under consideration are food constituents or previously used pharmaceutical products. Evaluation of new agents not in these classes will be very difficult and probably will have to be carried out in high-risk individuals with lesions very likely to progress to invasive cancer. Such a strategy could miss important compounds that only are effective at an earlier stage, when lesions are less fully programmed to become cancerous. A major challenge is to develop new agents for commonly used indications such as oral contraception, hormone replacement therapy, or analgesia which have other important benefits (e.g., reductions in cancer, cardiovascular disease, osteoporosis) and few serious side effects.

Safety, acceptability and cost

Safety is a crucial issue in dealing with healthy individuals. It must always be remembered that, as with screening, one is dealing with members of a healthy population who have not come to the clinician for treatment and in many cases have not actively sought out any advice or help. In such a case one is not obliged to do anything, and the potential benefits should substantially outweigh any potential risks for the individual involved before a preventive agent is recommended.

For these reasons there is a requirement to fully evaluate potential chemopreventive agents in trials, both to establish efficacy and to evaluate side effects in a quantitative manner. There is a tension between safety and efficacy, since most active compounds are likely to have some side effects, and these are the only ones most likely to show benefit in a reasonable amount of time in a trial setting. Benefits of mild agents that need to be taken for a very long time will be very difficult to assess until well-validated biomarkers and intermediate endpoints are established. High-risk populations offer a useful population for study since their increased risk makes side effects somewhat more tolerable and, in general, shift the risk-benefit ratio in a positive direction. Acceptability of an intervention is also likely to be better in a high-risk group, especially if risk is based on prior disease or family history so that they have some personal experience with the disease in question.

Cost is clearly important, especially if the agent is to be recommended for general usage. The acceptable cost for a chemopreventive agent will depend on its effectiveness, the individual's risk for the specific cancer, and a range of sociological factors related to the perception of risk and anxiety about disease. In some cases the costs associated with screening for a specific cancer can provide some idea about the willingness to pay for chemoprevention.

References

1. Kelloff GJ, Boone CW. Cancer Chemopreventive agents: drug development status and future prospects. J Cell Biochem 1994;Suppl 20.
2. Kelloff GJ, Boone CW. Cancer chemopreventive agents: drug development status and future prospects. J Cell Biochem 1995;Suppl 22.
3. De Palo G, Sporn M, Veronesi U. Progress and Perspectives in Chemoprevention of Cancer. New York: Serono Symposia Publ, Raven Press, 1992;79.
4. Miller AB. Fundamental Issues in Screening in Cancer Epidemiology and Prevention. In: Schottenfeld D, Fraumeni JF (eds) Philadelphia: W.B. Saunders, 1982;1064–1074.
5. Parkin DM, Pisani P, Ferlay J. Estimates of the worldwide incidence of eighteen major cancers in 1985. Int J Cancer 1993;54:594–606.
6. Pisani P, Parkin DM, Ferlay J. Estimates of the worldwide mortality from eighteen major cancers in 1985. Implications for prevention and projections of future burden. Int J Cancer 1993;55:891–903.
7. Heinonen OP, Albanes D. The effect of vitamin E and β-carotene on the incidence of lung cancer and other cancers in male smokers. N Engl J Med 1994;330:1029–1035.

The Scientific Bases of Cancer Chemoprevention.
C. Maltoni, M. Soffritti and W. Davis, editors.

In vitro/ex vivo studies using primary cells of tumor target tissues for studying aspects of cancer prevention

Beatrice L. Pool-Zobel

Institute of Nutritional Physiology, Federal Research Center for Nutrition, Karlsruhe, Germany

Abstract. Freshly isolated, primary cells closely resemble the cells of adult, intact, and nontransformed tumor-target tissues more closely than any cultured embryonic or tumor cell line in several ways. Foreign compound metabolism, DNA repair, membrane receptors and protein composition are expected to be retained in an in vivo like condition for a few hours after isolation. Therefore, these cells are relevant in vitro models to study chemicals for diverse biological activities, including genotoxicity and antigeno-toxicity. Using the technique of microelectrophoresis, it is possible to rapidly and economically detect DNA damage in freshly isolated cells of numerous rat tissues and of human biopsy samples. Cells are embedded into agar on microscopical slides, where the DNA is freed from the remaining cell components. Electrophoresis and staining with fluorescent dyes reveals images resembling comets, if DNA damage has occurred. Using N-methyl-N′-nitro-N-nitrosoguanidine (MNNG) and 1,2-dimethylhydrazine (DMH) as inducers of DNA damage an experimental model has been developed to study chemoprevention in the colon of rats. Sixteen hours after oral application of the carcinogen, DNA damage is detectable in various regions of the gastrointestinal tract. For the example of several strains of lactic acid bacteria (LAB), effective inhibition of DNA damage can be achieved if the LAB are applied 8 h before application of the carcinogen.

The studies can be supplemented by in vitro investigations with colon cells of human and rat, to more closely elucidate the responsible factors of protection. This is done by incubating the cells for 30 min with a carcinogen, such as MNNG, together with the potential chemopreventive agent. The assay can be performed within a day, and since only few cells are needed, it is very versatile in respect to the tissue types which can be studied.

Key words: antigenotoxicity, colon, genotoxicity, microelectrophoresis, "comet assay".

Introduction

Our knowledge on the molecular mechanisms of cancer induction has grown immensely in the past few years. For the example of colon cancer, Vogelstein and Fearon have reviewed their own work and that of others in a most noted paper on involved mechanisms [1]. Several mutations in tumor-suppressor genes and in proto-oncogens are jointly necessary during the development of normal cells to transformed cells and subsequently for tumor formation. Induced cell death, including apoptosis, and stimulation of cell proliferation are further important events which may either lead to the elimination of an initiated cell or to its survival. Chemical carcinogens induce the processes, and the best-known examples are carcinogens of inhaled

---

Address for correspondence: Prof Dr B.L. Pool-Zobel, Institute of Nutritional Physiology, Federal Research Center for Nutrition, Engesser Str. 20, 76131 Karlsruhe, Germany.

tobacco smoke causing a high incidence of lung tumors by promoting some of the lesions briefly outlined above [2].

For the example of colon cancer we assume that not single environmental agents but rathermore complex functional consequences of imbalanced diets are the decisive risk factors [3–5]. In this context physiological products or certain specific food contaminants have been identified which may be involved [6–8]. These compounds include heterocyclic amines which are contaminants and may be formed in proteinous food at high temperatures. Other risk factors may be endogenous physiological products formed during digestion and cellular processing of foods, such a peroxides of lipid peroxidation or nitroso compounds from amines and bacterial catalysis. These compounds have been identified in part by their ability to induce tumors in the rat colon [9–11].

Genotoxicity is often used as a surrogate for carcinogenic activity, since it is much quicker and easier to detect in standard short-term assay systems and since mutations are important initiating events in the process of carcinogenesis. However, the difficulties of interpreting results of mutagenicity testing using bacteria or cultivated cells of different sources has been an issue of much controversy in the past [12,13]. It is now generally accepted that the relevancy of such results are questionable, since neither the genetic end points nor the target tissues of such tests reflect the situation of tumor induction [14]. Meanwhile, we have increased our knowledge on the processes of chemical carcinogenesis, as described above and, thus the possibilities have increased to devise sensible methods, with which it is possible to assess chemicals for preventing these alterations.

The methods we have been developing are based on using primary cells derived from tumor-target tissues and assessing chemicals from preventing DNA damage, cytotoxicity or modulating cell proliferation. The endpoints may be studied in vitro, or ex vivo, thereby allowing the analysis of pharmacological influences [15]. Also, in addition to using cells of experimental animals, cells from human biopsies may be included in the evaluation [16]. This report summarizes some of the studies enabling detection of DNA damage in the gastrointestinal tract of the rat in vivo. Subsequently, for the example of prevention of this damage by lactic acid bacteria, the applicability of the assay for chemoprevention studies will be presented.

Microelectrophoresis assay

DNA damage is detected with the single-cell microelectrophoresis assay which involves embedding cell suspensions into agar on microscopical slides [17]. The slides are submerged into lysis and DNA unwinding solution (EDTA, Triton-X 100) and then placed into an electrophoresis chamber (25 V, 300 mA, 20 min). Subsequently, the DNA is stained with ethidium bromide and the slides are evaluated with image analysis. Round images signifying intact cells are distinguished from comet forms, indicative of damaged DNA.

Various evaluation criteria may be used, depending on the type and extent of induced DNA damage. Usually 50–100 cells per slide are analyzed for "image length", "% DNA in tail" (tail intensity) or "tail moment", last of which is a factor of both criteria (tail length and tail intensity). The cells can be classified according to the extent of damage and the results transformed into units [18,19]. Also, direct values such as "% cells intact" or "median image lengths" are valid parameters. Statistical analysis is dependent on type of evaluation and several tests have been used. Aliquots of the cells may be processed for cytotoxicity (trypan blue exclusion, intracellular Ca^{2+} levels) or proliferation (BrDU incorporation, PCNA) [20].

Detection of DNA damage in the gastrointestinal tract in vivo

For the elucidation of nutrition and cancer prevention, we have been looking at the genotoxicity of compounds which may induce tumors in the gastrointestinal tract (GI-tract). MNNG was chosen as representative of N-nitroso compounds which may be formed endogenously in the GI tract [21,22]. It is a direct-acting compound which is expected to decompose at the site of application to yield the DNA-reactive species. DMH is a model carcinogen with strong potential to induce tumors and preneoplastic lesions, specifically in the colon of rats. Its activity in the colon is expected to arise systemically after activation in the liver and transport of conjugated intermediates via blood stream to the colon cells [23]. Both compounds give rise to electrophilic intermediates with methylating capacity.

MNNG and DMH have been investigated for their potential to induce DNA damage in different sections of the GI-tract following oral application. As we have described in more detail previously, MNNG induces DNA damage throughout the GI-tract [24]. Short-exposure periods of 1 h are more effective in the upper regions (gastric mucosa, duodenum), whereas longer exposures of 16 h are needed for inducing optimal effects in the colon. With these conditions 3 mg MNNG /kg b.w. results in 43% intact cells (Table 1). Similarly, DMH induces its optimal effect when the colon cells are isolated 16 h after application of the compound. A detailed dose-time response is presented in Fig. 1. DNA damage is not seen after longer exposure periods. This may be due to exfoliation of damaged cells or to DNA repair. In any case the localization of the major DNA-damage correlates well to the sites of tumor formation [20]. Thus, both compounds have been used as inducing agents to study protective, antigenotoxic effects of food components such as lactic acid bacteria (LAB), lactulose, short-chain fatty acids and anthocyanides or anthocyanidines [24–26]. This paper will mainly focus on the work with LAB.

Table 1. DNA damage in gastric and colon mucosa by MNNG (5 mg/kg b.w., p.o.). Cells were isolated 1 or 16 h after gavage in NaCl (10 ml/kg b.w.). Values are % intact cells with image lengths <40 μm (means ± SD, n = 6). Data is from [24].

Tissue	Exposure time (hours)	Control	MNNG
Gastric mucosa	1	92 ± 1	42 ± 8
Colon mucosa	16	70 ± 10	43 ± 5

114

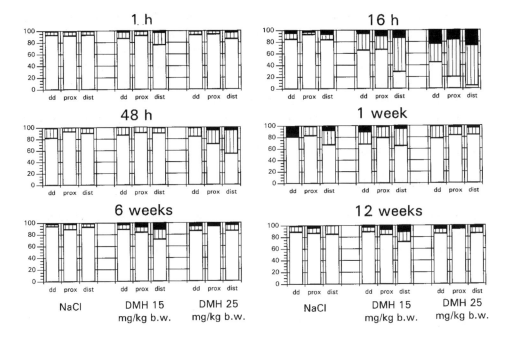

Fig. 1. Course of DMH-induced genotoxicity throughout the gastrointestinal tract. Each bar signifies 100% cells (200 cells per animal, two to four animals per experimental point), proportions of which remained intact (white area, image length <40 μm), moderately damaged (shaded area, image length 40–80 μm), or severely damaged (black solid area, image length >80 μm). (dd, duodenum; upco, upper colon; loco, lower colon). *Type of treatment chosen for assessing protective effects by LAB.

Antigenotoxicity of lactic acid bacteria in vivo

This technique has been utilized to study the protective effects of LAB in vivo [24]. LAB may be endogenous to the GI tract or to be ingested with fermented food products. Their numbers or metabolism in the gut may be increased by resistant starch or disaccharides [27]. They have been associated with many health benefits including the prevention of cancer. In animal studies simultaneous application of specific LAB has lead to a reduction of tumors or preneoplastic lesions induced by DMH-analogs [28–30]. We have performed some studies with a number of different strains of bacteria and with yoghurt products to determine whether DNA damage induced by MNNG or DMH could be inhibited [20,31]. Antigenotoxic effects are assessed in colon cells of animals which have been pretreated with the protective agent being studied and subsequently with MNNG or DMH. Colon cells are isolated after short-term exposure and subjected to microelectrophoresis. In vivo, it has been shown that lactic acid bacteria may prevent DNA damage induced by MNNG more efficiently if the LAB are applied 8 h before the carcinogen than if a treatment schedule with simultaneous application is chosen [20]. Using these treatment conditions yoghurt containing LAB were effective against MNNG-induced damage (Table 2). They were fermented by *Lactobacillus delbrueckeii* ssp. *bulgaricus* and *Streptococcus thermophilus*, or *L. acidophilus* and *Bifidobacterium longum*, respectively. Isolates of these strains have since been also tested against MNNG and DMH [20]. *L. acidophilus* (isolated from the yoghurt Y9) and *B. longum* (from human infant faeces) were efficiently antigenotoxic in the colon (Table 3). Selected strains, but not all, of *S. thermophilus* and *L. delbrueckeii* ssp. *bulgaricus* were also effective [20]. These results show that the same strains, but of different origin may have different potentials of protective activities.

Antigenotoxicity in vitro

Alternatively to the in vivo approach, the genotoxic agent and the protective agent are incubated with the colon cells in vitro [16]. The cells may be incubated with the carcinogen together with the protective agent or a sequential treatment protocol may

Table 2. DNA damage in colon of rats 16 h after application of single doses of yoghurt and 8 h after application of MNNG (7.5 mg/kg b.w.).

Treatment 1 per kg b.w.	Treatment 2 per kg b.w.	n =	% intact cells
7.5 mg MNNG	10 ml NaCl	8	—
7.5 mg MNNG	10 ml Y1	7	20**
7.5 mg MNNG	10 ml Y9	3	38**

**Raw data is significantly different from positive control group [20].
Shown are mean and SD of % intact cells (IL, 40 μm). Y1, yoghurt fermented with *Lactobacillus delbrueckeii* ssp. *bulgaricus* and *Streptococcus thermophilus*; Y9, yoghurt fermented with *L. acidophilus* and *Bifidobacterium longum*. (Data is from [20]).

Table 3. DNA damage in colon of rats 16 h after application of single or multiple doses of LAB (10^{10} cells) and 8 h after application of MNNG (7.5 mg/kg b.w.) or DMH, respectively.

Treatment 1 per kg b.w.	Treatment 2 per kg b.w.	n =	% intact cells
7.5 mg MNNG	10 ml NaCl	4	—
7.5 mg MNNG	10^{10} acid	4	42.5**
7.5 mg MNNG	10^{10} long	4	33.5**
7.5 mg MNNG	10^{10} therm	4	24.5**
15 mg DMH	10 ml NaCl	6	—
15 mg DMH	4×10^{10} acid	4	44.3**
15 mg DMH	4×10^{10} long	6	40** b)
15 mg DMH	4×10^{10} delbr	4	46** b)
15 mg DMH	4×10^{10} therm	6	38**

**Raw data is significantly different from positive control group [20].
% inhibition is defined as "% intact cells" of treatment group minus corresponding positive control group (carcinogen + NaCl). delbr, *Lactobacillus delbrueckeii* ssp. *bulgaricus*; therm, *Streptococcus thermophilus*; acid, *L. acidophilus*; long, *Bifidobacterium longum*. (Original data is from [20]).

be chosen. For the analysis of LAB, the bacterial cells (whole cultures, supernatants, pellets supplemented with medium) were incubated with the carcinogen. Aliquots were then added to the colon cells, since direct incubation with colon cells is not feasible due to toxic effects of the bacteria. Using this approach, it has been shown that pellets supplemented with growth medium, but not with NaCl or buffer may produce intermediates which may inactivate MNNG, resulting in a reduced degree of DNA damage in rat colon cells. Apparently, a short-lived metabolic fraction is produced which may deactivate the carcinogen [24].

Other in vitro active antigenotoxic substances are an acetone extract of a *L. acidophilus* pellet, butyrate, and acetate [20,26].

Conclusions

With this combined ex vivo/in vitro approach, we have been able to detect a variety of LAB strains which may be beneficial, and also to identify the metabolites which may contribute to their protective effects in colon cells. The technique is rapid and economical. A special merit is its versatility, since many other target tissues can be monitored in addition to the GI-tract.

Acknowledgements

The work has in part been supported by ECAIR AIR-1-CT92-256. The excellent technical assistance of Ms R. Lambertz, M. Knoll and B. Mathony-Holschuh is greatly appreciated. We are much obliged to Ms Lindner for competent secretarial work.

References

1. Tacchi AM, Bertram B, Pool BL, Wiessler M. The formation of methyldiethyldithiocarbamate from the reaction of disulfiram with different nitroso compounds — evidence for a scavenging action of disulfiram. J Cancer Res Clin Oncol 1983;105:(Abstract).
2. IARC. IARC Monographs on the Evaluation of Carcinogenic Risks to Humans, vol. 38, Tobacco Smoking. Lyon: IARC, 1986.
3. Hill MJ. Diet and cancer: A review of scientific evidence. Eur J Cancer Prev 1995;4(Suppl 2):3—42.
4. Schatzkin A, Friedman LS, Lanza E, Tungrea J. Diet and colorectal cancer: Still an open question. J Natl Cancer Inst 1995;87:1733—1735.
5. Giovannucci E, Willett WC. Dietary factors and risk of colon cancer. Ann Med 1994;26:443—452.
6. Abbot PJ. Carcinogenic chemicals in food: Evaluating the health risk. Fd Chem Toxicol 1992;30:327—332.
7. Scheuplein RJ. Perspectives on toxicological risk — an example: Foodborne carcinogenic risk. Crit Rev Food Sci Nutr 1992;32:105—121.
8. Wakabayashi K, Nagao M, Esumi H, Sugimura T. Food-derived mutagens and carcinogens. Cancer Res 1992;52(Suppl):2092s—2098s.
9. Gangolli SD, van den Brandt PA, Feron VJ et al. Assessment, Nitrate, nitrite and N-nitroso compounds. Eur J Pharmacol Environ Toxicol Pharmacol Sect 1994;292:1—38.
10. Hill MJ. Dietary fat and cancer. ECP-News 1995;27:4—5.
11. Kune GA, Vitetta L. Alcohol consumption and the etiology of colorectal cancer: A review of the

scientific evidence from 1957 to 1991. Nutr Cancer 1992;18:97—111.

12. Caderni G, Bianchini F, Dolara P, Lodovici M, Quattrucci E. Effect of dietary lipids on hepatic and intestinal monooxygenases in mice. Nutr Cancer 1990;13:111—117.

13. Sobels FH. Evaluating the mutagenic potential of chemicals. The minimal battery and extrapolation problems. Arch Toxicol 1980;46:21—30.

14. Pool BL. Short term tests as a tool in the identification of combinations in carcinogenesis. In: Anonymous Combination Effects in Chemical Carcinogens. Weinheim: Verlag Chemie, 1988:45—64.

15. Pool BL, Brendler SY, Liegibel UM, Tompa A, Schmezer P. Employment of adult mammalian primary cells in toxicology: In vivo and in vitro genotoxic effects of environmentally significant N-nitrosodialkylamines in cells of the liver, lung and kidney. Environ Molec Mutagen 1990;15:24—35.

16. Pool-Zobel BL, Lotzmann N, Knoll M et al. Detection of genotoxic effects in human gastric and nasal mucosa cells isolated from biopsy samples. Environ Molec Mutagen 1994;24:23—45.

17. Singh NP, McCoy MT, Tice RR, Schneider EL. A simple technique for quantitation of low levels of DNA damage in individual cells. Exp Cell Res 1988;175:184—191.

18. Collins AR, Duthie SJ, Dobson VL. Direct enzymic detection of endogenous oxidative base damage in human lymphocyted DNA. Carcinogenesis 1995;14:1733—1735.

19. Collins AR, Ai-guo M, Duthie SJ. The kinetics of repair of oxidative DNA damage (strand breaks and oxidised pyrimidines) in human cells. Mutat Res 1995;336:69—77.

20. Pool-Zobel BL, Neudecker C, Domizlaff I et al. *Lactobacillus-* and *Bifidobacterium*-mediated antigenotoxicity in colon cells of rats: Prevention of carcinogen-induced damage in vivo and elucidation of involved mechanisms. 1996;(Unpublished).

21. Bingham SA, Pignatelli B, Pollock JRA et al. Does increased endogenous formation of N-nitroso compounds in the human colon explain the association between red meat and colon cancer? Carcinogenesis 1996;17:515—523.

22. Rowland IR, Granli T, Bockman OC, Key PE, Massey RC. Endogenous N-nitrosation in man assessed by measurement of apparent total N-nitroso compounds in feces. Carcinogenesis 1991;12:1395—1401.

23. Fiala ES. Investigations into the metabolism and mode of action of the colon carcinogens 1,2-dimethylhydrazine and azoxymethane. Cancer 1977;40:2436—2445.

24. Pool-Zobel BL, Bertram B, Knoll M et al. Antigenotoxic properties of lactic acid bacteria in vivo in the gastrointestinal tract of rats. Nutr Cancer 1993;20:271—282.

25. Rowland IR, Fischer R, Pool-Zobel BL. The effect of lactulose on DNA damage indued by 1,2-dimethylhydrazine in the colon of human-flora-associated rats. 1996;(Unpublished).

26. Pool-Zobel BL, Abrahamse SL, Rechkemmer G. Protective effects of short-chain fatty acids on early events of carcinogenesis: Antigenotoxic effects of butyrate in rat and human colon cells. 1995;(Unpublished).

27. Gibson GR. In vivo effects of oligofructose and inulin on the colonic microbiota. Ingredients 1995;35—38.

28. Goldin BR, Gorbach SL. Effect of Lactobacillus acidophilus dietary supplements on 1,2-dimethylhydrazine-dihydrochloride-induced intestinal cancer in rats. J Natl Cancer Inst 1980;64:263—265.

29. Koo M, Rao V. Long-term effect of *Bifidobacteria* and neosugar on precursor lesions of colonic cancer in CF$_1$ mice. Nutr Cancer 1991;16:249—257.

30. Reddy BS, Rivenson A. Inhibitory Effect of *Bifidobacterium longum* on colon, mammary and liver carcinogenesis induced by 2-amino-3-methylimidazo[4,5-*f*]quinoline, a food mutagen. Cancer Res 1993;53:3914—3918.

31. Felton JS, Knize MG, Roper M, Fultz E, Shen NH, Turteltaub KW. Chemical analysis, prevention, and low-level dosimetry of heterocyclic amines from cooked food. Cancer Res 1992;52:2103s—2107s.

In vivo studies, their strengths and weaknesses

Robert Kroes

Research Institute Toxicology, Utrecht University, The Netherlands

Abstract. Tumour models are used for several purposes, amongst which: 1) the study of the genesis of cancer; 2) the study of modulating factors on the genesis of cancer and the development of cancer; and 3) the study of therapeutic or treatment modalities are the most important.

The models are used to investigate etiological and/or physiological properties or processes which usually cannot be studied in humans for practical and/or ethical reasons.

The experimental tumour models used are spontaneous tumour models, chemically induced tumour models, or models bearing transplanted tumours, each model having its own advantages and disadvantages.

In cancer chemoprevention research, both spontaneous and induced models are used. The use of transplanted tumour models in cancer chemoprevention is as yet quite limited. The requirements which should be met to be able to use spontaneous and induced tumour models will be discussed as well as the advantages and disadvantages of the use of the particular model.

To understand the experimental set-up of experiments for the investigation of possible chemopreventive properties of substances or conditions, a simplified scheme of the carcinogenesis process will be put forward. This scheme will allow the researcher to explain the possible impact of modulating and/or inhibiting factors or substances in the primary and secondary prevention and in the treatment of specific cancers.

Animal models do have considerable advantages over human studies but their weaknesses should be recognised at the same time in that they are rarely, if ever, identical to the human cancer they imitate. The integration of animal and human data in this area of research will in the end provide us with the best insight in the potential of suspected chemopreventive agents.

Key words: chemopreventive agent, induced tumour model, mechanisms, spontaneous tumour model.

Introduction

Experimental tumour model systems are used for several purposes among which the study of: 1) the genesis of cancer, 2) the study of modulating factors on the genesis and development of cancer, and 3) the study of treatment modalities are the most important.

When studies are performed to investigate chemopreventive potential, usually a programmed systematic approach is used [1]. In this systematic approach in vivo testing follows in vitro screening and is primarily focussed on prioritisation and characterisation of the agents. Chemoprevention can be defined as the use of substances to prevent the occurrence of precancerous lesions or markers, e.g.,

---

Address for correspondence: Robert Kroes, Research Institute Toxicology, Utrecht University, P.O. Box 80176, 3508 TD Utrecht, The Netherlands.

intraepithelial neoplasia or to delay or reverse progression to invasive disease.

In this paper several issues pertaining to the availability and use of models, their advantages and disadvantages in detecting chemopreventive potential, and the strengths and weaknesses of their use are discussed.

Relevant issues in relation to the model

When using tumour model systems an important feature is to have sufficient data available which characterise the model. The animal species and strain should be easily available from a respected breeding facility. The species should have a sufficient reproduction rate, preferably have a specific pathogen-free status, should be easy to manipulate and have ideally a reasonable flat survival curve within the period of experiment. This latter feature pertains specifically to spontaneous tumour models which may show tumours not earlier than later in the lifetime when the survival curve is starting to descend. The dietary modalities which may influence tumour incidence, tumour growth, metastasis and behaviour should preferably be known. In this respect it is important, besides tumour characteristics, to possess data concerning the latency period of the tumours, the incidence, its morphology and behaviour, and its reproducibility.

Latency periods may vary considerably and are usually long and show considerable spread when spontaneous tumour models are used. Since the time of initiation in such models cannot be defined, the time of occurrence of the tumour is usually registered and may be used as a surrogate for latency. In induced models the standardisation of the cancer induction procedure may lead to a more constant, usually shorter latency period, with a limited deviation amongst the experimental animals. It should be emphasised that for many tumours the latency period cannot be established properly since tumours cannot be seen or detected easily.

The incidence of the tumour being studied should be sufficiently high to allow statistical evaluation on the results but, of course, a larger number of animals per treatment group could overcome the potential problem of relatively low incidences. However, in terms of animal welfare the use of unlimited numbers of animals is not justified.

Of extreme importance is that tumour incidences are reproducible since considerable variations over time or seasonal variations may hamper results of experiments and their statistical power. As with incidence, tumour morphology should be consistent and behaviour, growth and metastasis should be constant over time.

The tumour model used should be as similar as possible to the human tumour type it is supposed to imitate in terms of morphology, behaviour, growth pattern, metastasis and comparable latency period.

A point of discussion, which will only be marginally mentioned here, is if inbred or outbred strains of laboratory animals should be preferred [2].

The choice of pure, genetically homogeneous strains for experimentation assures increased reliability in comparison between groups, but at the same time may decrease the validity of such experiments as useful models for humans.

The argument, however, that outbred strains in this respect may be more appropriate seems false since genetic variation in outbred stocks of laboratory rodents is usually quite limited because most stocks are maintained as relatively small colonies.

Good experimental design requires the control of variation. In this respect, inbred strain may be considered as clones of genetically identical individuals, thus providing a means of controlling the effects of genotype in laboratory rodents [3].

Relevant issues in relation to the tumour

The tumour studied should be well-characterised. As stated earlier, aspects such as morphology, differentiation, invasion, (early) necrosis should be well-known and fairly stable. Data concerning other growth characteristics and behaviour of the tumour including metastasis and pattern of metastasis are also pertinent.

The possibility of investigating early hyperplastic and/or premalignant lesions offers additional parameters to be followed when modulating factors are investigated.

Most important, and not yet fully developed, is the use of intermediate endpoints or biomarkers of cancer. Intermediate biomarkers of cancer are of extreme value in the studies of potential effects of chemopreventive agents. One may discern genetic markers (nuclear aberrations and mutations), cellular markers (proliferation, differentiation), histological markers (hyperplasia, premalignant lesions such as intraepithelial neoplasia) and biochemical and pharmacological markers (i.e., enzyme activity).

Metabolic changes due to the development of a lesion may sometimes be a good indicator of stages of development of lesions but possible other causes for such metabolic changes should be excluded when data are evaluated and interpreted.

Carcinogenesis is a multipath process and the use of single biomarkers as surrogate endpoints may be difficult to evaluate since they may present only one of the many possible pathways. Therefore, panels of biomarkers especially those representing a whole range of carcinogenesis pathways may be more appropriate [4,5].

Since carcinogenesis is a complex process the researcher should have insight in this process which is given below in a simplified scheme.

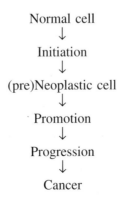

Normal cell
↓
Initiation
↓
(pre)Neoplastic cell
↓
Promotion
↓
Progression
↓
Cancer

In this scheme the arrows represent the events when enhancing or inhibiting factors may modulate the process. It is evident that in the experimental set-up this simplified scheme should be taken into consideration in order to best assess in what stage of the carcinogenic process changes occur in the event that a substance seems to modulate the process. Information derived from studies of multistep carcinogenesis has added considerably to the knowledge of chemoprevention.

Modulating factors which may influence the genesis and development of cancer

Carcinogenesis is a very complex, multifactorially controlled process which can be influenced by numerous endogenous or exogenous factors. Endogenous factors are among others: genetic predisposition, endocrine status, immune status and metabolic processes, which in turn can also be influenced by different exogenous factors.

The most important exogenous factors are those which influence proliferation, endocrine balance or modulate immune response, metabolic processes [6] or intracellular signalling [7]. Such factors can be chemically, physically, microbially, nutritionally and/or psychosocially derived.

As an example, in bladder carcinogenesis irritation and inflammation as precursors of proliferation are important [8]. A variety of factors may cause irritation and inflammation: bladder stones, long-term indwelling catheterisation (physical factors), chronic inflammation (i.e., schistosomiasis), chemicals which may produce bladder stones (diethylene glycol and derivatives), or microcrystalluria or other urinary precipitates (i.e., sodium saccharin, sodium ascorbate and others). Proliferation enhances the probability of converting DNA lesions to mutation (i.e., preneoplastic cells) [9].

Immunomodulation influences the carcinogenesis process in many different ways. The classic example that immunosuppression increases human cancer occurrence, for example, in kidney transplantation is well-known [10].

A last example, and a very relevant one for the subject discussed in this paper, is the modulating effect of dietary constituents in the carcinogenesis process. This may entail the diet as a whole or individual substituents such as individual macro- and/or micronutrients. Evidence in humans as well as in experimental animals is abundant although the impact of individual substances in the process in relation to other dietary substituents is difficult to assess [11].

Of similar importance is dietary restriction. A recent update concerning this issue was published by Hart, Neumann and Robertsen [12]. From this book it becomes evident that the present custom to allow animals to eat ad libitum is certainly a promoting factor in the occurrence of spontaneous and induced tumours and causes a shorter lifetime.

In chemoprevention numerous possibilities exist to influence the carcinogenesis process. Largely three important mechanisms may be involved: 1) carcinogen blocking activities, 2) antioxidant activities, and 3) antiproliferation and/or anti-progression activities [1].

Examples of carcinogen-blocking activities are amongst others inhibition of carcinogen uptake, inhibition of formation or activation, deactivation, inhibition of binding to DNA or increased efficacy (fidelity) of DNA repair.

Certain chemopreventive agents have antioxidant activities in that they scavenge electrophiles, oxygen radicals or inhibit arachidonic acid metabolism.

Agents may have antiproliferative properties evoked by, amongst others, the inhibition, induction or modulation of numerous processes involving signal transduction, endocrine-, immune- and growth parameters and intracellular communication.

Investigations for chemopreventive potential

Experimental and spontaneous tumour model systems can effectively be used for investigations for chemopreventive potential. Whereas, on the one hand the models can be used to screen chemopreventive potential of numerous substances, on the other hand specific models may be used to investigate in detail chemopreventive properties.

For screening purposes spontaneous tumour models may primarily be used to investigate the chemopreventive potential with the focus not necessarily on one specific tumour type.

Usually groups of 50 males and 50 females are used with two to three different dosages and a control group. The doses should be in a range of no overt toxicity and descending dosages by a decrement of two or less. Total tumour incidences and incidences of specific tumours are calculated and where possible time of occurrence of the tumours. Tumours should always be examined histologically to assess the neoplastic status, and to define if the tumour is benign or malignant.

More appropriate for screening purposes are induced tumour models, especially when chemopreventive potential is suspected to occur in specific organs. Such studies are shorter in duration, less costly and may later be followed by more detailed studies in the same system.

Usually substances are first screened in in vitro essays for its chemopreventive potential [1]. Depending on the information from in vitro essays more detailed studies can be designed to investigate in which stage or step of carcinogenesis the chemopreventive potency is expected. Such studies can almost exclusively be carried out in induced tumour models for which the initiation moment or period is exactly known and the period of development of hyperplastic, preneoplastic, benign and malignant lesions is usually well-characterised.

In the NCI Chemoprevention Drug Development Programme [13] doses of 0.4 and 0.8 maximum tolerated dose (MTD) up to 2% in the diet are usually used. The MTD, established in a range finding study, is defined as the highest dose which does not cause more than 10% reduction in weight gains or final weight after 6 weeks of administration.

Treatment schedules may vary: 1) starting 1 week prior to the initial carcinogen dose to the end of the study, 2) administration only before (1 week) and during (usually 4 weeks) carcinogen treatment, or 3) 4 weeks after the last treatment with the carcinogen for 4 or more weeks.

Sometimes a multiorgan carcinogenesis model is used in which different carcinogens are used to induce different tumours in the same model [14].

Apart from information about the period in which an agent may exert its chemo-preventive action, in such controlled studies information can be obtained concerning the dose/response, mechanisms involved and possible interactions with other factors including other interventions (surgery and physical or chemical means).

The design of such studies should be prepared with great care and detail in order to obtain an optimum of information from performed studies. The saying that the planning process of a study may take almost as much time as carrying it out may not be believed by those who never performed such studies but is well-recognised by those who did.

When studies are planned with more substances given together, it is appropriate to follow designs as used in combination toxicology experiments and to assume additivity of toxicity for effects in the same target organ. All in all, models are used to investigate aetiological and/or physiopathological properties or processes which for practical and/or ethical reasons cannot directly be studied in humans.

Available models, their advantages and disadvantages

As depicted earlier, four types of tumour models are available: spontaneous tumour models, induced tumour models, tumour transplantation models and in vitro tumour models.

Spontaneous tumour models are with a few exceptions, not similar to common human tumours. They are usually used to measure total tumour response of benign and/or malignant tumours and may, where tumour incidences are sufficiently high, be used for the investigation of effects on specific tumours. This may especially be the case for breast tumours (rat), lung tumours (mouse) and liver tumours (mouse).

For all common human tumours experimental models have been developed and are available. This concerns amongst others, lung tumours (hamster), colorectal tumours (rat, mouse), breast tumours (rat), skin tumours (mouse), pancreatic tumours (hamster, rat), prostate tumours (rat), skin (mouse) and bladder tumours (mouse).

Other available tumour models may concern organs or tissues, e.g., oral cavity, oesophagus, bones, adrenals, ovaries, thyroid, testis, endometrium, kidney and liver.

In the NCI Chemopreventive Drug Development Programme [13] all animal models which are used are chemically induced models. They concern tumours induced by:
— N-methyl N-nitrosourea (MNU) in hamster trachea;
— N-nitrosodiethylamine (DEN) in hamster lungs;
— Azoxymethane (AOM) in rat colon;
— Methylazoxymethane (MAM) in mouse colon;
— 7,12-dimethylbenz(alpha)anthracene promoted by 12-O-tetradecanoylphorbol 13-acetate (TPA) in mouse skin; and
— N-butyl N-(4-hydroxybutyl)nitrosamine (BBN) in mouse bladder.

All these models are well-validated and are perfectly fitted for the evaluation of potential chemopreventive agents. Moreover, they are representative for the high incidence of human cancers. An extensive summary of the evaluation of results of 144 agents tested has been published recently [13].

The use of tumour transplantation models in chemopreventive studies is limited. However, the interest in tumour transplantation has increased since T-cell devoid animals or even T-cell and B-cell deprived animals are now available. In the past, laboratory animals were immunologically deprived by irradiation.

The lifetime of tumour transplants as tissue or as a cell population was usually limited. T-cell devoid mice or rats are very adequate to study tumour implant behaviour. Advantages are properly standardised dosing and tumour growth. Major disadvantages, however, are the deprived immune status of the animal since this does not only influence the growth of the tumour (cells) but also interferes with many other physiological functions of the model, thus making it less prone to the investigation of tumour-modulating factors.

Advantages and disadvantages of spontaneous tumour models

It has been claimed that the use of spontaneous tumour models imitates the "reality" of life better than induced models do since the "natural" occurrence of tumours may be better compared to the circumstances in humans.

The animals are not treated with relatively high doses of carcinogen, thus preventing possible other interactions of the carcinogen with the system. One may also consider the spontaneous tumour model more animal friendly but since incidences are, with some exceptions, quite low the need to use substantial numbers of animals to achieve interpretable results seems to counteract this argument.

Moreover, the common human tumours are usually not common in spontaneous models (colon, lung, pancreas, prostate), the tumours are usually not similar to humans, do seldom metastasize, show long latency periods, show multiplicity when they occur and may interact with other age-related spontaneous tumours and chronic diseases which occur late in life, thus making the model less representative.

In addition, the model is less economical due to longer experimentation time and the large number of animals used. Finally, the model does not allow studies to define in which stage or step of the carcinogenesis process the interaction with a chemopreventive agent occurs.

Advantages and disadvantages of induced tumour models

In general, induced models are preferred to spontaneous models. Possible disadvantages are the relatively short experimentation times in relation to lifetime, which does not adequately imitate the circumstances in humans. The animals are treated with relatively high doses of carcinogens, which also may lead to additional undesired interactions of the carcinogen with other processes.

However, tumour type and behaviour are much more comparable to humans. The models can be adequately standardised and validated, thus leading to reproducible results. Latency periods are relatively short and known, and time to tumour occurrence usually prevents interaction with other chronic diseases which occur at a

126

later age. The model is more economical and enables the researcher to investigate behaviour, growth and metastasis in more detail, and provides more insight into the mechanism of action of the chemopreventive agent since the study design can be focused on different stages/steps in the carcinogenesis process.

Finally, it provides the possibility of combined studies, in which therapeutic action such as surgery and chemotherapy can be investigated with chemopreventive potential.

The ideal animal tumour model

As described earlier, the ideal tumour model should histologically be similar to the human tumour type which it represents. Growth pattern, metastasis pattern and speed of growth should ideally be similar as well. The model should be reproducible in terms of incidence and latency period, should be cost efficient and well-validated. In this respect, in certain tumours the use of athymic mice inoculated with human tumour cells may be preferred.

The induced animal model provides a perfect tool to investigate individual factors in a system with controlled variables. Research on combinations of factors or agents is possible as well. The different stages in the carcinogenesis process can be studied in detail, thus enabling all types of mechanistic studies. The model can be standardised and validated according to the necessary standards and is biologically well-characterised.

Finally, it is relatively cost efficient in its use and it overcomes ethical implications which may occur in human studies. Nevertheless, any animal tumour model is only a tool for approximations. It is rarely completely identical to human disease. Metabolism and clinical features are usually quite different. They generally provide information in experiments using considerable doses both of the carcinogen to provoke the tumour and of the modulating factor, which is investigated. Such results should be interpreted with care.

Animal models are not sufficient on their own. They only provide leads to and/or support for further studies, which in the end have to be performed on humans. Epidemiological intervention studies may then give the conclusive information as to whether an agent can effectively be used in the general population or more likely in identified high-risk groups as a subset of the population.

It is the integration of animal and epidemiological studies which provides us with the best insight in the development of cancer, in the cancer growth, its aetiology, its treatment and its prevention by chemopreventive means. Epidemiological and laboratory animal research should go hand-in-hand since in this way we will obtain a wealth of information necessary to understand the complex multifactorial disease, which is called cancer.

Acknowledgements

The author acknowledged Mrs Machteld Schmidt for the skilful preparation of the manuscript.

References

1. Kelloff GJ, Johnson JR, Cromwell JA, Boone CW, De George JJ, Steele VE, Mehta MU, Temeck JW, Schmidt WJ, Burke G, Greenwald P, Temple RJ. Approaches to the development and marketing approval of drugs that prevent cancer. Cancer Epidem Biomark Prev 1995;4:1—10.
2. Abramovici A, Wolman M. Inbred strains of laboratory animals: superior to outbred mice? J Natl Cancer Inst 1995;87:933.
3. Festing MF. Use of genetically heterogeneous rats and mice in toxicological research: a personal perspective. Toxicol Appl Pharmacol 1990;102;197—204.
4. Kelloff GJ, Boone CW, Crowell JA, Nayfield SG, Hawk E, Steele VE, Lubet RA, Sigman CC. Strategies for phase II cancer prevention trials: cervix, endometrium and ovary. J Cell Biochem 1995;59(Suppl 23):1—9.
5. Lipkon M. Strategies for intervention with chemopreventive agents. Int J Cancer 1996;69:64—67.
6. Kroes R. Contribution of toxicology towards assessment of carcinogens. Arch Toxicol 1987;60: 224—228.
7. Powis G, Alberts DS. Inhibiting intracellular signalling as a strategy for cancer chemoprevention. Eur J Cancer 1995;30A:1138—1144.
8. Rodent Bladder Carcinogenesis Working Group. Urinary bladder carcinogenesis: implications for risk assessment. Fed Chem Toxic 1995;33:797—802.
9. Ames BN, Gold LS, Willett WC. The causes and prevention of cancer. Proc Natl Acad Sci USA 1995;92(12):5258—5265.
10. Kinlen LJ. Immunosuppressive therapy and cancer. In: Penn I (ed) Cancer Surveys. 1982;1:565—583.
11. Hill MJ. Diet and cancer: a review of scientific evidence. Eur J Cancer Prev 1995;4(Suppl 2):3—42.
12. Hart RW, Neumann DA, Robertson RT (eds) Dietary Restriction: Implications for the Design and Interpretation of Toxicity and Carcinogenicity Studies. Washington DC: ILSI Press, 1995.
13. Steele VE, Moon RC, Lubet RA, Grubbs GJ, Reddy BS, Wargovich M, McCormick DL, Pereira MA, Crowll JA, Bagheri D. Preclinical efficacy evaluation of potential chemoprevention agents in animal carcinogenesis models: methods and results from the NCI Chemoprevention Drug Development Program. J Cell Biochem 1994;(Suppl 20):32—54.
14. Shibata M et al. Chemoprevention by dehydroepiandrosterone and indomethacin in a rat multiorgan carcinogenesis model. Cancer Res 1995;55:4870—4874.

The Scientific Bases of Cancer Chemoprevention.
C. Maltoni, M. Soffritti and W. Davis, editors.

Methodology of intervention trials and programs for cancer prevention

H. Sancho-Garnier

Hôpital G, Doumergue CHU, Nîmes, France

Key words: benefits, intervention trials, methods, population, risks, size.

The aim of cancer prevention is either to reduce the incidence of the disease or to lessen its pathological consequences (mortality in particular). Action may be directed towards:
— removing or reducing exposure to risk factors (i.e., reducing nicotine addiction);
— counterbalancing the effect of exposure through the use of protective factors (vitamins, medicines, vaccination, diet);
— treating precancerous lesions with a considerable likelihood of developing into cancers (polyps of the colon, cervical dysplasia); and
— cancer screening and treatment at a more curable stage (breast cancers).
The first type of action uses informational, educational and even legislative resources, while the other forms of intervention are based on diagnostic and therapeutic medical activities. These are the activities in the field of cancer prevention research that are of interest to us here.

The studies are based on the results of epidemiological surveys and experimental work and are aimed at reducing the incidence of the cancer locations targeted. Such approaches should not, however, threaten the physical, mental and social wellbeing of the individuals concerned. Prevention is usually directed at subjects who consider themselves to be "in good health", in other words at populations that are not seeking medical care and for whom, in most cases, there is no direct benefit. The random nature, or at any event the delayed effect, of any benefit to be derived from such intervention activities means that the methodological choices are governed by particular ethical considerations. The principles governing the establishment of such interventions in a population are based on voluntary participation, demonstration of a sufficiently large collective benefit and the inacceptability of serious and/or frequent adverse effects of a physical or psychological nature. For all such actions, it is clearly essential to have a stage of rigorous evaluation. It may seem trivial to say that healthcare actions, whether of a curative or a preventive nature, should be of proven effectiveness before being put to widespread use. Unfortunately, in the prevention

---

Address for correspondence: H. Sancho-Garnier, Hôpital G, Doumergue CHU, Nîmes 3000, France.

field in particular, too few of those promoting healthcare actions are concerned with demonstrating the effectiveness of the programs they propose!

Principles and Methods

Two different situations can always be identified, regardless of the measures being tested or the populations targeted [1]:
1. Experimentation; where the aim is to demonstrate the effectiveness of the projected action (a new preventive agent) or compare it with another one.
2. Transfer to general application for a wide population, where the program undertaken should follow the guidelines previously established and guarantee maximum benefits at minimum cost in this situation.

In either case, two levels of evaluation can be identified:
1. Evaluation of the procedure to be used, so that the action's feasibility, acceptability and costs can be assessed.
2. Evaluation of the results in terms of the objectives chosen, these having previously been defined and quantified.

The two levels are complementary and both, therefore, indispensable.

As with any scientific approach, the need for evaluation makes it necessary, after formulation of the hypothesis to be tested, to specify the strategy (or experimental design) used, the populations targeted, details of the actions planned and their quality control, the assessment criteria selected and the way they will be measured, the number of subjects required to provide interpretable results, the way in which consent will be obtained from subjects, their on-going surveillance, etc., in the context of a written protocol.

Strategy

The contents of the proposed program should be assessed by outside experts before the action is put into operation. They should analyze the knowledge already available, the methods and resources to be used in the program's implementation, and the ethical considerations involved.

The procedure should be evaluated while the program is actually in operation, so that actions can be adjusted to meet conditions in the field. On-going interactive evaluation can be conducted by a multidisciplinary steering committee independent of anyone involved in the program and having access to all data concerning the action's operation. Conformance with the protocol, the continuing involvement of subjects, the quality of procedures, any anticipated or unexpected side effects, and costs will be examined at regular intervals. Analysis of these different factors will aid reproducibility and may also explain the reasons behind a setback or success.

Results are evaluated in order to generate knowledge that will help decide whether the intervention tested should be used in a widespread application.

In experimental situations, the effects of an action can be demonstrated if the results observed for the group undergoing the action are compared with those of a group either not subject to it or subject to a reference action (control group). There are several ways of constituting groups. To obtain an a priori unbiased assessment, each subject (or group of subjects) in the target population should be allocated to one of the two groups (test or control) by random selection. If this procedure is used, the possible change observed (decline in incidence) can then be associated with the action carried out. With chemoprevention trials, as with therapeutic trials, causal conclusions on the value of a particular preventive measure can only be reached if the strategy involves random selection.

In routine situations, only actions tested in experimental studies should be undertaken. The procedure used and the results obtained should both be evaluated with equal care, but a random selection strategy is no longer necessary. The aim of evaluation will be to ensure that the result obtained is the same as with experimental actions, with a good level of effectiveness, i.e., a definite improvement in health, at a lower cost, so as to serve users better.

Populations subject to these actions

Such populations may be samples taken from the general population: in Gambia, for instance, hepatitis B vaccinations, which have a secondary effect of hepatocarcinoma prevention, are carried out on the entire population of particular geographical areas.

More frequently, they are high-risk populations either subject to heavy and prolonged exposure or having presented an initial cancer that has been cured (cancers in the ENT sphere, breast cancer) or, lastly, subjects presenting anomalies with a considerable likelihood of malignant transformation (benign lesions, cancers in situ, tumor markers, etc.)

Subjects in this second group have a much greater likelihood of presenting the event under study in the course of surveillance, which makes it possible to include a reasonable number of individuals in the trial, with sufficient power to test the hypothesis. These subjects are, moreover, readier to accept the idea of repetitive examination, permanent treatment, even side effects.

There are a number of difficulties inherent in selecting certain populations, however: The lesions on which inclusion in the study is based must be clearly defined and the treatments proposed must be capable of acting on the late stage of carcinogenic development: i.e., can antioxidants act on already existing cytological anomalies?

It also hardly seems ethical to leave in place lesions with a considerable likelihood of malignant transformation (carcinoma in situ) when they can be removed surgically.

Finally, can the results obtained for these populations be applied to the general population? This question still remains to be answered.

Treatments

Chemoprevention uses nutriments or pharmacological agents (Table 1) to stimulate endogenous physiological mechanisms protecting the organism against the develop-

Table 1. Chemopreventive agents under trial from Buiatti [2].

Agents[a]	Tumor sites
Vitamin C	Colon, stomach
Vitamin A	Oral cavity, esophagus, skin, lung
Vitamin E	Esophagus
Vitamin B12	Lung
β-carotene	Oral cavity, esophagus, lung, colon, cervix, skin, stomach
Retinoids	Skin, head and neck, lung, breast
Calcium	Colon, esophagus
Selenium	Lung, liver, skin
Zinc	Esophagus
Tamoxifen	Breast
Fernetidine	Colon, esophagus
NSAIDS	Colon
Antivirus vaccine	Liver, cervix

[a]Alone or in association.

ment of clones of malignant cells.

Such agents are selected on the basis of epidemiological observations or experimental studies, which means that the substances are often not well-defined chemically and that information on effective doses, duration, routes of administration and action mechanisms is rare and even more complex when mixtures of various substances are used. The protective effect of fruit and vegetable consumption on various types of cancer found in many epidemiological studies is not currently demonstrated in most supplementation trials for various nutriments [2].

In most cases we do not know at what stage of carcinogenesis these agents act, which consequently makes it difficult to select the populations to include. As far as nutriments are concerned, the question can be raised as to whether their activity will be the same with regard to populations suffering from malnutrition (cancer of the esophagus in China) and those close to normality (cancers in smokers in Western countries).

Vaccination is obviously an attractive type of intervention because of its effectiveness for infectious diseases. Unfortunately, cancers for which there exist both a pathogenic agent and an effective vaccine are rare. At present only the hepatitis B vaccine is undergoing experimental study. A papillomavirus vaccine should soon be undergoing expert evaluation for use in treating cervical cancer. As with chemoprevention trials, trials of carcinogenesis vaccines clearly require a very long surveillance period.

Assessment criteria

The "ideal" criterion is clearly a reduced incidence of the disease. Cancer is a rare event, however, in terms of a population, even in populations at risk (except for families with a genetic risk).

A very long surveillance period is thus required to observe the events (incidence or mortality).

What is more, differences in incidence between groups subject to the action and those not subject to it are usually slight, and there is also frequently a "contamination" effect on the control group: in other words, the subjects in this group "spontaneously" undergo the examinations or treatments of the "treated" group, which reduces the possible differences.

These various reasons lead to an increase in the numbers of subjects, the time and the expense required for these studies. A lot of trials use other assessment criteria (Table 2), as they are obtained more rapidly and are thought to be markers for intermediate stages of carcinogenesis.

Some of these criteria are, however, simply markers of exposure or of very early stages and the results obtained with such markers cannot be used to conclude that the cancer risk has been reduced.

Several criteria can be used in the same trial, and some may serve as indicators for stopping the action. When the treatment includes several substances (in some cases four to six vitamins and trace elements are involved), the conclusions will be difficult to interpret and to extrapolate to an entire population if results are positive. It will, in fact, always be impossible to distinguish between active ingredients and toxic substances except if an experimental design, possibly a factorial one, has been drawn up.

Lastly, several cancer sites or even disease sites (trials focussing jointly on cardiovascular diseases and cancers) may be targeted in one and the same trial, the agent tested being thought to act on a common mechanism [2].

Number of subjects

The number of subjects required depends on the "acceptable" error risk (α) where it would be wrong to conclude that a difference exists, the required power ($1 - \beta$) enabling an existing difference to be indicated, the number of events usually observed

Table 2. Intervention trials — criteria of assessment.

Direct criteria

Cancer incidence (or second primary)
Mortality
Adverse reactions (physical or sociophysiological)
Quality of life

Indirect criteria

Tumor regression, or lack of recurrence of precancerous lesions
DNA markers (micronuclei, unscheduled DNA synthesis, sister chromatid exchange)
Cell proliferation (mitotic index...)

in the target population and the minimum difference one wishes to observe between the group subject to the action and the control group.

Given the rarity of the events, this calculation always indicates a very large number of subjects to be included. Several "special characteristics" of these trials also add to the number of subjects to be included [3]. If it is a matter of randomized testing, random selection is sometimes carried out "in blocks", with one block corresponding to the clientele of certain doctors, a geographical area, etc. This type of strategy facilitates intervention in organizational terms, avoids ethical problems, reduces contamination of the control group and keeps costs down. On the other hand, this strategy involves an increase in the number of subjects as the individuals in a block are not independent: members of the same family are usually assigned to the same group.

A dependency term (ρ) should, therefore, be included in the estimate of N, equal to $(1 + (n-1) \rho)$, where n is the number of individuals in the family and ρ the assessment criterion's intrafamily correlation coefficient [4]. In addition, only volunteers are enrolled in these studies, and numerous works show that volunteers are low risk subjects, which reduces the number of events that will be observed. Lastly, as we have already noted, there is also a "contamination" effect on the control group with a danger of reducing the difference noted in the trial between the two groups and thus reducing the power.

In addition, given the length of treatment necessary to obtain a result, many problems arise concerning patient compliance and surveillance. Poor patient compliance and too great a number of subjects lost track of can also lead to a major reduction in the expected difference and the power of the trial.

Summary of risks and benefits

Preventive medicine is not neutral. Preventive medical activities are aimed at people subjectively in good health and they are a priori seen as a constraint [5]. The risks of side effects are very often not known at all or only slightly known and these risks are run by a whole population, whereas the danger one is attempting to prevent will affect only a certain number, usually a small number, of individuals in this population. Even if the activity is of slight advantage to a large number of subjects, any high risk of side effects for a minority of them is difficult to accept. Obviously one can compare this situation to that of smallpox vaccination, where rare fatal accidents have been accepted as the price for the effective protection of a population a large number of which were previously in danger of contracting the disease.

Any intervention, thus requires prior consideration with regard to the advantages and disadvantages involved, even before starting. Trials should only be undertaken if the potential advantages are a priori considerably greater that any side effects.

Benefits are represented by a reduced incidence of the disease and, where appropriate, by an improved quality of life. One notes, however, that a large number of actions are launched without their effectiveness being properly demonstrated (vitamin therapy, tamoxifen to prevent breast cancers, etc.) or in inadequate conditions for obtaining results (poor methodology, absence of quality control, poor target population, etc.)

Risks of harm are varied: they are either of a medical nature, such as the deleterious effects of preventive medicines or vaccines, or of a psychosocial nature. We can cite among other effects the increased degree of anxiety in the population as a result of widespread information on the target disease, permanent medical treatment for the rest of one's life, the false hopes of subjects who will contract the disease despite preventive action, the blame attributed to victims who have not followed advice on how to avoid the disease and whose illness becomes a burden to society, reduction in free will when subjects are strongly encouraged to join a program, the inequality of access to medical care as a result of activities being poorly suited to the underprivileged classes of society, etc. [6].

If it is demonstrated, for instance, that tamoxifen can be used to reduce the incidence of breast cancer by 35%, the administration of this medicine over a 10-year period to 100,000 50-year-old women who are twice as much at risk from breast cancer as the overall population could prevent 600 deaths caused by this cancer. But 98,800 women will have absorbed this substance every day for 10 years to no purpose, 2,000 of them will still have breast cancer and 1,000 of them will die from it. And, lastly, 1,000 women will suffer from serious or fatal side effects. One might add that the cost would be 1.5 billion francs, or 2.5 million francs for every life prolonged. Such a summary fails to take into account all the harmful effects that are difficult to quantify, such as the daily awareness of the possibility of contracting cancer, the anxiety of forgetting to take the medicine and the consequences that might result from this, culpabilization if the treatment is stopped prematurely, etc. It seems to us necessary to summarize all the "fors and againsts" before promoting any intervention trial.

Such a summary should be repeated once the results of any trial have been obtained, incorporating the data observed, in order to extrapolate the results to the whole target population and assess the possibility of carrying out this action on a large scale.

In this type of public health intervention, the likelihood of benefit accruing to any given subject is very low and remote, and the latter must admit the primacy of the collective interest over that of the individual. In prevention actions, the doctor-patient relationship is reversed: doctors ask individuals to look after their own health and become their own doctor. It is a complete social turnaround. Intervention trials can only be accepted if they are a constituent element of a finalized collective action, the effectiveness of which has already been proven [5,6].

These considerations also imply that such actions are based on the voluntary and informed participation of the target population [7]. "Individual" consent can be difficult to achieve in the field of public health: one might, for instance, cite the case for compulsory vaccinations or the addition of fluoride to drinking water.

An alternative to individual consent is provided by R.J. Levine [6], who uses the term "community consent" in the context of certain research activities such as those affecting an entire population, and this may be the case where prevention is

136

concerned. It would thus be a matter of consulting the community to assess how it sees the action's risk-benefit ratio. On a practical level, such a consultation might be conducted by means of consultation by delegation, negotiated with a group representing the preventive action's target population. In conclusion, the ethical problems in intervention trials, as in all actions involving a large number of people, cannot be resolved within the framework of the traditional contract between patient and doctor but are rather a matter of bioethics and should be incorporated within the framework for collective action, the objectives and various consequences of which have been carefully studied and evaluated. The psychosocial consequences of such actions are still not studied to any great extent and research in this area needs to be promoted.

References

1. Sancho-Garnier H. Evaluation des programs de prévention du tabagisme. Rev Prat 1993;43(Suppl 10):1252–1255.
2. Bouvier P, Doucet H, Jeanneret O, Strasse T. Aspects éthiques du dépistage: réflexions à partir du cancer du sein. Cahier médico-sociaux. Ed. Médecine Hygiène 1994;38:1.
3. Buiatti E. Intervention trials of cancer prevention: Results and new research programs. IARC technical report 1994;(Report No. 8).
4. Byar DP. Some statistical considerations for design of cancer prevention trials. Prev Med 1989;18: 688–699.
5. Ederer F, Church T, Manderl LS. Sample sizes for Prevention Trials have been too small. AJE 1993; 137(Suppl 7):787–810.
6. Agora — Ethique Médecine, Société. Idéologies de la prévention. 1994;30.
7. Jeanneret O, Raymond L. Aspects éthiques des études d'intervention. Rev Epidem Santé Publ 1981; 29:269–279.

Vitamins, oligo-elements and cancer prevention: epidemiological evidence

P. van 't Veer[1], E. Guallar[2], F.J. Kok[1] and J.M. Martin-Moreno[2]
[1]Department of Epidemiology and Public Health, Agricultural University, Wageningen, The Netherlands; and [2]Escuela Nacional de Sanidad, Madrid, Spain

Abstract. Vitamins, minerals and trace elements have been proposed as cancer chemopreventives. Focusing on antioxidants, epidemiological studies on cancer of the lung and gastro-intestinal tract are summarized.

Regarding lung cancer, observational studies suggest that selenium might reduce risk at low exposures, while it might increase risk at high levels. Decreased risk with fruits and vegetables was attributed to β-carotene, but population trials using high doses in high risk groups suggest a risk increase by about 20%. Combined use of β-carotene, vitamin E and selenium at moderate doses reduced stomach cancer incidence, without clear effects for esophageal cancer, whereas subjects with esophageal dysplasia seemed to benefit from a multivitamin/mineral supplement. For colorectal cancer, recurrence of adenomatous polyps after polypectomy was not reduced after antioxidant supplementation, and some increase in risk was suggested.

Overall, there is no clear evidence for cancer chemoprevention by antioxidant supplements exceeding dietary intake levels in populations without dietary deficiencies. Adverse effects in some of the trials could be attributed to duration of supplementation and/or stage of carcinogenesis. While further research in this field is warranted, guidelines like the "European Code Against Cancer" are considered the most sensible public health approach to cancer prevention.

Key words: β-carotene, antioxidant, colorectal, lung, selenium, stomach.

Introduction

Cancer chemoprevention, a specific form of cancer prevention and control, can be defined as prevention of cancer by the administration of one of more chemical compounds, either as individual substances or as naturally occurring constituents of the diet [1,2]. On the basis of mechanistic considerations and animal experimentation, chemopreventive agents can be classified as inhibitors of carcinogen formation, blocking agents and suppressing agents [2]. The basic cancer-related chemical and biological sciences and epidemiology have contributed to the understanding that antimutagenesis and antiproliferation are the important general mechanisms of chemoprevention and to the identification and development of potentially chemopreventive agents. These agents might prevent oxidant-stress (e.g., carotenoids, tocopherols), block formation of carcinogens directly or indirectly (e.g., vitamin C,

---

Address for correspondence: P. van 't Veer, Department of Epidemiology and Public Health, Agricultural University, PO Box 238, 6700 AE Wageningen, The Netherlands.

cruciferae), block proliferative stimuli (e.g., calcium), act as cofactors of (antioxidant) enzymes (e.g., Zn, Cu, Se), or modulate gene expression (e.g., folate). At the tissue level, steroidlike vitamins affect differentiation (e.g., retinoids, vitamin D), while nonsteroidal anti-inflammatory drugs (e.g., NSAIDs, aspirin) may also reduce risk.

During life, human beings are constantly exposed to a large diversity of carcinogens, suppressors and promotors, exerting different effects depending on genetic susceptibility, amount of accumulated genetic damage, clonal selection, stage of carcinogenesis, and presence of precursor lesions and/or subclinical disease. Epidemiological research can yield direct quantitative estimates of (relative and attributable) risk. In this respect, the type of target population for chemoprevention is especially relevant, i.e., high-risk groups characterized by: 1) lifestyle, 2) occupation, 3) premalignant lesions, 4) genetic predisposition, 5) previous treatment with chemotherapy and/or radiation therapy, and 6) survivors of cancer at high risk of recurrence.

This paper will focus on the epidemiological evidence obtained from observational and experimental studies among the three groups mentioned first (lifestyle, occupation, premalignant lesions). Based on observational epidemiological studies it has been concluded that high consumption of fruits and vegetables may appreciably reduce cancer risk [3,4]. This is most convincing for cancers of the respiratory and gastrointestinal tract, but less so for hormone-related cancers. With respect to cancer sites we will focus on cancer of the lung, upper- (esophagus and stomach) and lower gastro-intestinal tract (colon, rectum). With respect to the substances our attention will focus on diet-related substances such as selenium, β-carotene, vitamin C and folate. The epidemiological evidence on calcium, steroidlike retinoids and deltanoids, and nonsteroidal anti-inflammatory drugs will not be addressed in this overview.

Lung cancer

Smoking is the major cause of cancer at various sites, but especially so for lung cancer. However, dietary antioxidants may counteract the smoking-induced oxidant stress and depletion of antioxidant status.

Reviewing the observational evidence, four large-scale prospective cohort studies have specifically addressed selenium (Se) and lung cancer, taking into account the effect of smoking (Table 1). In a traditionally low selenium country like Finland, an inverse association between plasma selenium and lung cancer has been observed [5]. In the Netherlands, with intermediate Se levels (assessed in toenails) the association was inverse as well, but slightly weaker [6]. In the USA, with generally higher plasma Se levels, the association was U-shaped [7] or positive [8]. In line with animal experiments, this suggests that both marginally low and excessive Se levels may lead to increased cancer risk, but methodological reasons and population characteristics might also account for the diversity of associations [9].

A combination of antioxidants might be more effective than single substances in preventing cancer. In the Netherlands Cohort Study, the inverse association between Se and lung cancer was potentiated among subjects with high β-carotene or vitamin

Table 1. Smoking-adjusted association between biomarkers of selenium status and lung cancer in four large cohort studies [5—8].

Quintile of selenium	Knekt[a] (189/378)	Brandt (317/2459)	Menkes (99/196)	Garland (47/47)
Q1 (low)	3.33	1.00	0.68	1.00
Q2	2.26	0.71	0.49	
Q3	1.93	0.79	0.39	1.95
Q4	1.50	0.82	0.98	
Q5 (high)	1.00	0.50	1.00	4.33
p-value for trend	0.001	0.006	0.07	0.17
Mean selenium-level plasma (µg/L)	61	—	119	—
toenails (ppm)	—	0.561	—	0.897

[a]First author of publication (number of cases and referents in parentheses).

C intake [6]. A large number of observational studies on diet-related antioxidants have been summarized by Comstock [10]. The majority of results showed lower levels of serum retinol, β-carotene, vitamin E and/or selenium among subjects who subsequently developed cancer. This association was more marked for β-carotene, but there were differences by cancer site [10].

In the framework of the antioxidant hypothesis of cancer, several population trials have been initiated. The Finnish α-tocopherol β-carotene (ATBC) trial among heavy male smokers was the first one to report its results after 7 years of follow-up [11]. The ATBC trial is a double blind placebo controlled trial, with α-tocopherol (50 mg/day) and β-carotene (20 mg/day) supplementation in a two-by-two factorial design. In contrast to expectations, α-tocopherol showed no association with lung cancer, while β-carotene was associated with a statistically significant 18% increased risk (95% confidence interval (95% CI): 3—36%), independent of α-tocopherol treatment. For other cancer sites no significant effects were observed, and total mortality was increased in the β-carotene group by 8% (95% CI: 1—16%). Moreover, in the placebo group, an inverse association was observed between baseline levels of dietary and plasma β-carotene and incidence of lung cancer. These latter results were in line with observational epidemiology, but at the same time the trial results indicated that β-carotene is very unlikely to be the protective agent among these 75-year-old men who had smoked 20 cigarettes/day during 36 years on average.

At the end of 1995, the β-carotene arm of the Physicians Health Study (PHS) was completed without showing any beneficial effect of β-carotene on cancer or mortality, neither among smokers or nonsmokers [12]. At that time, preliminary results of the CARET trial among smokers and asbestos workers showed an increased lung cancer risk of 28% with β-carotene supplementation (including vitamin A), while total mortality was increased by 17%. In view of these results, it was decided to stop immediately the β-carotene arm of cancer chemoprevention trials among high-risk groups as well as the β-carotene arm of the Women's Health Study, conducted among 40,000 female health professionals [12]. The idea that one single nutrient, or a few of them combined, could compensate for high-risk behaviour, is in serious trouble; cancer stage may be of relevance, plasma β-carotene might be a marker of other essential dietary constituents or low-risk lifestyle [12].

Cancers of the upper gastro-intestinal tract

Risk factors for stomach cancer include *Helicobacter pylori* infection, nitrosamine formation from nitrites, and possibly a diet poor in fruits and vegetables. For oesophageal cancer, precursor lesions have been identified, giving extra opportunities for observational and experimental studies.

Chemoprevention of oesophageal cancer and stomach cancer was the major objective of the Linxian Nutrition Intervention Trial [13]. The study population consisted of 30,000 males and females 40–69 years of age, at high risk of stomach cancer, who were followed for 5 years. Four factors were tested, each consisting of a combination of various related compounds: vitamin A and zinc, riboflavin and niacin, vitamin C and molybdenum, and the three compounds β-carotene, vitamin E and selenium. Eight intervention groups were formed, consisting of the six possible combinations of two treatments, a placebo group and all treatments taken together. For the β-carotene, vitamin E and selenium group, results showed an overall reduction in mortality of 9% (95% CI: 1–16%), and a 13% (95% CI: 0–25%) reduction in cancer mortality. The latter was due to stomach cancer reduction by 21% (95% CI: 1–36%), while oesophageal cancer was not significantly reduced (4%). For total cancer incidence results pointed in the same direction (7% reduction), but only for stomach cancer the 95% CI excluded the null value (16% reduction, 0–29%). For all other combinations tested, no clear effects were observed on site specific cancer incidence or mortality.

In the same area, an intervention study was conducted among subjects who had oesophageal dysplasia. Here, a cocktail of 14 vitamins and 12 minerals was given and cytology and endoscopics after 2.5 and 6 years of follow-up served as endpoints [14]. Cancer incidence and death rates during this follow-up did not differ clearly between the groups. Although for oesophageal cancer incidence and death the risks seemed to be somewhat reduced, they were increased (though not beyond chance) for stomach cancer.

Colorectal cancer

Colorectal cancer has been associated with high-fat, low fruit and fibre diet in epidemiologic and experimental studies [15]. Also, laboratory animal model and epidemiologic studies have shown that certain dietary lipids and fibres influence risk of colon cancer [16]. Moreover, there is epidemiologic evidence to suggest that the increased intake of calcium or aspirin is associated with a reduced risk of colon cancer [17].

In the framework of the adenoma-carcinoma sequence, looking for informative and efficient approaches, adenomatous polyps have been studied endpoints in observational studies, while adenoma-recurrence in high-risk groups has been used as endpoint in chemoprevention studies (Table 2).

In a study among 58 patients with familial adenomatous polyps, DeCosse [18] reported a slightly lower number of polyps/visit in the group with prescribed vitamin C, E and fibre, although the effect was attributed primarily to fibre. McKeown-Eyssen [19] conducted a randomized trial to test the effect of a low-fat, high-fibre diet (as achieved by dietary counselling) on polyp recurrence among 201 polypectomized subjects. Despite successful dietary counselling, the 2-year risk of polyp recurrence was increased by 20%, though this was not statistically significant (the confidence interval was wide: 40% reduction to 120% increase). The Polyp Prevention Study Group [20] reported a clinical trial of antioxidant vitamins on polypectomized subjects (without a history of familial adenomatous polyps) on polyp-recurrence 1—4 years after the initial examination. The relative risk for β-carotene was 1.01 (95% CI: 0.85—1.20), for vitamins C and E combined it was 1.08 (95% CI: 0.91—1.29), and there was no evidence for interaction. Moreover, subgroups according to polyp size or location, did not suggest reduced risks either. Recently, the Australian Polyp Prevention Project [21] reported results on 411 polypectomized subjects after 2 and 4 years of follow-up. No statistically significant risk reduction was found with any of the three intervention groups (25% of energy from fat, 25 g of wheat bran, 20 mg of β-carotene). Nonsignificant reduced risks were observed for large adenomas (>1 cm) with the low-fat treatment. Among the combined low-fat, high-fibre diet, no large adenomas were observed (p = 0.03). Similar to the study reported by Greenberg [20],

Table 2. Main characteristics and results of four intervention trials on adenoma recurrence [18—21]

Author	Population (size)	Intervention	Main results
DeCosse	Familial Adenomatous Polyp Patients (n = 58)	Vitamin C + E (4 g and 400 mg) Grain Fiber (22.5 g extra).	Weak indication for some benefit due to grain fiber.
McKeown-Eyssen	Postpolypectomy (n = 201)	LFHF[1] (25% of energy and 35 g grain fiber) vs. (33% of energy and 16 g).	RR[3] of recurrence = 1.2; gender possibly a modifier.
Greenberg	Postpolypectomy (n = 751)	β-car (25 mg). Vitamin C and E (1 g and 400 mg). Both treatments, placebo.	RR of recurrence = 1.0 for β-car and RR = 1.1 for vitamin C and E.
MacLennan	Postpolypectomy (n = 411)	LF[2] (25% of En), HF (25 g bran), β-car (20 mg). Combined/ no treatment.	LF OR = 0.3—0.4, HF OR = 0.8, LFHF: no large adenomas found. β-car OR -1.3—1.4 for large adenomas.

[a]LFHF: Low-fat, high-fiber diet, contrasted to normal diet; [b]LF: low fat; HF: high fiber; and OR[3] (RR): odds ratio (relative risk) for treatment indicated.

β-carotene actually seemed to be associated with a slight deleterious effect, although the results are compatible with chance variation [22]. New studies should be considerably larger, and should further develop the idea of comprehensively testing the overall effect of changes in consumption of several nutrients or foods, rather than testing individual components [22]. Another way out is to focus on more precisely defined target tissue endpoints, like mucosal proliferation, and conducting trials of longer duration, begin earlier in life and focus on mechanisms and specific stage of abnormal cell development [23].

A relatively recent potential chemopreventive in colorectal carcinogenesis is dietary folate. Among other possible mechanisms, folate plays a role in the availability of methyldonors, relevant to DNA-methylation. Although it is not at all clear how this might influence cancer risk [24], epidemiological studies among American men and women showed clearly increased risk of colorectal adenomas and of colorectal cancer among subjects at a "methyldeficient diet", which is characterized by low folate and either low methionine or high alcohol (or all three of them) [25,26]. The attractiveness of this hypothesis is its potential generalizibility to some other cancer sites, such as the cervix [27], and that the combination of dietary factors is based on a mechanistic concept. Although calcium has been implicated in preventing colon cancer by forming insoluble calcium soaps with secondary bile acids, this hypothesis is beyond the scope of this review.

Discussion

The overall picture emerging from this overview is that antioxidants are indeed indicators of a low-risk dietary pattern. Assuming that the results from observational studies have been sufficiently adjusted for confounding by smoking habits, a diet rich in fruit and vegetables seems beneficial and safe. For selenium, the question on risk or protection has not yet been elucidated. High levels of intake of antioxidants, however, may not be advisable.

In fact, supplementation beyond the natural dietary range in randomized trials has not fulfilled the initially high expectations. For lung cancer and colorectal cancer no beneficial effects of vitamin E have been observed, while β-carotene supplementation has become suspicious for adverse effects among subjects at high risk because of exposure to smoking or asbestos, or because of colorectal adenomas as precursor lesions. To the extent that these statements can be generalized to other sites, the effects of moderate (1–2 times US-RDA) supplementation with vitamin E, β-carotene and selenium in the Linxian trial might mainly result from selenium, which was supplied at 50 μg/day only. We need to keep in mind, however, that the Linxian population had marginal deficiencies regarding those vitamins, and the actual results may not be generalizable to Western populations.

With respect to the observational and intervention studies, it is relevant to recognize that time plays an important role as well. First, in terms of age, time is related to the stage of carcinogenesis in the population. Intervention measures are, therefore, imposed on subjects with a large variety of unidentifiable precursor lesions of cancer. The effect of such an intervention on cancer risk will become evident relatively quickly (e.g., 5—10 years) if a late stage event is affected, and it may last many decades if early stage events are involved. The effects seen after relatively short periods of follow-up suggest that late stages may be involved, but these effects were opposite to expectations. As observational studies addressing habitual diet have clearly suggested reduced risks, the duration of follow-up in the trials may have been insufficient to observe these later effects.

With respect to dose and time taken together, we should be aware that their effects cannot be distinguished in the studies that have been discussed in this overview. Observational studies with moderate dietary exposures did show inverse associations. On the other hand, experimental studies among high-risk groups — either because of carcinogen exposure, or the presence of a precancerous lesion — used relatively high doses, most of them far beyond the dietary range, and the results suggested risk enhancement. Basic sciences could help us distinguish whether this apparently conflicting evidence results from a U-shaped exposure-disease association, from different effects depending on the stage in the carcinogenic process, or both.

Conclusion

Given the complexity of living organisms like humans and of exposures like diet, it seems unlikely that any single substance could exert a general cancer protective effect. Nevertheless, for subjects at high risk for certain cancers, either because of exposure history or because of the presence of precursor lesions, it might be possible to identify some stage- and site-specific chemopreventive agents. Large trials of considerable duration in defined groups are needed to reliably quantify the potential health effects of chemopreventives or other risk reducing factors. Before embarking on large population trials, however, there should be a considerable degree of consistency between laboratory research, observational epidemiology and clinical studies. The public health potential for reducing cancer incidence and mortality through chemopreventive interventions provides a promising opportunity, and this approach to cancer prevention should remain as a high research priority. However, the results from trials conducted so far have indicated that we should be very modest with advocating any specific compound as being chemopreventive. As far as clear nutritional deficiencies in large segments of the population are concerned, a mild enrichment of foods via industrial means might be considered. However, net risk reductions derived from supplements in human populations without dietary deficiencies are generally moderate or may even become adverse at high dose levels. Therefore, and in general, the guidelines as laid down in the "European Code Against Cancer" seem currently to be the most sensible approach to control the cancer epidemic.

References

1. Miller AB. Perspectives on cancer prevention. Risk Analysis 1995;15:655—660.
2. Morse MA, Stoner GD. Cancer chemoprevention: principles and prospects. Carcinogenesis

144

1993;14:1737—1746.

3. Block G, Patterson B, Subar A. Fruit, vegetables and cancer prevention: A review of the epidemiological evidence. Nutr Cancer 1992;18:1—29.

4. Steinmetz KA, Potter JD. Vegetables, fruit, and cancer. I. Epidemiology. Cancer Cause Control 1991;2:325—357.

5. Knekt P, Aromaa A, Maatela J, Alfthan G, Aaran RK, Hakama M, Hakulinen T, Peto R, Teppo L. Serum selenium and subsequent risk of cancer among Finnish men and women. J Natl Cancer Inst 1990;82:864—868.

6. Van den Brandt PA, Goldbohm RA, Van 't Veer P, Bode P, Dorant E, Hermus RJJ, Sturmans F. A prospective study on selenium status and the risk of lung cancer. Cancer Res 1993;53:4860—4865.

7. Menkes MS, Comstock GW, Veilleumier JP, Helsing KJ, Rider AA, Brookmeyer R. Serum beta-carotene, vitamins A and E, selenium and the risk of lung cancer. N Engl J Med 1986;315: 1250—1254.

8. Garland M, Morris JS, Stampfer MJ, Colditz GA, Spate VL, Baskett CK, Rosner B, Speizer FE, Willett WC, Hunter DJ. Prospective study of toenail selenium levels and cancer among women. J Natl Cancer Inst 1995;87:497—505.

9. Clarck LC, Alberts DS. Selenium and cancer: risk or protection? J Natl Cancer Inst 1995;87: 473—475.

10. Comstock GW, Bush TL, Helzlsouer K. Serum retinol, beta-carotene, vitamin E, and selenium as related to subsequent cancer of specific sites. Am J Epidemiol 1992;135:115—121.

11. Alpha-Tocopherol, Beta Carotene Cancer Prevention Study Group. The effect of vitamin E and beta-carotene on the incidence of lung cancer and other cancers in male smokers. N Engl J Med 1994;330:1029—1035.

12. Rowe PM. Beta-carotene takes a collective beating. Lancet 1996;347:249.

13. Blott WJ, Li JY, Taylor PR, Guo W, Dawsey S, Wang GQ, Yang CS, Zheng SF, Gail M, Li GY, Yu Y, Liu B, Tangrea J, Sun Y, Liu F, Fraumeni JF Jr, Zhang YH, Li B. Nutrition intervention trials in Linxian, China: Supplementation with specific vitamin/mineral combinations, cancer incidence, and disease-specific mortality in the general population. J Natl Cancer Inst 1993;85:1483—1492.

14. Li JY, Taylor PR, Li B, Dawsey S, Wang GQ, Ershow AG, Guo W, Liu SF, Yang CS, Shen Q, Wang W, Mark SD, Zou XN, Greenwald P, Wu YP, Blot WJ. Nutrition intervention trials in Linxian, China: Multiple vitamin/mineral supplementation, cancer incidence, and disease-specific mortality among adults with espohageal dysplasia. J Natl Cancer Inst 1993;85:1492—1498.

15. Greenwald P. Colon cancer overview. Cancr 1992;70(Suppl 5):1206—1215.

16. Reddy BS. Chemoprevention of colon cancer by dietary fatty acids. Cancer Metast Rev 1994;13: 285—302.

17. Pence BC, Dunn DM, Zhao C, Landers M, Wargovich MJ. Chemopreventive effects of calcium but not aspirin supplementation in cholic acid-promoted colon cancer carcinogenesis: correlation with intermediate endpoints. Carcinogenesis 1995;16:757—765.

18. DeCosse JJ, Miller HH, Lesser ML. Effect of wheat fiber and vitamins C and E on rectal polyps in patients with familial adenomatous polyposis. J Natl Cancer Inst 1989;81:1290—1297.

19. McKeown-Eijssen GE, Bright-See E, Bruce WR, Jazmaji V, The Toronto Polyp Prevention Group. A randomized trial of a low fat high fibre diet in the recurrence of colorectal polyps. J Clin Epidemiol 1993;47:525—536.

20. Greenberg ER, Baron JA, Tosteson TD, Freeman DH, Beck GJ, Bond JH, Colacchio TA, Coller JA, Frankl HD, Haile RW, Mandel JS, Nierenberg DW, Rothstein R, Snover DC, Stevens MM, Summers RW, Van Stolk RU for the Polyp Prevention Study Group. A clinical trial of antioxidant vitamins to prevent colorectal adenoma. N Engl J Med 1994;331:141—147.

21. MacLennan R, Macrae F, Bain C, Battistutta D, Chapuis P, Gratten H, Lambert J, Newland RC, Ngu M, Russel A, Ward M, Wahlqvist ML, The Australian Polyp Prevention Project. Randomized trial of intake of fat, fiber, and beta-carotene to prevent colorectal adenomas. J Natl Cancer Inst 1995;87:1760—1766.

22. Schatzkin A, Freedman LS, Lanza E, Tangrea J. Diet and colorectal cancer: Still an open question.

J Natl Cancer Inst 1995;87:1733—1735.

23. Lipkin M, Newmark H. Development of clinical chemoprevention trial. J Natl Cancer Inst 1995;87:1275—1277.

24. Balmain A. Exploring the bowels of DNA-methylation. Curr Biol 1995;5:1013—1016.

25. Giovanucci E, Stampfer MJ, Colditz GA, Rimm EB, Trichopoulos D, Rosner BA, Speizer FE, Willett WC. Folate, methionine, and alcohol intake and risk of colorectal adenoma. J natl Cancer Inst 1993;85:875—884.

26. Giovanucci E, Rimm EB, Ascherio A, Stampfer MJ, Colditz GA, Willett WC. Alcohol, low-methionine-low-folate diets, and risk of colon cancer in men. J Natl Cancer Inst 1995;87:265—273.

27. Butterworth CE, Hatch KD, Macaluso M, Cole P, Sauberlich HE, Soong SJ, Borst M, Baker VV. Folate deficiency and cervical dysplasia. JAMA 1992;267:528—533.

Prevention of hormone-related cancers

Brian E. Henderson

University of South California, Los Angeles, California, USA

Experimental, clinical, and epidemiologic evidence indicates that hormones play a major role in the etiology of several human cancers [1]. Specific epidemiologic hypotheses based on the premise that hormones cause cancer relate specific hormones to breast, endometrial, and prostate cancer and the process of ovulation induced by gonadotropin release to ovarian cancer. A key element of these hypotheses is that excessive hormonal stimulation of the particular target organ increases cell division which increases the likelihood that random genetic errors accumulate and lead to neoplastic phenotypes [2,3].

Cancers of hormone-responsive tissues currently account for more than 25% of all newly diagnosed male and more than 40% of all newly diagnosed female cancers in the USA. Because of the evidence that endogenous hormones directly affect the risk for these cancers, chemoprevention through administration of "antihormones" has become an important focus of cancer prevention research. A summary of chemopreventive agents for hormone-induced cancers is shown in Table 1. The acceptability of agents such as these for widespread use in cancer prevention relies on the balance of the health benefits vs. the health risks of such usage.

The prototype antihormone is progesterone, which has a natural antiestrogenic effect on endometrial cell proliferation. During the follicular phase of an ovulatory menstrual cycle, endometrial cells divide in response to estrogen stimulation that is unopposed by progesterone. During the luteal phase, further estrogen-induced endometrial cell proliferation ceases in the presence of progesterone. Epidemiologic evidence shows that events or circumstances that increase estrogen stimulation in the absence of progesterone increase endometrial cancer risk, whereas those that decrease unopposed estrogen exposure decrease risk [4]. The application of these principles to the chemoprevention of endometrial cancer has been amply demonstrated through the use of combination type oral contraceptives and through the addition of progestogens to estrogen replacement therapy.

Oral contraceptives

Endometrial cancer

During the time when the association of prolonged use of estrogen replacement therapy and increased risk of endometrial cancer was being established, case series reports suggested a similar association between sequential oral contraceptives and

148

Table 1. Hormone chemopreventive agents currently in clinical use.

Chemopreventive agent	Cancer site	Mechanism of action
Oral contraceptives	Endometrium	Antiestrogen
	Ovary	Cease ovulation
Progestogens (HRT)	Endometrium	Antiestrogen
LHRH agonist	Breast	Eliminate ovarian steroid
	Endometrium	hormone production
	Ovary	Cease ovulation
Tamoxifen	Breast	Antiestrogen
Finasteride	Prostate	5α-reductase inhibition

Note: HRT = hormone replacement therapy; LHRH = luteinizing-hormone-releasing-hormone.

endometrial cancer [5]. It is not surprising that sequential formulations had this effect on the endometrium, because they induced a menstrual cycle that began with a 14- to 16-day proliferation phase (administration of unopposed estrogen), followed by a short 7-day secretory phase (administration of estrogen-progestogen combination), and ended with a 5- to 7-day period without treatment. Three case-control studies that accumulated sufficient data on the use of sequential type oral contraceptives and the risk of subsequent endometrial cancer showed that endometrial cancer risk of women who had used these preparations was 2-fold greater than that of women who had not used them [6–8].

In contrast to the adverse effects on the endometrium of sequential oral contraceptives, use of combination oral contraceptives substantially reduces the risk of endometrial cancer [9]. These preparations contain an estrogen and high-dose progestin which are given in combination for 21 days during the 28-day cycle. As a result, the endometrium is only exposed to unopposed (endogenous) estrogen at low levels during the 7-day period without treatment, thereby minimizing endometrial mitotic activity. Overall, case-control studies show that endometrial cancer risk among users of combination oral contraceptives is decreased by approximately 11.7%/year [9]. Prospective cohort studies have demonstrated similar decreases in risk [10,11].

In the large cancer and steroid hormone (CASH) study sponsored by the Centers for Disease Control and the National Institute of Child Health and Human Development, the protective effect of combination oral contraceptives on endometrial cancer risk was the same for both short-term users (<5 years) and longer term users (>5 years) [6]. In contrast, Henderson and colleagues observed a clear decrease in risk with increasing duration of use [7]. Among women with 6 or more years of use, the risk of endometrial cancer was less than one-sixth that of women who had never used oral contraceptives. In combination, these two studies show a reduction in endometrial cancer risk of approximately 12%/year of combination oral contraceptive use [9].

Whether the protective effect of combination oral contraceptives is long lasting is an important question and study results have been mixed. In the CASH study, the protective effect of pill use persisted for women who discontinued using oral contraceptives 15 years before participation in the study [6]. Similarly, another multicentered study, conducted more recently, showed persistence of a protective effect up to 20 years since last oral contraceptive use [12].

Henderson and colleagues [13] have illustrated the protective effect of use of combination oral contraceptives on the age-specific incidence curve for endometrial cancer (Fig. 1A). The results of the studies summarized in Pike and Spicer [9] suggest that the slope of the age-specific incidence curve is reduced during combination oral contraceptive use, but once use is discontinued, the slope increases again to the precombination-oral-contraceptive rate. As shown in Fig. 1A, the protective effect of combination oral contraceptives under this model will be lifelong, consistent with the persistent protective effect observed in epidemiologic studies.

Ovarian cancer

In addition to their chemoprotective action on the endometrium, combination oral contraceptives reduce a woman's risk of epithelial ovarian cancer. Hankinson and

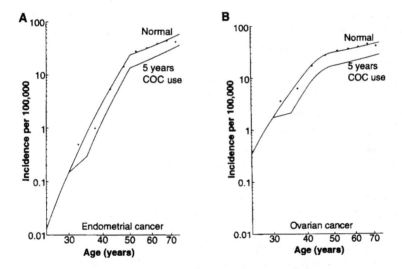

Fig. 1. A: Age-specific incidence rates for cancer of the endometrium in "normal" women and in women using combination oral contraceptives for 5 years. These curves are based on data from the Birmingham Cancer Registry for 1968–1972, where high hysterectomy and oophorectomy rates (prominent in the USA) do not distort the rates. The dots are the actual incidence data and the solid lines marked "normal" represent mathematical models predicting incidence rates from the major known risk factors for these cancers [23]. On the basis of these models and the reduction in cancer risk associated with COC use observed in epidemiological studies, it is possible to calculate how these age-incidence curves will be altered by COC use; these predicted age-incidence curves are also shown (lower solid lines in A and B). Abbreviations — COC = combination oral contraceptives. B: Age-specific incidence rates for cancer of the ovary in "normal" women and in women using combination oral contraceptives for 5 years. These curves are based on data from the Birmingham Cancer Registry for 1968–1972, where high hysterectomy and oophorectomy rates (prominent in the USA) do not distort the rates. Abbreviations — COC = combination oral contraceptives.

colleagues [14] provide an overview of 20 studies (hospital- and community-based case-control studies and cohort studies) which have assessed the relationship between previous use of combination oral contraceptives and subsequent risk of ovarian cancer. Based on the data provided in these reports, Hankinson and colleagues have estimated that the summary relative risk of ovarian cancer associated with any use of combination oral contraceptives is 0.64 (95% confidence interval = 0.57–0.73). The risk of ovarian cancer decreases with longer duration of use; for each year of oral contraceptive use, risk is estimated to decline by 7.5% [9]. This reduced risk appears to persist for at least 10 years after women discontinue use. Women whose last use of oral contraceptives was 10 or more years earlier had a 40% reduction in risk of ovarian cancer (relative risk = 0.60; 95% confidence interval = 0.42–0.86) [14].

The epidemiologic results relating combination oral contraceptive use to reduced risk of ovarian cancer can be illustrated in terms of the effects of such use on the age-specific incidence rates of ovarian cancer (Fig. 1B). The pattern observed is comparable to that for endometrial cancer shown in Fig. 1A, again suggesting a persistent reduction in risk following cessation of use.

Many of the studies in the report of Hankinson and colleagues [14] were conducted when the majority of experience with oral contraceptives was with higher dose preparations; thus, the question arises as to whether newer, lower dose preparations confer similar protection against ovarian cancer. Rosenberg and colleagues [15] evaluated various types of formulations and their effects on ovarian cancer risk; their case-control study results suggest that both higher and lower dose preparations are protective. The experience with the newer biphasic and triphasic pills, as well as with the progestogen-only pills, is still limited; and no conclusions can be drawn as to whether such formulations are protective against ovarian cancer.

Two hypotheses are currently under consideration to explain the protective effect of oral contraceptives on ovarian cancer risk [9]. One is that ovarian cancer is the result of cell replication occurring in the repair of ovarian surface epithelium following ovulation. Any factor, such as oral contraceptive use, months of pregnancy, or earlier onset of menopause, that reduces a woman's cumulative number of ovulatory cycles should then reduce her ovarian cancer risk. However, inconsistent with this hypothesis is the fact that early age at menopause has a limited effect on ovarian cancer risk in most epidemiologic studies.

An alternative hypothesis is that follicle development may be the critical risk factor rather than ovulation, per se. In this case, ovarian cancers might be expected to arise in nonsurface epithelial cells. Currently, it is not known whether ovarian cancers arise in the surface or the nonsurface epithelium.

Breast cancer

Unlike the antiestrogenic effects of progesterone on the endometrium, evidence is accumulating that progesterone increases the rate of cell division in the breast beyond that induced by estrogen [16,17]. Studies relating endogenous hormone levels to breast cell proliferation show that proliferation is lowest during the follicular phase when levels of ovarian sex steroids are low, and that proliferation increases 2-fold to peak in the midluteal to late luteal phase when progesterone reaches its maximum [17]. Thus, the combination of estrogen and progesterone appears to have a greater stimulatory effect on breast cell division than estrogen alone. The simultaneous presence of estrogen and progesterone in combination oral contraceptives might be expected to have similar effects on breast cell proliferation rates and this is the case [17]. Therefore, oral contraceptive use is not protective against breast cancer as it is against cancers of the endometrium and ovary.

Use of oral contraceptives at particular ages actually may increase breast cancer risk. During the postmenarcheal period the naturally produced levels of estrogen and progesterone may be lower than those supplied by oral contraceptive formulations; use of oral contraceptives at this time may be associated with an increased risk of breast cancer [18,19].

Secular changes in cancer risk

The annual age-adjusted incidence rate of endometrial and ovarian cancer had fallen over the period 1972–1987 in women below the age of 50 in the USA [13]. These secular decreases are consistent with the widespread use of oral contraceptives in American women since the introduction of OCs in the early 1970s. It is estimated that an average 60% of American women have used OCs for an average of 5 years. The reduction in rate of these two cancers was entirely consistent with the predicted impact of OC use on these two cancers. As predicted, the incidence rates of breast cancer have not fallen [13] and, in fact, have shown a small increase.

Hormone replacement therapy

Endometrial cancer

The use of hormone replacement therapy (HRT) to provide short-term relief of symptoms related to menopause and long-term protection from the consequences of estrogen deficiency constitutes the other major setting in which exogenous steroid hormones are widely used in essentially healthy women. As with combination oral contraceptives, use of HRT has had a remarkable impact on cancer incidence and mortality. As strategies for delivering HRT have evolved, however, the nature of this impact has dramatically changed. In particular, the ever-expanding use of a combination regimen, in which a progestogen is added continuously or sequentially to estrogen during a monthly cycle, has not only highlighted the importance of progestogens but also raised important issues concerning the risk-benefit balance of various HRT formulations.

A strong association exists between estrogen replacement therapy (ERT) and endometrial cancer risk that is related both to dose and to duration of therapy [20–22]. The endometrial cell mitotic activity in a woman on continuous high-dose ERT is approximately equal to that observed during the follicular phase of the menstrual cycle; thus, the total mitotic activity over a 28-day period is roughly double

152

that of a premenopausal woman because the ERT is not opposed by progesterone at any time. On the basis of this mitotic rate, 5 years of ERT use starting at menopause is predicted to extend the premenopausal portion of the endometrial cancer incidence curve for the 5 years of ERT use (Fig. 2A) [23]. As a result, endometrial cancer risk would increase by a factor of ~3.5 and would be of long-term (lifelong) duration after 5 years of such ERT use, in agreement with actual epidemiologic observations.

The benefit of adding a progestogen to ERT in reducing endometrial mitotic activity has been clearly established. Therefore, in response to the "epidemic" of endometrial cancer that followed the rise in estrogen prescriptions in the 1960s and 1970s, progestogens were added to the estrogen in various doses and schedules (typically 5–10 mg of medroxyprogesterone acetate for 10–12 days/month). Such combination therapy has been shown to reduce the estrogen-enhanced risk of endometrial cancer [24]. As a second response, the average daily dose of the most commonly used form of estrogen, conjugated equine estrogen, was lowered from 1.25 mg to 0.625 mg. Noncontraceptive estrogen prescriptions in the USA declined almost 50% in the mid-1970s as it became clear that ERT caused endometrial cancer. This decline led to a decrease in endometrial cancer incidence and mortality in the late 1970s, after the substantial increases that had occurred in the preceding decade. The reduced dosages of ERT and the addition of a progestogen to HRT have sustained these decreases into the 1980s. Incidence and mortality from endometrial cancer in postmenopausal women declined 27.9 and 14.4%, respectively, between 1973 and 1987.

Breast cancer

The addition of a progestogen to ERT has implications not only for endometrial

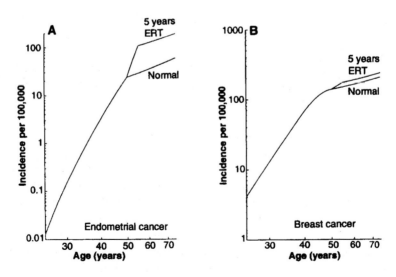

Fig. 2. A and B: Age-specific incidence rates for endometrial cancer (A) and breast cancer (B) in "normal" women and in women using ERT for 5 years. Calculation of the effects of ERT follows the same logic as that described in Fig. 1A,B.

cancer, but also for other components of the risk-benefit equation. Because of the importance of these other health effects, we discuss them in detail below, together with comparative data for ERT alone.

Breast cancer incidence increases with age at ~2.1%/year in postmenopausal women. If this rise is attributable solely to endogenous estrogens, as appears likely, the risk of breast cancer associated with ERT use can be predicted by comparing endogenous serum estrogen levels with the serum estrogen levels achieved while a woman uses ERT. In postmenopausal American women, the serum level of bioavailable estradiol (E_2), the fraction of E_2 that is not bound to sex hormone binding globulin (SHBG), is ~12 pg/ml [16]. The serum level of non-SHBG-bound E_2 in women receiving 0.625 mg CEE per day is approximately double the normal postmenopausal level (~26 pg/ml). On the assumption that E_2 is the most important estrogen both from endogenous serum and from ERT, the incremental increase in breast cancer risk due to ERT should be approximately equal to that due to endogenous estrogens (an additional 2.1%/year). The risk estimates from population-based epidemiologic studies show an increase in breast cancer risk of 3.1%/year of ERT use, for all formulations combined. When only conjugated equine estrogen in a dose of 0.625 mg is considered, however, the increase in breast cancer risk is estimated to be slightly less than 2%/year of ERT use (Fig. 2B) [25], almost precisely as predicted.

Nearly all breast cancer studies to date have evaluated risk attributable to ERT alone, not to combination HRT. Data from a prospective study in Sweden have suggested that risk associated with combination HRT is higher than any found for ERT alone [26], as the breast mitotic rate data would suggest. Other studies have not confirmed this observation although the number of subjects with more than 5 years of use was small [27,28].

The most important long-term health effect of ERT is to lower cardiovascular disease morbidity and mortality [29]. Largely because of this profound effect, the reduction in overall mortality (from all causes) for ERT users is 20% or more in some populations, with an even greater reduction in mortality for current long-term users. In addition to their possible adverse effects on breast cancer risk, progestogens may negate some of this cardiovascular benefit of ERT.

Luteinizing-hormone-releasing-hormone agonists

Among premenopausal women, a proposed strategy for retaining the benefit of oral contraceptives on the risk for endometrial and ovarian cancer while possibly preventing breast cancer is to eliminate ovarian estrogen and progesterone production by using luteinizing-hormone-releasing-hormone (LHRH) agonists. Experimentally, these drugs cause regression of estrogen-dependent dimethylbenzanthracene-induced rat mammary tumors [30]; clinically, they suppress ovulation and cause regression of metastatic breast cancer in premenopausal women [31–33].

As a primary means for preventing breast cancer, the use of LHRH agonists is designed to exploit the preventive aspect of early menopause on breast cancer risk

[34]. By totally eliminating ovarian steroid hormone production, LHRH agonists induce a reversible "bilateral oophorectomy". It is predicted that such a regimen taken for 5 years during the premenopausal years would lead to a reduction in breast cancer risk of 38%, and such a regimen taken for 15 years could reduce risk by as much as 80% [34]. By preventing ovulation, as in the case with combination oral contraceptives, such a regimen markedly reduces endometrial and ovarian cancer risk.

The beneficial effect of eliminating ovarian steroid hormone production is associated with adverse side effects. These adverse consequences are primarily those related to a hypoestrogenic state, both acutely and in the long term. Particular examples are hot flushes, bone loss, and probably a significantly increased risk for cardiovascular disease resulting at least in part from an increase in low-density lipoprotein cholesterol [35]. Extensive experience suggests that these harmful side effects can be eliminated by the addition of low-dose estrogen replacement therapy to the regimen. Such a regimen (LHRH agonist plus low-dose estrogen replacement therapy) does not affect the protective effect of LHRH agonists alone on ovarian cancer risk; Pike and colleagues have argued that the estrogen replacement therapy dose required to eliminate these side effects is sufficiently low to retain the major part of the benefit on breast cancer risk [34]. Intermittent regular addition of a progestogen to the regimen could avoid any increased risk for endometrial hyperplasia (or carcinoma) associated with low-dose estrogen replacement therapy. Medroxyprogesterone acetate given every 3–4 months for 13 days of one monthly cycle at a dose of 5–10 mg/day is one possible regimen. Addition of a small amount of testosterone to replace that normally produced by the ovary, in conjunction with the estrogen, reduces the risk of bone loss.

In addition to the advantages related to breast cancer risk, such a regimen may provide other notable advantages over low-dose oral contraceptives in terms of long-term health effects. Although data are sparse, the addition of a low-dose estrogen replacement therapy to the LHRH regimen would appear to create a favorable lipid profile, particularly with regard to high-density lipoprotein cholesterol levels, and would be expected to have a favorable influence on cardiovascular disease risk [34].

This proposed regimen is a highly effective hormonal contraceptive method. It has been tested in a small, 2-year, pilot clinical trial among premenopausal women with an extremely high risk of breast cancer. At the end of the 1st year, relatively few side effects were noted [36] and potentially beneficial mammographic changes, measured as reductions in mammographic densities, were observed [37].

Tamoxifen

The first proposal for the hormonal chemoprevention of breast cancer was introduced by Cuzick and colleagues in 1986 [38]. The goal was to treat healthy postmenopausal women at high risk for breast cancer using the antiestrogenic drug, tamoxifen. The rationale for this proposal was based partly on the extensive evidence that the amount of estrogen available to breast tissue is a critical factor in the cause of human breast cancer. Two years later, a summary analysis of 28 ongoing USA, Canadian and

European randomized clinical trials showed a significant reduction in the mortality from breast cancer of women older than 50 years of age treated with tamoxifen [39]. This beneficial effect appears to extend to women regardless of lymph node status at diagnosis and regardless of the initial estrogen receptor status of their tumors.

The most compelling argument to extend the use of tamoxifen to healthy women at high risk for breast cancer is the lower risk for contralateral primary breast cancer observed among women receiving adjuvant tamoxifen therapy for breast cancer. Nayfield and colleagues [40] have summarized data from eight randomized trials of tamoxifen vs. a control regimen which show a 35% reduction in risk for contralateral breast cancer among tamoxifen treated women.

Breast cancer chemoprevention trials are currently ongoing in the USA, Canada, UK and Italy. The goal of these trials is to provide information on the magnitude of breast-cancer risk reduction, and to clarify other benefits, such as a possible cardiovascular disease reduction, and risks associated with tamoxifen use. The USA trial, the Breast Cancer Prevention Trial, was begun in April, 1992 at 270 centers in the USA and Canada. A total of 16,000 eligible women are being recruited who are at least 35 years of age and whose risk of breast cancer is at least that of a 60-year-old woman. Tamoxifen treatment or placebo is being administered for 5 years. Although accrual of participants was to have been completed during the first 2 years, recruitment was somewhat slower than expected and accrual was halted briefly during 1994.

The possible adverse effects of tamoxifen on other organ systems has restrained optimism about its efficacy in primary breast cancer prevention [41–44]. Tamoxifen shows highly selective antiestrogenic properties; it appears to be an estrogen agonist in most tissues other than breast and to create a somewhat favorable lipid profile. As part of a 2-year randomized, double-blind, placebo-controlled toxicity trial of tamoxifen in postmenopausal women with a history of node-negative breast cancer, Love and colleagues found that low-density lipoprotein cholesterol levels declined approximately 18% and that this decline persisted for at least 1 year of treatment [45]. High-density lipoprotein cholesterol levels remained unchanged for the first 6 months of therapy, but, compared with baseline values, were reduced significantly by 7% at 1 year. Total cholesterol was reduced significantly in the tamoxifen-treated group. Overall, because of the large declines in low-density lipoprotein cholesterol, the relative amount of high-density lipoprotein cholesterol (i.e., high-density lipoprotein/total cholesterol ratio) increased among women treated with tamoxifen.

Nonetheless, the effect of long-term tamoxifen use with regard to heart disease risk remains uncertain; the pattern of lipid changes with tamoxifen is different from that induced by ERT and mechanisms other than lipid changes may be involved in the cardioprotective effect of ERT. Furthermore, few data are available for women regarding the potential benefits for cardiovascular disease risk of reducing low-density lipoprotein cholesterol.

The Scottish Adjuvant Tamoxifen Trial provides some preliminary evidence that tamoxifen may have a beneficial effect on coronary heart disease risk [46]. In this randomized trial, a group of women received 20 mg tamoxifen daily for at least 5 years and follow-up ranged from 5–11 years. Among postmenopausal women, those treated with tamoxifen had a statistically significant reduction in mortality due to acute myocardial infarction compared with control patients.

Available evidence on the effects of tamoxifen on bone mineral density is encouraging. Two studies evaluating this issue have reported slight increases in the density of the lumbar spine during tamoxifen treatment for postmenopausal breast cancer [47,48]. Although osteoporotic fracture rates have not been studied after tamoxifen use, these data suggest that, as with ERT, fracture risk may be reduced.

Among the breast cancer clinical trials, some [49–54], but not all [55,56] find an increased risk of endometrial cancer associated with tamoxifen therapy. Caveats to consider in interpreting these trial results are that they were not designed to assess endometrial cancer risk and hence do not adequately deal with problems of confounding by prior hysterectomy and use of ERT. Further, following the initial concern that tamoxifen increased the risk of endometrial cancer, women undergoing tamoxifen treatment as part of these trials may have undergone greater detection efforts than those receiving other treatment modalities. Although the evidence from the positive trials is generally taken as conclusive, two of the three major positive studies appear to have a deficit of endometrial cancer among their comparison groups [49,52] and the results of the third study were not statistically significant [50]. Therefore, the magnitude of increased risk is not well-quantitated from these trials.

Another concern is that tamoxifen may have estrogen-like effects on the liver. In rats, estrogens act as promoters of liver carcinogenesis [57]. In large doses or with extended exposure, tamoxifen can produce rat liver tumors [58]. No increase in liver tumor incidence has been reported among tamoxifen-treated patients in any clinical trial, although Fornander and colleagues observed two cases of hepatocellular carcinoma among their patients receiving tamoxifen [49].

A possible increased risk of thromboembolic disease has been suggested [59], but has not been well-documented. Among postmenopausal women receiving long-term adjuvant tamoxifen therapy, small decreases in the levels of antithrombin III have been reported [60], although these values are generally within the normal range. As a result, a history of clotting disorders may be a contraindication to tamoxifen treatment.

Although tamoxifen probably reduces certain acute menopausal effects, such as vaginal dryness, the drug has no beneficial effect on hot flushes (some data suggest the opposite may be true) and the relation between tamoxifen and other acute menopausal symptoms is largely unstudied.

Chemoprevention of prostate cancer

Testosterone is essential for the maintenance of prostatic tissue, but there are no studies in men relating variation in circulating testosterone levels to the rate of cell proliferation in the prostate. Epidemiologic support for an association of increased testosterone levels and increased prostatic cancer risk is inconsistent [61]. Prostatic adenocarcinomas can be produced by testosterone administration in rats and such treatment increases proliferation of the glandular cells in the prostate, which give rise to prostatic cancer [62]. Testosterone may increase the mitotic activity of prostatic cells in men and such an increase in mitotic activity would increase the risk of prostatic cancer.

Diethylstilbestrol and LHRH agonists are effective therapeutically in metastatic prostate cancer, presumably because of their indirect effect on testosterone production, by decreasing luteinizing hormone secretion. These drugs in their usual therapeutic doses produce impotence and other side effects that are unacceptable when considered as chemopreventive agents.

Despite the dependence of the prostate on testosterone for normal growth and maintenance, testosterone has no strong direct effect on prostatic epithelium, requiring metabolic activation to dihydrotestosterone for these functions. Dihydrotestosterone has much stronger affinity than testosterone for the androgen receptor, a molecule required to transport androgens to the DNA of prostate cells for activation of androgen-responsive genes, including those which regulate cell division. Conversion of testosterone to dihydrotestosterone in the prostate requires activity of the enzyme 5-α-reductase.

Japanese and Chinese men have among the lowest prostate cancer rates in the world. Recent data strongly suggest that both of these populations have much reduced 5-α-reductase activity relative to American blacks and whites [63,64]. These findings may provide a hormonal basis for the low levels of prostate cancer in these Asian populations and emphasize the need to clarify further the role of 5-α-reductase activity in prostatic carcinogenesis. If such enzymatic activity proves crucial, then chemoprevention of prostate cancer using the 5-α-reductase inhibitor category of drugs may be feasible. These drugs, which selectively block production of dihydrotestosterone from testosterone in the prostate, reduce prostatic size without affecting testosterone-dependent processes such as fertility, muscle strength, and libido.

Finasteride, a 5-α-reductase inhibitor, is used in the treatment of benign prostatic hyperplasia. In clinical trials, it has been shown to reduce prostate size and improve urinary flow [65]. Preliminary studies in a rat model of finasteride and of casodex, a pure antiandrogen preparation, suggest that these drugs are effective in reducing the incidence of prostate tumors induced by the combined exposure to testosterone and a carcinogen [66]. Recently, a nationwide, 7-year prostate cancer chemoprevention trial of 5-α-reductase inhibitors has been instituted in the USA. [67]. The primary endpoint is biopsy-proven presence or absence of prostate cancer. A total of 18,000 healthy men, aged 55 years or more will be randomized to receive either finasteride 5 mg/day or placebo for 7 years.

Future directions

The proven effectiveness of tamoxifen in preventing contralateral breast cancer and the potential promise of finasteride in the prevention of prostate cancer have prompted the systematic search for other compounds that might decrease intracellular estradiol or dihydrotestosterone and thereby reduce the risk of breast and prostate cancer. Potential targets for breast cancer prevention include the enzymes that synthesize estradiol. In the premenopausal period, the major enzyme appears to be a member of the 17 hydroxysteroid dehydrogenase (17HSD) family, most probably 17HSD type I [68]. This enzyme converts estrone to estradiol in the ovary and in the breast and presumably is at least partly responsible for the increased concentration of estradiol in the breast compared to the circulation [68]. In the postmenopausal period, the major route of estradiol production is through peripheral conversion of androstenedione to estrone and then to estradiol [69]. The cytochrome p450 aromatase enzyme responsible for this conversion is concentrated in adipose tissue and is also a candidate enzyme for pharmacologic intervention in breast cancer [70].

Not only are these enzymes themselves potential targets but the genes that encode these enzymes are of considerable interest [71]. There is speculation that there are sequence variations and functional polymorphisms in such "metabolic" genes that might alter plasma or intracellular steroid levels sufficiently to confer individual variation in risk to the hormone-related cancers [71].

References

1. Henderson BE, Ross RK, Pike MC et al. Endogenous hormones as a major factor in human cancer. Cancer Res 1982;43:3232–3239.
2. Henderson BE, Ross RK, Bernstein L. Estrogens as a cause of human cancer: The Richard and Hinda Rosenthal Foundation Award Lecture. Cancer Res 1988;48:246–253.
3. Preston-Martin S, Pike MC, Ross RK et al. Increased cell division as a cause of human cancer. Cancer Res 1990;50:7415–7421.
4. Key TJA, Pike MC. The role of estrogens and progestagens in the epidemiology and prevention of breast cancer. Eur J Cancer Clin Oncol 1988;24:29–43.
5. Silverberg SG, Makowski EL. Endometrial carcinoma in young women taking oral contraceptive agents. Obstet Gynecol 1975;46:503–506.
6. Centers for Disease Control. Oral contraceptive use and the risk of endometrial cancer. JAMA 1983;249:1600–1604.
7. Henderson BE, Casagrande JT, Pike MC et al. The epidemiology of endometrial cancer in young women. Br J Cancer 1983;47:749–756.
8. Weiss NS, Sayvetz TA. Incidence of endometrial cancer in relation to the use of oral contraceptives. N Engl J Med 1980;302:551–554.
9. Pike MC, Spicer DV. Oral contraceptives and cancer. In: Shoupe D, Haseltine F (eds) Contraception. New York: Springer-Verlag, 1993;.
10. Ramcharan S, Pellegrin FA, Ray R et al. A prospective study of the side effects of oral contraceptive use. Washington, DC: U.S. Government Printing Office, 1981.
11. Beral V, Hannaford P, Kay C. Oral contraceptive use and malignancies of the genital tract. Lancet 1988;2:1331–1335.
12. Stanford JL, Brinton LA, Berman ML et al. Oral contraceptives and endometrial cancer: Do other risk factors modify the association? Int J Cancer 1993;54:242–248.
13. Henderson BE, Ross RK, Pike MC. Hormonal chemoprevention of cancer in women. Science 1993;259:633–638.
14. Hankinson SE, Colditz GA, Hunter DJ et al. A quantitative assessment of oral contraceptive use and risk of ovarian cancer. Obstet Gynecol 1992;80:708–714.
15. Rosenberg L, Palmer JR, Zauber AG et al. A case-control study of oral contraceptive use and

invasive epithelial ovarian cancer. Am J Epidemiol 1994;139:654—661.

16. Key TJA, Pike MC. The dose-effect relationship between "unopposed" oestrogens and endometrial mitotic rate: Its central role in explaining and predicting endometrial cancer risk. Br J Cancer 1988;57:205—212.

17. Pike MC, Spicer DV, Dahmoush L et al. Estrogens, progestogens, normal breast cell proliferation and breast cancer risk. Epidemiol Rev 1993;15:17—35.

18. Bernstein L, Henderson BE. Hormone intake: Relationship to cancer risk. In: DeVita VT, Hellman S, Rosenberg SA (eds) Cancer prevention. Philadelphia: JB Lippincott, 1990;1—17.

19. Brinton LA, Daling JR, Liff JM et al. Oral contraceptives and breast cancer risk among younger women. J Natl Cancer Inst 1995;87:827—835.

20. Smith DC, Prentice R, Thompson DJ et al. Association of exogenous estrogen and endometrial cancer. N Engl J Med 1975;293:1164—1167.

21. Ziel HK, Finkle WD. Increased risk of endometrial carcinoma among users of conjugated estrogens. N Engl J Med 1975;293:1167—1170.

22. Mack TM, Pike MC, Henderson BE et al. Estrogens and endometrial cancer in a retirement community. N Engl J Med 1976;294:1262—1267.

23. Pike MC. Age-related factors in cancers of the breast, ovary and endometrium. J Chronic Dis 1987;40(Suppl 2):595—695.

24. Voigt LF, Weiss NS, Chu J et al. Progestogen supplementation of exogenous oestrogens and risk of endometrial cancer. Lancet 1991;338:274—277.

25. Pike MC, Bernstein L, Spicer DV. The relationship of exogenous hormones to breast cancer risk. In: Niederhuber JE (ed) Current therapy in oncology. St. Louis: Dekker, Mosby-Year Book, 1993;292—303.

26. Persson I, Yuen J, Bergkvist L et al. Combined oestrogen-progestogen replacement and breast cancer risk (letter). Lancet 1992;340:1044.

27. Colditz GA, Hankinson SE, Hunter DJ et al. The use of estrogens and progestins and the risk of breast cancer in postmenopausal women. N Engl J Med 1995;332:1589—1593.

28. Stanford JL, Weiss NS, Voigt LF et al. Combined estrogen and progestin hormone replacement therapy in relation to risk of breast cancer in middle-aged women. JAMA 1995;274:137—142.

29. Henderson BE, Paganini—Hill A, Ross RK. Decreased mortality in users of estrogen replacement therapy. Arch Int Med 1991;151:75—78.

30. Nicholson RI, Walker KJ, Maynard PV. Anti-tumor potential of a new potent luteinizing hormone releasing hormone analogue, ICI 118630. Eur J Cancer 1980;1(Suppl):295—299.

31. Harvey HA, Lipton A, Max DT et al. Medical castration produced by the GnRH analogue leuprolide to treat metastatic breast cancer. J Clin Oncol 1985;3:1068—1072.

32. Williams MR, Walker KJ, Turkes A et al. The use of an LH-RH agonist (ICI118360, Zoladex) in advanced premenopausal breast cancer. Br J Cancer 1986;53:629—636.

33. Dixon AR, Robertson JFR, Jackson L et al. Goserelin (Zoladex) in premenopausal advanced breast cancer: Duration of response and survival. Br J Cancer 1990;62:868—870.

34. Pike MC, Ross RK, Lobo RA et al. LHRH agonists and the prevention of breast and ovarian cancer. Br J Cancer 1989;60:142—148.

35. Henderson BE, Ross RK, Lobo RA et al. Re-evaluating the role of progestogen therapy after the menopause. Fertil Steril 1988;49(Suppl):9s—15s.

36. Spicer DV, Pike MC, Pike A et al. Pilot trial of a gonadotropin hormone agonist with replacement hormones as a prototype contraceptive to prevent breast cancer. Contraception 1993;47:427—444.

37. Spicer DV, Ursin G, Parisky YR et al. Changes in mammographic densities induced by a hormonal contraceptive designed to reduce breast cancer risk. J Natl Cancer Inst 1994;86:431—436.

38. Cuzick J, Wang DY, Bulbrook RD. The prevention of breast cancer. Lancet 1986;1:83—86.

39. Early Breast Cancer Trialists' Collaborative Group. Effects of adjuvant tamoxifen and cytotoxic therapy on mortality in early breast cancer. N Engl J Med 1988;319:1681—1692.

40. Nayfield SG, Karp JE, Ford LG et al. Potential role of tamoxifen in prevention of breast cancer. J Natl Cancer Inst 1991;83:1450—1459.

41. Bernstein L, Ross RK, Henderson BE. Prospects for the primary prevention of breast cancer. Am J Epidemiol 1992;135:142–152.
42. Bush TL, Helzlsouer KJ. Tamoxifen for the primary prevention of breast cancer: A review and critique of the concept and trial. Epidemiol Rev 1993;15:223–243.
43. Love RR. The National Surgical Adjuvant Breast Project (NSABP) Breast Cancer Prevention Trial revisited. Cancer Epidemiol Biomarkers Prev 1993;2:403–407.
44. King CM. Tamoxifen and the induction of cancer. Carcinogenesis 1995;16:1449–1454.
45. Love RR, Newcomb PA, Wiebe DA et al. Effects of tamoxifen therapy on lipid and lipoprotein levels in postmenopausal patients with node-negative breast cancer. J Natl Cancer Inst 1990;82:1327–1332.
46. McDonald CG, Stewart HJ. Fatal myocardial infarction in the Scottish adjuvant tamoxifen trial. Br Med J 1991;303:435–437.
47. Love RR, Mazess RB, Torney DC et al. Bone mineral density in women with breast cancer treated with adjuvant tamoxifen for at least two years. Breast Cancer Res Treat 1988;12:297–301.
48. Turken S, Siris E, Seldin D et al. Effects of tamoxifen on spinal bone density in women with breast cancer. J Natl Cancer Inst 1989;81:1086–1088.
49. Fornander T, Rutqvist LE, Cedermark B et al. Adjuvant tamoxifen in early breast cancer: Occurrence of new primary cancers. Lancet 1989;1:117–120.
50. Andersson M, Storm HH, Mouridsen T. Carcinogenic effects of adjuvant tamoxifen treatment and radiotherapy for early breast cancer. Acta Oncol 1992;31:259–263.
51. Ryden S, Ferno M, Moller T et al. Long-term effects of adjuvant tamoxifen and/or radiotherapy. The South Sweden Breast Cancer Trial. Acta Oncol 1992;31:271–274.
52. Fisher B, Constantino JP, Redmond CK et al. Endometrial cancer in tamoxifen-treated breast cancer patients: Findings from the National Surgical Adjuvant Breast and Bowel Project (NSABP) B-14. J Natl Cancer Inst 1994;86:527–537.
53. Rutqvist LE, Johansson H, Signomklao T et al. Adjuvant tamoxifen therapy for early stage breast cancer and second primary malignancies. J Natl Cancer Inst 1995;87:645–651.
54. Boccardo F, Rubagotti A, Amoroso D et al. Chemotherapy versus tamoxifen versus chemotherapy plus tamoxifen in node-positive, oestrogen-receptor positive breast cancer patients. An update at 7 years of the 1st GROCTA (Breast Cancer Adjuvant Chemo-hormone Therapy Cooperative Group) trial. Eur J Cancer 1992;28:673–680.
55. Ribeiro G, Swindell R. The Christie Hospital adjuvant tamoxifen trial. Natl Cancer Inst Monogr 1992;11:121–125.
56. Stewart HJ for the Scottish Cancer Trials Breast Group. The Scottish trial of adjuvant tamoxifen in node-negative breast cancer. Natl Cancer Inst Monogr 1992;11:117–120.
57. Yager JD, Yager R. Oral contraceptive steroids as promoters of hepatocarcinogenesis in female Sprague-Dawley rats. Cancer Res 1980;40:3680–3685.
58. Jordan VC. Tamoxifen for the prevention of breast cancer. In: DeVita VT, Hellman S, Rosenberg SA (eds) Cancer prevention. Philadelphia: J.B. Lippincott, 1990;1–16.
59. Lipton A, Harvey HA, Hamilton RW. Venous thrombosis as a side effect of tamoxifen treatment. Cancer Treat Rep 1984;68:887–889.
60. Jordan VC, Fritz NF, Tormey DC. Long-term adjuvant therapy with tamoxifen effects on sex hormone binding globulin and antithrombin III. Cancer Res 1987;47:4517–4519.
61. Ross RK. Prostate cancer. In: Schottenfeld D, Fraumeni J (eds) Cancer epidemiology and prevention, 2nd edn. Cambridge, England: Oxford University Press, 1996;(In press).
62. Noble RL. The development of prostatic adenocarcinoma in Nb rats following prolonged sex hormone administration. Cancer Res 1977;37:1929–1933.
63. Ross RK, Bernstein L, Lobo RA et al. Evidence for reduced 5-alpha-reductase activity in Japanese compared to U.S. white and black males: Implications for prostate cancer risk. Lancet 1992;339:887–889.
64. Lookingbill DP, Demers LM, Wang C et al. Clinical and biological parameters of androgen action in normal healthy Caucasian versus Chinese subjects. J Clin Endocrinol Metab 1991;72:1242–1248.

65. Andersen JT. Alpha 1-blockers vs 5-alpha-reductase inhibitors in benign prostatic hyperplasia. A comparative review. Drugs Aging 1995;6:388–396.

66. Tsukamoto S, Akaza H, Imada S et al. Chemoprevention of rat prostate carcinogenesis by use of finasteride or casodex. J Natl Cancer Inst 1995;87:842–843.

67. Brawley OW, Ford LD, Thompson I et al. 5α-reductase inhibition and prostate cancer prevention. Cancer Epidemiol Biomarkers Prev 1994;3:177–182.

68. Poutanen M, Isomaa V, Peltoketo H et al. Role of 17β-hydroxysteroid dehydrogenase type 1 in endocrine and intracrine estradiol biosynthesis. J Steroid Biochem Molec Biol 1995;55:525–532.

69. Harada N, Utsumi T, Takagi Y. Molecular and epidemiological analyses of abnormal expression of aromatase in breast cancer. Pharmacogenetics 1995;5:S59–S64.

70. Vermeulen A, Deslypere JP, Paridaens R et al. Aromatase, 17β-hydroxysteroid dehydrogenase and intratissular sex hormone concentrations in cancerous and normal glandular breast tissue in postmenopausal women. Eur J Cancer Clin Oncol 1986;22:515–525.

71. Feigelson HS, Ross RK, Yu MC et al. Genetic susceptibility to cancer from exogenous and endogenous exposures. J Cell Biochem (In press).

1996 Elsevier Science B.V.
The Scientific Bases of Cancer Chemoprevention.
C. Maltoni, M. Soffritti and W. Davis, editors.

Immunological and other active agents

O.C. Leeksma, G.J.A. ten Bosch and C.J.M. Melief

Department of Immunohaematology and Blood Bank, Leiden University Hospital, Leiden, The Netherlands

Abstract. Recent years have witnessed a tremendous increase in our understanding of the way the immune system works as well as of the molecular genetics of cancer.

The challenge we are facing now is to apply this knowledge for the benefit of patients suffering from all sorts of malignancies.

The potential of the immune system to control cancer is perhaps best illustrated by the effects donor T cells can have in patients relapsing after allogeneic bone marrow transplantation. Progress in delineating the precise target molecules, primarily peptides presented within major histocompatibility complex molecules, is rapid and bound to result in hopefully highly specific nontoxic immunotherapies, which can be applied in both the prevention of the recurrence as well as the treatment of neoplasias.

A very intriguing issue is the demonstration by sensitive RT-PCR of, e.g., gene translocations (like t 14; 18; t 8; 21 and t 9; 22) in apparently healthy individuals. Assuming a predisposition in these people for malignancies associated with these genes immunotherapy might even play a role in primary disease prevention.

We have only just begun to explore the potential of, for instance, synthetic antigenic peptides (based on amino acid sequences of oncoproteins) to modulate the immune system, but already exciting data have been obtained. These developments coincide with the introduction of other potentially specific treatment strategies based among others on a functional inhibition of oncoproteins.

Key words: BCR-ABL, oncoprotein inhibitors, oncoproteins, peptides, T cells.

Introduction

Major histocompatibility complex molecules on the cell surface present peptides derived from endogenous or exogenous proteins to the immune system. Insights into how such peptides are generated are rapidly growing and different processing pathways have been discerned (Fig. 1). A key element in the generation of peptides from endogenous, e.g., cytoplasmic or nuclear, proteins by cells is a proteolytic machinery called the proteasome [1]. Ubiquitination of various proteins precedes their proteasomal degradation [2,3]. Peptides are subsequently translocated to the endoplasmic reticulum by the transporters associated with antigen processing (Tap), a complex formed from two subunits Tap-1 and Tap-2 [4,5]. Alternatively, as has been demonstrated for certain viral envelope proteins, i.e., Tap independent cotranslational translocation into the ER may occur with subsequent proteolysis presumably within the ER. [6] Peptide delivery from Tap's to nascent MHC

Address for correspondence: Dr O.C. Leeksma, Department of Immunohematology and Blood Bank, Leiden University Hospital, Building 1-E3-50, P.O. Box 9600, 2300 RC Leiden, The Netherlands.

A

B

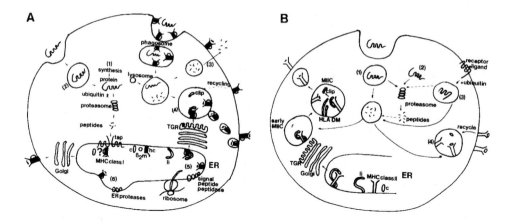

Fig. 1. **A**: Antigen processing pathways MHC class I; ER = endoplasmic reticulum, c = calnexin, hc = heavy chain, li = invariant chain. (1) The presumably most important way peptides are generated from endogenous proteins through digestion by the proteasome. Peptides transported to the ER bind to MHC class I and reach the cell membrane via exocytosis. The question mark refers to as yet unidentified additional player(s) facilitating MHC class I Tap interaction [8]. (2) Proteasome-dependent degradation of exogenous proteins transferred from endocytic vesicles to the cytosol [18]. (3) Possible alternative pathway in which exogenous protein is taken up and degraded in a phagosome. Peptides after regurgitation into the extracellular fluid bind to MHC class I on the plasma membrane. (4) Binding of peptides generated via [3] may also occur within the phagosome either by newly synthesized class I with [12] or without associated invariant chain or by class I recycling from the plasma membrane. (5) Signal peptides cleaved from newly synthesized polypeptides by signal peptide peptidase bind MHC class I within the ER especially in Tap deficient cells. (6) Proteins cotranslationally translocated into the ER can be degraded by ER proteases. Occurs primarily in cells lacking Tap with more empty class I available for peptide binding. Perhaps important for certain viral envelope proteins [6]. **B**: Antigen processing pathways MHC class II. (1) Classically class II peptides were thought to be generated from exogenous proteins degraded in the endosome contributing peptides to the MIIC in which HLA DM mediated Clip removal allowed peptide binding. (2) Whether cleavage of endogenous, e.g., cytosolic proteins by the proteasome also yields class II binding peptides is at present unknown. (3)Internalization of membrane bound receptor proteins upon ligand binding induced ubiquitination with subsequent endosomal degradation. Cytosolic proteins associated with these receptors or with tyrosine kinase receptor like properties themselves might follow a similar pathway. (4) Recycling class II [19] and self-release of associated clip [20] may also facilitate peptide loading.

molecules requires physical Tap MHC interactions with the involvement of additional accessory molecule(s) [7,8]. Traditionally MHC molecules have been divided into so-called class I and II proteins. Two similar, yet not identical heterodimeric structures. class I molecules consist of a membrane glycoprotein heavy chain, that contains all peptide binding features [9,10], noncovalently associated with the light chain $\beta 2$ microglobulin. Class II molecules consist of two MHC encoded membrane glycoprotein chains α and β. The class II $\alpha\beta$ heterodimer assembles in the ER with a third chain, the invariant chain. [11]. The invariant chain serves to prohibit binding of (endogenous) peptide to class II molecules in the ER. It also functions as a targeting signal directing class II molecules to the endocytic route and may fulfil similar tasks for a subset of MHC class I molecules. [12].

Peptide ligands for MHC class II molecules are presumably generated in a special endocytic compartment, the so-called MHC class II compartment (MIIC) [13]. Proteolysis of the invariant chain followed by the removal of a class II associated invariant chain peptide (clip) from class II molecules by HLA DM molecules within the MIIC allows for peptide ligand binding [14–16]. Although ubiquitination may promote the endosomal degradation of cell membrane receptor proteins [17] evidence for a role for the proteasome in the generation of class II binding peptides has not been presented to date. However, when protein-coated latex beads are taken up by macrophages the subsequent generation of peptides presented within class I molecules appears to be proteasome-dependent [18]. Therefore, the precise way these different processing pathways intersect remains to be determined.

In spite of the still unresolved issues regarding protein processing by cells our present knowledge on how peptides derived from virtually all cellular proteins can be presented to the immune system by MHC molecules has led to a tremendous revival of tumor immunology. The key question that is addressed now is whether proteins which malignant cells synthesize in a qualitatively or even quantitatively different manner compared to nonmalignant cells may generate more or less tumor-specific peptides as potential targets for the immune system. In the case of melanoma such target molecules have already to some extent been unravelled, i.e., peptides derived from MAGE, melan A/MART-1, BAGE, GAGE [21] and a rare cyclin-dependent kinase mutant [22]. Viral oncoproteins like E6 and E7 of the human papilloma virus associated with cervical carcinoma are likely candidates [23–25]. In general, mutated proteins involved in tumorigenesis or oncoproteins originating from gene fusions are examples of attractive targets.

The polymorphic MHC molecules differ with respect to their ability to bind peptides. Peptide length and amino acid composition determine whether HLA alleles can accommodate peptides within their binding groove [26]. Sequencing of peptides eluted from different HLA alleles as well as peptide binding studies have revealed motifs in peptides showing HLA allele specificity [27]. This knowledge combined with insights in proteasomal cleavage preferences allows for a certain degree of epitope prediction within given oncoproteins. For instance an effort was recently made to map HLA class I binding motifs in the fusion regions of 44 fusion proteins involved in human cancers [28].

The specificity of T (or B) cell responses will depend on the uniqueness of the actual epitope which consists presumably of a combination of a few amino acids from the peptide sequence with a few amino acids from the MHC molecule [29].

Our group has studied primarily T cell responses to different peptides derived from proteins involved in oncogenesis both in mice and man. T cell responses, cytotoxic as well as helper, have been successfully generated in vivo and in vitro. Peptide vaccinations in vivo were shown in murine models to elicit protective immunity against tumors expressing viral oncoproteins [30,31]. Established tumors could be eradicated by adoptive transfer of peptide specific CTLs [32]. These encouraging results in animal models, have led to Phase I in vivo studies in women with endstage cervical carcinoma in which two HLA*0201-binding peptides encoded by HPV16E7 are currently tested as a potential cervical cancer vaccine (in collaboration with the Cytel Company, San Diego).

Depending on the mode of administration, peptides may instead of inducing an immune response lead to tolerance and hence to tumor outgrowth as we have recently observed in animal models [33,34]. Furthermore, subtle (i.e., single amino acid) changes in the composition of peptides may induce T cell anergy instead of activation [35–37].

Although we have obtained T cell responses to peptides corresponding to sequences in (mutated) p53 and ras proteins [38,39] we will confine ourselves in this overview to what appears to be a highly tumor-specific T cell target, namely peptides corresponding to fusion regions in the BCR-ABL hybrid oncoproteins in chronic myelogenous leukemia (CML) and acute lymphoblastic leukemia (ALL).

BCR-ABL peptide specific T cells

Fusion region sequences of the BCR-ABL$_{b3-a2}$ oncoprotein can induce BCR-ABL peptide specific T cells upon in vivo immunization in mice [40]. As we have shown, similar T cells can be generated by primary in vitro immunization with BCR-ABL peptides in human volunteers [41]. The fine specificity and HLA-DR2 restriction of such T cells were analyzed (Fig. 2 and Table 1).

Since this original publication we have been able to obtain several other BCR-ABL peptide specific T cell lines and clones not only directed to the b3-a2 but to the b2-a2 fusion as well. One of these BCR-ABL$_{b3-a2}$ peptide specific T cell lines showed a HLA-DR4 restriction and was induced to proliferate by DR4 and BCR-ABL$_{b3-a2}$ mRNA positive blasts from a CML patient in blast crisis [42]. No responses were observed with DR4 positive p210$^{BCR-ABL}$ negative cells or with p210^{b3-a2} positive leukemic cells with absent or insufficient expression of DR4. These data provided a first suggestion of potential processing of endogenous BCR-ABL protein by CML cells into MHC peptide ligands. More recently, we have also been able to elicit, via primary in vitro BCR-ABL, peptide immunization cytotoxic T cell clones, showing lysis of partially HLA matched BCR-ABL$_{b3-a2}$ transfected but not of nontransfected control fibroblasts (data not shown).

Other active agents

Immunological agents ideally constitute highly specific nontoxic interventions. Both antisense and ribozyme strategies also potentially have this virtue and therefore, are currently explored. Apart from ex vivo application of antisense for purging purposes, i.e., of autologous marrow in CML the in vivo use of these approaches in man is still hampered by pharmacodynamic problems.

Based on insights in growth regulation and transformation by oncoproteins in malignancy new promising compounds have recently been developed. A selective inhibitor of the ABL tyrosine kinase (CGP 57148) appears to induce specific killing

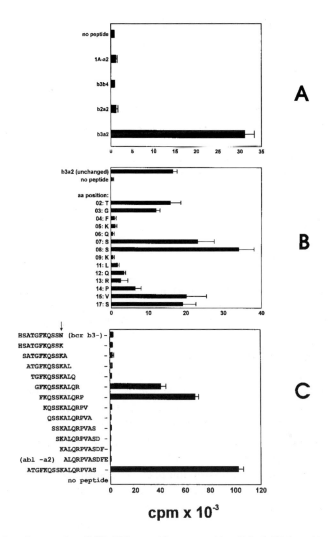

Fig. 2. Specificity of an against BCR-ABL $_{b3\text{-}a2}$ 17 mer peptide elicited CD4 positive T cell P1. **A**: Proliferation of P1 is only induced by the BCR-ABL b3-a2 peptide upon presentation by antigen presenting cells (APC), not by physiological 17 mer ABL 1A-a2 and BCR b3-b4 counterparts or a 17 mer BCR-ABL b2-a2 peptide. **B**: Replacement by alanine of eight individual amino acids (aa) within the BCR-ABL $_{b3\text{-}a2}$ peptide (F at position 4, K at 5, Q at 6, K at 9, L at 11, Q at 12 and R at position 13) led to a complete loss of reactivity of P1, substitution of P at 14 to a substantially reduced proliferation of P1. **C**: Reactivity of P1 with a panel of 11 mer peptides overlapping by 10 aa and together encompassing a 22 aa long b3-a2 joining region sequence (including the BCR b3 and ABL a2 sequence adjacent to the joining point of BCR and ABL). Only two of the peptides, containing all seven aa which could not be replaced by alanine (for recognition by P1) induced a response. Reproduced with permission from the publishers from [37].

of BCR-ABL-expressing cells and could provide a new therapeutic option in CML and other BCR-ABL positive leukemias [43]. Constitutive activation of JAK-2 kinase

Table 1. HLA DR restriction of BCR-ABL b3-a2 peptide specific T cell line P1.

APC	HLA DR type	Proliferation index
Autologous	$2^b,4^b$	11
Ko0403886	2^b	221
B10408389	$4^b,13$	2
G10405258	1,13	1
Be0408807	1,8	39
Ku6360502	$4^b,5$	28
V10407655	2^b	704
Te0406980	10,13	0
Ru0414215	7,13	3
K10402841	13	1
Br0405060	11,13	1
Ko0408109	13,52	2
Ve0403669	10,13	2
Aa0410314	3,13	2
Gee6719603[a]	$1,2^b$	0

Donor identification codes of HLA typed panel APC are given. DR2 represents DRB1*1501/DR-B5*0101. [a]Gee cells express the DRB5*0101 gene (DR2a) in association with the DR1 (DRB1*0101) gene instead of the DRB1*1501 gene (DR2b). [b]Indicates DR compatibility with P1. Responses of the T cell line to different APC loaded with b3a2 peptide are shown as proliferation indices. Reproduced with permission from the publishers from ten Bosch et al. [42].

in ALL can be inhibited by another specific tyrosine kinase blocker leading to leukemic cell apoptosis in vitro and in vivo without affecting normal hematopoiesis [44].

Even, more or less selective, ras inhibition has been accomplished [45,46]. Side effects of these cytostatic farnesyl transferase inhibitors, in view of the role of ras in T cell anergy perhaps immunosuppression [47], are conceivable and might limit their in vivo applicability in man. Effective doses of such an inhibitor, however, did not appear to elicit systemic toxicity in mice [46].

Concluding remarks

As it stands, we are closer than ever to specific immunotherapy in cancer. Trials based on vaccination with peptides, with protein loaded dendritic cells or yet other antigen delivery systems like viral vectors are in progress and all aim at somehow augmenting the autologous immune response.

Although some optimism seems justified, tumors will no doubt create obstacles on the road to immunotherapeutic success.

The generation of escape variants, e.g., by alternative splicing of oncoprotein mRNAs, interference with antigen processing, or down regulation of MHC expression are only a few of the many possible hurdles one can envisage.

Also, qualitative abnormalities in the host's immune system, i.e., in heterozygotes of genetic instability disorders like Ataxia Telangiectasia might compromise effective immunotherapy. The feasibility of specific antiviral adoptive immunotherapy post-bone marrow transplantation has been demonstrated and refinements of present day donor buffycoat therapies in post-BMT relapses in disorders like CML appear within reach.

New cytotoxic or cytostatic drugs with tumor selectivity based on specific oncoprotein function inhibition are anticipated and may prove to be a simple, more generally applicable, alternative to immunotherapy, although such therapies will not have the memory or presumably the degree of specificity of, e.g., cytotoxic T lymphocytes.

Acknowledgements

Supported by the Dutch Cancer Society.

References

1. Rock KL, Gramm C, Rothstein L, Clark K, Stein R, Dick L, Hwang D, Goldberg AL. Inhibitors of the proteasome block the degradation of most cell proteins and the generation of peptides presented on MHC class I molecules. Cell 1994;78:761–771.
2. Michalek MT, Grant EP, Gramm C, Goldberg AL, Rock KL. A role for the ubiquitin-dependent proteolytic pathway in MHC class I-restricted antigen presentation. Nature 1993;363:552–554.
3. Seufert W, Futcher B, Jeutsch S. Role of a ubiquitin-conjugating enzyme in degradation of S-and M-phase cyclins. Nature 1995;373:78–81.
4. Spies T, Cerundolo V, Colonna M, Cresswell P, Townsend A, De Mars R. Presentation of viral antigen by MHC class I molecules is dependent on a putative peptide transporter heterodimer. Nature 1992;355:644–646.
5. Kelly A, Powis SH, Kerr LA, Mockridge I, Elliott T, Nastin J, Uchauska-Ziegler B, Ziegler A, Trowsdale J, Townsend A. Assembly and function of the two ABC transporter proteins encoded in human major histocompatibility complex. Nature 1992;355:641–644.
6. Hammond SA, Bollinger RC, Tobery TW, Siliciano RF. Transporter independent processing of HIV-I envelope protein for recognition by CD8[+] T cells. Nature 1993;364:158–160.
7. Ortmann B, Androlewicz MJ, Creswell P. MHC class I/β-microglobulin complexes associate with TAP transporters before peptide binding. Nature 1994;368:864–867.
8. Grandea AG, Androlewicz MJ, Athwal RS, Geraghty DE, Spies T. Dependence of peptide binding by MHC class I molecules on their interaction with TAP. Science 1995;270:105–108.
9. Bjorkman PJ, Saper MA, Samraoui B, Bennett WS, Strominger JL, Wiley DC. Structure of human class I histocompatibility antigen HLA-A2. Nature 1987;329:506–512.
10. Townsend A, Ohlen C, Bastin J, Ljunggren HG, Foster L, Kärre K. Association of class I major histocompatibility heavy and light chains induced by viral peptides. Nature 1989;340:443–448.
11. Ghosh P, Amaya M, Mellins E, Wiley DC. The structure of an intermediate in class II MHC maturation: CLIP bound to HLA-DR3. Nature 1996;378:457–462.
12. Sugita M, Brenner MB. Association of the invariant chain with major histocompatibility complex class I molecules directs trafficking to endocytic compartments. J Biol Chem 1995;270:1443–1448.
13. Peters PJ, Neefjes JJ, Oorschot V, Ploegh HL, Geuze HJ. Segregation of MHC class II molecules from MHC class I molecules in the Golgi complex for transport to lysosomal compartments. Nature 1991;349:669–675.
14. Moris P, Shaman J, Attaya M, Goodman S, Bergman C, Monaco JJ, Mellins E. An essential role for HLA-DM in antigen presentation by class II major histocompatibility molecules. Nature 1994;368:551–554.
15. Fling SP, Arp B, Pious D. HLA-DMA and-DMB genes are both required for MHC class II/peptide

complex formation in antigen-presenting cells. Nature 1994;368:554—558.

16. Sloan VS, Cameron P, Porter G, Gammon M, Amaya M, Mellins E, Zaller DM. Mediation by HLA-DM of dissociation of peptides from HLA-DR. Nature 1995;375:802—806.

17. Hicke L, Riezman H. Ubiquitination of a yeast plasma membrane receptor signals its ligand-stimulated endocytosis. Cell 1996;84:277—287.

18. Rock KL. A new foreign policy: MHC class I molecules monitor the outside world. Immunol Today 1996;17:131—137.

19. Pinet V, Vergelli M, Martin R, Bakke O, Long EO. Antigen presentation mediated by recycling of surface HLA-DR molecules. Nature 1995;375:603—606.

20. Kropshofer H, Vogt AB, Stern LJ, Hämmerling GJ. Self release of Cip in peptide loading of HLA-DR molecules. Science 1995;270:1357—1359.

21. Van Pel A, Van der Bruggen P, Coulie PG, Brichard VG, Lethé B, Van den Eynde B, Uyttenhove C, Renauld JC, Boon T. Genes coding for tumor antigens recognized by cytolytic T lymphocytes. Immunol Rev 1995;145:229—250.

22. Wölfel T, Hauer M, Schneider J, Serrano M, Wölfel C, Klehman-Hieb E, De Plaen E, Hankeln T, Meyer zum Büschenfelde K-H, Beach D. A p16 [INK 4a] — insensitive CDK4 mutant targeted by cytolytic T lymphocytes in a human melanoma. Science 1995;269:1281—1284.

23. Kast WM, Brandt RMP, Sidney J, Drijfhout JW, Kubo RT, Grey HM, Melief CJM, Sette A. The role of HLA-A motifs in identification of potential CTL epitopes in human papillomavirus type E6 and E7 proteins. J Immunol 1994;152:3904—3912.

24. Ressing ME, Sette A, Brandt RMP, Ruppert J, Wenthworth PA, Hartman M, Oseroff C, Grey HM, Melief CJM, Kast WM. Human CTL epitopes encoded by human papillomavirus type E6 and E7 identified through in vivo and in vitro immunogenicity studies of HLA-A*0201-binding peptides. J Immunol 1995;154:5934—5943.

25. Ressing ME, Van Driel WJ, Celis E, Sette A, Brandt RMP, Hartman M, Anholts JDH, Schreuder GMT, ter Harmsel WB, Fleuren GJ, Trimbos BJ, Kast WM, Melief CJM. Occasional memory cytotoxic T cell responses of patients with human papillomavirus type 16-positive cervical lesions against HLA-A*0201-restricted E7-encoded epitope. Cancer Res 1996;56:1—7.

26. Schumacher TNM, De Bruijn M, Vernie LN, Kast WM, Melief CJM, Neefjes JJ, Ploegh HL. Peptide selection by MHC class I molecules. Nature 1991;350:703—706.

27. Rammensee HG, Friede H, Stevanovic S. MHC ligands and peptide motifs; first listing. Immunogenetics 1995;41:178—228.

28. Gambacorti Passerini C, Bertazzoli C, Dermime S, Stefanovic S, Appella E, Parmiani G. Mapping HLA class I binding motifs in forty four fusion proteins involved in human cancers. Blood (In press).

29. Fu XT, Bono CP, Woulfe SL, Swearingen C, Summers NL, Sinigaglia F, Sette A, Schwartz BD, Karr RW. Pocket of the HLA-DR (α,β1*0401) molecule is a major determinant of T cell recognition of peptide. J Exp Med 1995;181:915 926.

30. Feltkamp M, Vreugdenhil GR, Vierboom MPM, Ras L, Van der Burg SH, ter Scheffer J, Melief CJM, Kast WM. Cytotoxic T lymphocytes raised against a subdominant epitope offered as a synthetic peptide eradicate human papilloma virus type 16-induced tumors. Eur J Immunol 1995;25:2638—2642.

31. Feltkamp MCW, Smits HL, Vierboom MPM, Minnaar RP, de Jong BM, Drijfhout JW, Ter Schegget J, Melief CJM, Kast WM. Vaccination with a cytotoxic T lymphocyte epitope containing peptide protects against tumor induced by human papilloma virus type 16 transformed cells. Eur J Immunol 1993;23:2242—2249.

32. Kast WM, Offringa R, Peters PJ, Voordouw AC, Meloen RH, Van der Eb AJ, Melief CJM. Eradication of adenovirus E1-induced tumors by E1A-specific cytotoxic T lymphocytes. Cell 1989;59:603—614.

33. Toes REM, Offringa R, Blom JJ, Melief CJM, Kast WM. Functional deletion of tumor specific cytotoxic T lymphocytes induced by peptide vaccination can lead to the inability to reject tumors. J Immunol (In press).

34. Toes REM, Offringa R, Blom RJJ, Melief CJM, Kast WM. Peptide vaccination can lead to enhanced

tumor growth through specific T cell tolerance induction. PNAS (In press).

35. Sloan-Lancaster J, Evavold BD, Allen PM. Induction of T cell anergy by altered T cell-receptor ligand on live antigen presenting cells. Nature 1993;363:156—159.

36. Sloan-Lancaster J, Shaw AS, Rothbard JB, Allen PM. Partial T cell signaling: altered phopho-ς and lack of zap 70 recruitment in APL-induced T cell anergy. Cell 1994;79:913—922.

37. Höllsberg P, Weber WEJ, Dangond F, Batra V, Sette A, Hafler DA. Differential activation of proliferation and cytotoxicity in human T-cell lymphotropic virus type I Tax-specific CD8 T cells by an altered peptide ligand. PNAS 1995;92:4036—4040.

38. Houbiers JGA, Nijman HW, Van der Burg SH, Vierboom MPM, Kenemans P, Kast WM, Melief CJM. In vitro induction of human cytotoxic T lymphocyte responses against peptides of mutant and wild type p53. Eur J Immunol 1993;23:2072—2077.

39. Van Elsas A, Nijman HW, Van der Minne CE, Mourer JS, Kast WM, Melief CJM, Schrier PI. Induction and characterization of cytotoxic T lymphocytes recognizing a mutated p21 ras peptide presented by HLA-A* 0201. Int J Cancer 1995;61:389—396.

40. Chen W, Peace DJ, Rovira DK, You SG, Cheever MA. T cell immunity to the joining region of p210 $_{BCR-ABL}$ protein. PNAS 1992;89:1468—1472.

41. Ten Bosch GJA, Toornvliet AC, Friede T, Melief CJM, Leeksma OC.Recognition of peptides corresponding to the joining region of p210 $^{BCR-ABL}$ protein by human T cells. Leukemia 1995;9: 1344—1348.

42. Ten Bosch GJA, Joosten AM, Melief CJM, Leeksma OC. Specific recognition of CML blasts by BCR-ABL breakpoint peptide specific human T cells. Blood 1995;86:619a.

43. Druker BJ, Tumura S, Buchdinger E, Ohno S, Bagby GC, Lydon NB. Preclinical evaluation of a selective inhibitor of the abl tyrosine kinase as a therapeutic agent for chronic myelogenous leukemia. Blood 1995;86:2392a.

44. Meydam N, Grunberger T, Dadi H, Shahar M, Arpala E, Lapidot Z, Leeder JS, Freedman M, Cohen A, Gazit A, Levitzki A, Roifman CM. Inhibition of acute lymphoblastic leukaemia by a Jak-2 inhibitor. Nature 1996;379:645—648.

45. Gibbs JR, Oliff A, Kohl NE. Farnesyltransferase inhibitors: ras research yields a potential cancer therapeutic. Cell 1994;77:175—178.

46. Kohl NE, Omer CA, Conner MW, Anthony NJ, Davide JP, Jane de Solms S, Giuliani EA, Gomez RP, Graham SL, Hamilton K, Handt LK, Hartman GD, Koblan KS, Kral AM, Miller PJ, Mosser SD, O'Neill TJ, Rainds E, Schaber MD, Gibbs JB, Oliff A. Inhibition of farnesyltransferase induces regression of mammary and salivary carcinomas in Ras transgenic mice. Nature Med 1995;1: 792—797.

47. Fields PE, Gajewski TF, Fitch FW. Blocked ras activation in anergic CD4[+] T cells. Science 1996; 271:1276—1277.

Chemoprevention of mammary cancer: a selected model

Carcinogenesis, endocrine risk factors and natural history of breast cancer

Jan G.M. Klijn[1], Leon C. Verhoog[1], Cécile Brekelmans[1], Caroline Seynaeve[1], Peter Devilee*, Sonja C. Henzen° and Hanne J. Meijers-Heijboer[+] on behalf of the Rotterdam Committee for Genetic and Medical Counselling

[1]*Departments of Medical Oncology and °Pathology, Rotterdam Cancer Institute (Dr Daniel den Hoed Kliniek); [+]Department of Clinical Genetics, Erasmus University, Rotterdam; and *Department of Human Genetics, University of Leiden, The Netherlands*

Abstract. The incidence of breast cancer has doubled since 1940, but age-adjusted mortality rates remained remarkably stable, probably due to detection of tumors at an earlier stage, improvements in therapy and very recently, population-based screening. The prognosis is associated with tumor stage and a large series of cell biological characteristics. Multiple hereditary and acquired genetic alterations are involved in the development and progress of breast cancer but the exact etiology is still unclear. Presently known risk factors concern demographic, endocrine, hereditary and exogenic factors, such as carcinogens with or without estrogenic properties. In Rotterdam, we have registered more than 250 families with familial breast cancer, 20 of them with proven gene mutation. Most striking in these families is the occurrence of breast cancer at an earlier age in the youngest generation and a step-wise increase in mortality during this century which might be related to differences regarding reproductive factors, lifestyle, and exogenic factors during the last decades as compared with those in the beginning of this century. Interaction between genetic and environmental factors might be very important. An increasing number of women at risk opt for regular control and sometimes for preventive measures. Apart from surgical prevention, different options for chemoprevention are available, but prevention of death by cancer cannot be guaranteed.

Key words: breast cancer, counselling, etiology, prevention, risks, surveillance.

Overview

Incidence and prognosis of breast cancer

Breast cancer is a major public health problem of great interest and importance to physicians in a variety of specialties. The incidence of the disease has increased dramatically with a doubling since 1940, while the age-adjusted mortality rates remained remarkably stable [1]. This nonparallelism may be caused, on one hand, by diagnosis of breast cancer at an earlier stage with time — especially during the last 2 decades — and on the other hand by improved treatment results. Contributing to these

Address for correspondence: J.G.M. Klijn, Department Medical Oncology, Rotterdam Cancer Institute (DDHK), Groene Hilledijk 301, 3075 EA Rotterdam, The Netherlands. Tel.: +31-10-4391733. Fax: +31-10-4851618.

results, may have been the introduction of both adjuvant systemic therapy and new treatment modalities for primary, locally advanced and metastatic disease.

Breast cancer is the most common malignant tumor among women with an estimated 135,000 new cases and 58,000 recorded deaths per year in the European Community [2]. Presently, about 1,000 new cases per million women are registered each year in the Western world affecting 8–12% of all women during life. The disease is even the leading cause of death among all women who are 40–55 years of age [1]. Of all cancers in women 32% concern breast cancer.

At time of diagnosis manifest distant metastases are present in 5% and occult micrometastases in 50% of the patients. Regional deposits of the primary tumor in axillary lymph nodes are generally found in 40–50% of the cases at histologic examination. Ultimately, 40% of patients with node-negative disease and 70% of patients with node-positive disease will die due to macrometastasis within 10–15 years after diagnosis of primary disease. The median survival of patients with macrometastases is 2 years and nearly all will die of breast cancer. The disease-free survival, postrelapse survival, overall survival and type of response to therapy are associated with a series of cell biological prognostic and predictive factors [3,4].

Etiology and risk factors for breast cancer

Multiple hereditary and acquired genetic alterations are involved in the development and progress of breast cancer, but the exact etiology is still unclear. The elucidation of specific risk factors for breast cancer is important to understand the observed variation among and within countries, to identify women who could benefit from intensified surveillance or prophylactic treatment, to select subjects for participation in intervention studies, and to modify factors that will ultimately reduce risk. Several risk factors have been recognized such as demographic, endocrine, hereditary and exogenic factors [1,5,6]. Endocrine risk factors are summarized in Table 1. Exogenic risk factors are carcinogens, without or with estrogenic properties [7,8], radiation, dietary factors, possibly viral infections, etc. Most risk factors are relatively weak, i.e., between 1.1 and 2.0. A major risk factor, however, is a family history of breast cancer. Relative risks of 2–10 have been observed in first degree relatives depending

Table 1. Endocrine risk factors for breast cancer.

Type of risk factor	Relative risk
— early age of menarche (11 vs. 16 years)	1.3
— late age of menopause (>55 years)	1.5
— age at birth of first child (≥25–30 vs. <20 years)	1.6–1.9
— long-term breast feeding	↓
— early oophorectomy (<35–45 years)	0.4–0.7
— oral contraceptive (from young age)	1.5–2.0
— hormonal replacement therapy (HRT)	1.2–2.1
— use of DES by mother	1.4
— obesity (>50 years): total aromatase activity?	1.2

on the age and presence of bilateral cancer of the index patient [1,9–13]. Risk assessment can be performed with the help of genetic epidemiological tables, indicating absolute lifetime risks up to nearly 50% [13] or by DNA-analysis, indicating absolute lifetime risks up to 90% [14,15]. Hereditary factors are involved in about 5% of all cases when strict criteria are used, but might appear to be about 25% after future detection of gene mutations with lower penetrance.

Familial predisposition and breast cancer susceptibility genes

Genetic syndromes

Breast cancer patients in a family with hereditary breast cancer will generally show a significantly earlier age of onset and excess of bilaterality and multiple primary cancers; multiple generations are affected and transmission may be either paternal or maternal [16–18]. Another indicator for inherited breast cancer is a high frequency of other cancers in first and second degree relatives. Family studies suggest an autosomal dominant genetic model.

Breast cancer may be part of several inherited cancer syndromes. Most frequently familial clustering of predominantly breast cancer is seen, i.e., site-specific hereditary breast cancer (HBC). It also occurs in combination with ovarian cancer in about 20% of the families, called hereditary breast/ovarian cancer (HBOC). Less common autosomal dominant syndromes, all characterized by a specific combination of multiple types of malignancy including breast cancer, are Lynch type II syndrome, Li-Fraumeni syndrome, Cowden syndrome and Torre-Muir syndrome. The risk for breast cancer is also increased (relative risk of about 4) in heterozygous carriers of the ataxia-telangiectasia gene [19].

Breast cancer susceptibility genes

The first breast cancer susceptibility gene (BRCA-1) was localized by genetic linkage analysis on 17q21 in 1990 [20] and identified in 1994 [21]. Presently more than 100 distinct mutations in BRCA-1 have been described (Goldgar, this book). Mutations within BRCA-1 are associated with very high lifetime risks of breast and ovarian cancer (Table 2) due to high penetrance. Also an increased risk for colorectal (4.1) and prostate cancer (3.3) has been reported [15]. The gene frequency of BRCA-1 has been estimated to occur in 1 of 833 women [22,23], implying that 1.7% of all breast cancer patients disposed between the age of 20 and 70 years are carriers of such a mutation. This proportion increased to 7.5% in breast cancer patients younger than

Table 2. Estimated overall risks for BRCA-1 gene mutation carriers (in summary).

— Primary breast cancer	relative risk 10–200× dependent on age
	lifetime risk 85%
— Contralateral breast cancer	lifetime risk 64%
— Ovarian cancer	lifetime risk 63%
— Prostate cancer	relative risk 3.3× increased
— Colon cancer	relative risk 4.1× increased

30 years. Specific mutations have been found within certain populations such as the Jewish [24] and Dutch [25] population.

In 1994 the second breast cancer gene (BRCA-2) was mapped on chromosome 13q [26] and identified scarcely more than 1 year later [27,28]. Also mutations in this gene are associated with a high lifetime risk of breast cancer (85%) but with a lower risk of ovarian cancer (±20%). Strikingly, BRCA-2 mutations are associated with a relatively high risk of male breast cancer (100×), but the cumulative risk for men remains low (6%) in comparison with the absolute cumulative risk in women. This implies that the gene will remain nonpenetrant in most males, and that many families due to BRCA-2 will appear clinically with female breast cancer cases only.

Germline mutations in TP53, detected in about half of the families with the Li-Fraumeni syndrome, are very rare. Heterozygous mutations in the AT gene are expected to be present in 2–7% of all breast cancer cases, but they confer only moderately increased risk for the disease [22]. Approximately 5% of all breast cancer cases are estimated to be caused by highly penetrant gene alterations. Possibly, mutations in unknown genes with low penetrance are hereditary in families with less dramatic pedigrees, but with a higher frequency than BRCA-1 and -2 mutations. Therefore, it cannot be excluded that hereditary factors may play a role in the development of 15–25% of breast cancers. Indeed, up to 36% of cases diagnosed under the age of 30 years are expected to be genetic [12].

Surveillance and preventive therapy

The actual possibilities for molecular diagnosis and presymptomatic DNA-testing necessitate a multidisciplinary approach including extensive family studies, genetic counselling, molecular genetic studies on interfamilial heterogeneity, medical counselling regarding lifestyle, screening, development of preventive oncological strategies and psychological support during and after test and treatment periods. Such a comprehensive approach is required since a new field of medical intervention is now entered (Table 3).

Overall, screening reduces mortality from breast cancer by about 25–40% in women between the ages of 50–70 years, but there is no consensus with respect to younger women [1]. There is a lot of debate about the value of screening in premenopausal women in view of the lower incidence in this age group, lower sensitivity of mammography and a higher proliferation rate of tumors in young patients. However, one of the greatest potential benefits of genetic screening for breast cancer susceptibility may be the identification of younger women who may benefit from mammographic surveillance starting at an earlier age and done more frequently. The effectiveness of screening in this particular population is not yet known. The results of two small retrospective studies [29,30] suggest that mammographic screening (1× per year) in combination with regular physical examinations (once every 6 months) may lead to the detection of a greater proportion of smaller tumors and node-negative breast cancer.

Women with a high risk of breast cancer are increasingly seeking counselling

Table 3. Prevention of (death by) breast cancer.

I.	Avoidances of other risks for breast cancer
	Advices regarding lifestyle
II.	Early diagnosis
	— mammographic screening
	— regular physical examination
III.	Prevention measures (primary or secondary)
	1. Complete mastectomy
	2. Diet
	3. Chemoprevention
	a. tamoxifen
	b. retinoids
	c. for the future: synthetic BRAC1 and 2 gene proteins
IV.	Combination of measures (registration and follow-up)

N.B. Check on development of other tumor types, if applicable

about prophylactic mastectomy or other preventive measures. Women who receive subcutaneous mastectomy still have a risk of developing breast cancer since this procedure does not remove all cells at risk [17,31]. Until now, no evidence has existed that women remain at risk after prophylactic adequate total mastectomy. Women with an increased risk of breast cancer may also participate in the Tamoxifen Prevention Trial, if they do not opt for prophylactic surgery, but definite prevention can certainly not be guaranteed and the side effects of long-term treatment with tamoxifen are still a matter of debate [32–34]. A series of new endocrine agents are in development (such as LHRH analogues, antiprogestins, aromatase-inhibitors and vitamins) which potentially can be used in future prevention studies [35,36]. Future preventive strategies especially, may include retinoids or administration of synthetic peptides for which breast cancer suppressor genes encode (Table 3).

The Rotterdam and Dutch experience

In order to adequately comply with the increasing requests for professional advice, in 1990 we established a multidisciplinary Committee for Genetic and Medical Counselling and a family cancer clinic in Rotterdam, in close cooperation with laboratory researchers from Leiden (P. Devilee, C. Cornelisse). The present composition of this committee is indicated in Table 4. Within 5 years more than 250 families were registered (Fig. 1), most of them with HBC or HBOC. There was a striking peak of family accrual in 1994/1995 due to the extensive publicity in both the scientific and lay press regarding the detection and identification of the breast cancer genes BRCA-1 and BRCA-2.

Based on our first experience 75% of the family members are interested in a (presymptomatic) DNA-test, 15% are willing to participate in linkage studies but not immediately interested in their own personal test result (mainly men without children), while 10% refused DNA-testing. The first Dutch family with proven

Table 4. Committee for Genetic and Medical Counselling (chairman: Dr J.G.M. Klijn).

I. Clinical Departments
Familial Cancer Clinic/Medical Oncology/DDHK
    Dr J.G.M. Klijn, Dr C. Seynaeve, Drs L.C. Verhoog
Radiology/DDHK
    Drs C.C.M. Bartels, Drs M.M.A. Tilanus-Linthorst
Surgery/DDHK
    Dr A.N. Geel
Gynaecology/DDHK
    Drs A. Logmans
Clinical Genetics/EUR
    Drs E.J. Meijers-Heijboer, Prof Dr M.F. Niermeijer
Medical Psychology/EUR
    Dr P.G. Frets, Dr A. Tibben, Drs C. Dudok-de Wit

II. Laboratory Diagnostics
Pathology/Human Genetics/AZL
    Prof Dr C.J. Cornelisse, Dr. P Devilee
Clinical Genetics/EUR
    Dr D.J.J. Halley, Dr ir. A.M.W. v.d. Ouweland
Cell biology & Genetics/EUR
    Prof Dr A. Hagemeijer, Dr A. de Klein
Tumorendocrinology/DDHK
    Dr P.M.J.J. Berns, Dr J.A. Foekens
Pathology/DDHK
    Dr S.C. Henzen-Logmans

III. Epidemiology
Dr J.W.W. Coebergh/EUR, Dr C. Brekelmans/DDHK

BRCA-1 mutation was detected in 1994 [37,38]. Presently, in Rotterdam, 20 families and about 50 families in The Netherlands, have been found with a proven BRCA-1 or BRCA-2 mutation. Most markedly is the frequent finding of the 2803delAA mutation, which has never been reported elsewhere. The distribution of "Dutch" BRCA-1 mutations is thus quite distinct from the one derived from Northern American families, and might be typical for the Netherlands or Northern German Lowlands [25,39,40].

Most striking in our families is the occurrence of breast cancer at an earlier age in the youngest generation [41] and a step-wise increase in mortality during this century [42], which might be related to differences regarding reproductive factors, lifestyle and exogenic factors during the last decades as compared with those in the beginning of the century. Interaction between genetic and environmental factors might, therefore, be very important.

An increasing number of women from these families requests for advice, regular screening and physical examinations. Although the median follow-up is yet short (1–1.5 years), already eight breast cancers have been detected. Because screening cannot guarantee prevention of death by breast cancer, an increasing number of young

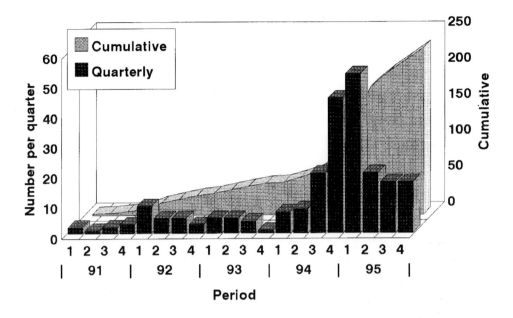

Fig. 1. Accrual Family Cancer Clinic Rotterdam (Dr Daniel den Hoed Kliniek/EUR).

women especially, opt for prophylactic bilateral mastectomy, mostly in combination with breast reconstruction. In case of HBOC, prophylactic oophorectomy is also frequently carried out, especially in the case of a proven gene mutation. In a number of 22 mastectomy specimens, a high frequency of fibrocystic changes and proliferative breast disease were observed [43], such as: florid (46%) and atypical (14%) hyperplasia, sclerosing adenosis (36%), adenosis in general (82%), fibroadenomas (23%), papillomatosis (14%) and microcalcifications (41%). Also, one invasive breast cancer (4%) with a diameter of 0.7 cm was found, not detected by physical examination and mammography before surgery. Also, in 28 pairs of ovaries prophylactically removed between 1993–1996, major histologic changes (1× multifocal ovarian endometroid adenocarcinoma, 1× mucinous cystadenoma, 1× a bilateral benign Brenner tumor, and 1× breast cancer metastasis) were found in 15% and minor changes in the majority of ovaries studied, which changes might be possibly signs of (early) premalignant lesions [44]. Thus, primary extraovarian peritoneal carcinoma has been diagnosed in one BRCA-1 gene mutation carrier 16 months after prophylactic oophorectomy.

Conclusions

1. Until recently, familial breast cancer was an underestimated problem, especially by physicians.
2. Several hereditary disorders and gene mutations are associated with an increased risk of breast cancer.

3. The majority of relatives in a family with hereditary breast cancer want to participate in (presymptomatic) DNA-testing.

4. Hereditary breast cancer warrants a multidisciplinary approach regarding genetic and medical counselling, early diagnosis, prevention and treatment.

5. Interactions between hereditary, reproductive and environmental factors may result in early onset of breast cancer and in a possible anticipation phenomenon.

6. At present, chemoprevention is less safe than surgical prevention of breast cancer.

7. Primary peritoneal carcinomas can occur after prophylactic oophorectomy ($\pm 2\%$ within 1—27 years of follow-up) [45].

Acknowledgements

First of all we would like to thank all members of our working group for hereditary tumors, Petra Bos for typing the manuscript, and the Dutch Cancer Society for financial support (grant DDHK 95-953).

References

1. Harris JR, Lippman ME, Veronesi U. Breast cancer (three parts). N Engl J Med 1992;327:319—328 (Part one), 390—398 (Part two), 473—480 (Part three).

2. Möller Jensen O, Estève J, Möller H, Renard H. Cancer in the European Community and its member status. Eur J Cancer 1990;26:1167—1256.

3. Klijn JGM, Berns PMJJ, Foekens JA. Prognostic factors and response to therapy in breast cancer. Cancer Surv 1993;18:165—198.

4. Klijn JGM, Berns PMJJ, Dorssers LCJ, Foekens JA. Molecular markers of resistance to endocrine treatment of breast cancer. In: Dickson RB, Lippman ME (eds) Drug and Hormonal Resistance in Breast Cancer: Cellular and Molecular Mechanisms. Chichester: Ellis Horwood, 1995;133—169.

5. Evans DGR, Fentiman IS, McPherson K, Asbury D, Ponder BAJ, Howel A. Familial breast cancer. Br Med J 1994;308:183—187.

6. Henderson IC. What can a woman do about her risk of dying of breast cancer. Curr Prob Cancer 1990;14(Suppl 4):165—230.

7. White R, Jolling S, Hoare SA, Sumpter JP, Parker MG. Environmentally persistant alkylphenolic compounds are estrogenic. Endocrinology 1994;135:175—182.

8. Krieger N, Wolff MS, Hiatt RA, Rivera M, Vogelman J, Orentreich N. Breast cancer and serum organochlorines: a prospective study among white, black and asian women. J Natl Cancer Inst 1994; 86:589—599.

9. Tulinius H, Sigvaldason H, Olofsdottir G, Tryggvadottir L. Epidemiology of breast cancer in families in Iceland. J Med Genet 1992;29:158—164.

10. Houlston RS, McCarter E, Parbhoo S, Scurr JH, Slack J. Family history and risk of breast cancer. J Med Genet 1992;29:154—157.

11. Houlston RS, Lemoine L, McCarter E, Harrington S, MacDermot K, Hinton J, Berger L, Slack J. Screening and genetic counselling for relatives of patients with breast cancer in a family cancer clinic. J Med Genet 1992;29:691—694.

12. Claus EB, Risch N, Thompson WD. Genetic analysis of breast cancer in the Cancer an Steroid Hormone Study. Am J Hum Genet 1991;48:232—242.

13. Claus EB, Risch N, and Thompson WD. Autosomal dominant inheritance of early onset breast cancer. Cancer 1994;73:643—651.

14. Easton DF, Bishop DT, Ford D, Crockford GP and The Breast Cancer Linkage Consortium. Genetic linkage analysis in familial breast and ovarian cancer: results from 214 families. Am J Hum Genet

1993;52:678–701.

15. Ford D, Easton DF, Bishop DT, Narod S, Goldgar DE and The Breast Cancer Linkage Consortium. Risks of cancer in BRCA1 mutation carriers. Lancet 1994;343:692–695.

16. Lynch HT, Harris RE, Guirgis HA, Maloney K, Carmody LL, Lynch JF. Familial association of breast/ovarian carcinoma. Cancer 1978;41:1543–1549.

17. King MC, Rowell S, Love SM. Inherited breast and ovarian cancer. What are the risks? What are the choices? JAMA 1993;269:1975–1980.

18. Offit K, Brown K. Quantitating familial cancer risk: a resource for clinical oncologists. J Clin Oncol 1994;12:1724–1736.

19. Swift M, Morrell D, Massey RB, Chase C. Incidence of cancer in 161 families affected by ataxia-telangiectasia. N Engl J Med 1991;325:1831–1836.

20. Hall JM, Lee MK, Morrow J, Newman B, Anderson L, Huey B, King MC. Linkage of early onset familial breast cancer to chromosome 17q21. Science 1990;250:1684–1689.

21. Miki Y, Swenson J, Shattuck-Eidens D, Futreal P, Harshman K, Tavtigian S, Liu Q, Cochran C, Bennett L, Ding W, Bell R, Rosenthal J, Hussey C, Tran T, McClure M, Frye C, Hattier T, Phelps R, Haugen-Strano A, Katcher H, Yakumo K, Gholami Z, Shaffer D, Stone S, Bayer S, Wray C, Bogden R, Dayananth P, Ward J, Tonin P, Narod S, Bristow P, Norris F, Helvering L, Morrison P, Rosteck P, Lai M, Barrett J, Lewis C, Neuhausen S, Cannon-Albright L, Goldgar R, Kamb A, Wiseman R, Skolnick M. A Strong candidate for the breast and ovarian cancer susceptibility gene BRCA1. Science 1994;266:66–71.

22. Ford D, Easton D. The genetics of breast cancer and ovarian cancer. Br J Cancer 1995;72:805–812.

23. Ford D, Easton D, Peto J. Estimates of the gene frequency of BRCA1 and its contribution to breast and ovarian cancer incidence. Am J Hum Genet 1995;57:1457–1462.

24. FitzGerald MG, MacDonald DJ, Krainer M, Hoover I, O'Neil E, Unsal H, Silva-Arrieto S, Finkelstein DM, Beer-Romero P, Englert C, Sgroi DC, Smith BL, Younger JW, Garber JE, Duda RB, Mayzel KA, Isselbacher KJ, Friend SH, Haber DA. Germ-line *BRCA1* mutations in Jewish and non-Jewish women with early onset breast cancer. N Engl J Med 1996;334:143–149.

25. Peelen T, Cornelis RS, van Vliet M, Petrij-Bosch A, Cleton-Jansen A, Meijers-Heijboer A-M, Meijers-Heijboer H, Klijn JGM, Vasen HFA, Cornelisse CJ, Devilee P. Genetic heterogeneity among 22 dutch high-risk breast cancer families; no evidence for a third susceptibility locus. Eur J Hum Genet (In press).

26. Wooster R, Neuhausen S, Mangion J, Quirk Y, Ford D, Collins N, Nguyen K, Seal S, Tran T, Averill D, Fields D, Marshall G, Narod S, Lenoir G, Lynch H, Feunteun J, Devilee P, Cornelisse C, Menko F, Daly P, Ormiston W, McManus R, Pye C, Lewis C, Cannon-Albright L, Peto J, Ponder B, Skolnick M, Easton D, Goldgar D, Stratton M. Localization of a breast cancer susceptibility gene BRCA2 to chromosome 13q12. Science 1994;265:2088–2090.

27. Wooster R, Bignell G, Lancaster J, Swift S, Seal S, Mangion J, Collins N, Gregory S, Gumbs C, Micklem G, Barfoot R, Hamoudi R, Patel S, Rice C, Biggs P, Hashim Y, Smith A, Connor F, Arason A, Gudmundsson J, Ficenec D, Kelsell D, Ford D, Tonin P, Bishop DT, Spurr NK, Ponder BAJ, Eeles R, Peto J, Devilee P, Cornelisse CJ, Lynch H, Narod S, Lenoir G, Egillson V, Barkardottir RB, Easton DF, Bentley DR, Futreal PA, Ashworth A, Stratton MR. Identification of the breast cancer susceptibility gene BRCA2. Nature 1995;378:789–792.

28. Tavtigan SV, Simard J, Rommens J, Couch F, Shattuck-Eidens D, Neuhausen S, Merajver S, Thorlacius S, Offit K, Stoppa-Lyonnet D, Belanger C, Bell R, Berry S, Bogden R, Chen Q, Davis T, Dumont M, Frye C, Hattier T, Jammulapati S, Janecki T, Jiang P, Kehrer R, Leblanc J-F, Mitchell JT, MacArthur-Morrison J, Nguyen K, Peng Y, Samson C, Schroeder M, Snyder SC, Steele L, Stringfellow M, Stroup C, Swedlund B, Swensen J, Teng D, Thomas A, Tran T, Tranchant M, Weaver-Feldhaus J, Wong AKC, Shizuya H, Eyfjord JE, Cannon-Albright L, Labrie F, Skolnick MH, Weber B, Kamb A, Goldgar DE. The complete BRCA2 gene and mutations in chromosome 13q-linked kindreds. Nature Genet 1996;12:333–337.

29. Vasen HFA, Beex LVAM, Cleton FJ, Collette HJA, Dongen JA van, Leeuwen FE van, Crommelin MA, Meera Khan P. Clinical heterogeneity of hereditary breast cancer and its impact on screening

protocols: the Dutch experience on 24 families under surveillance. Eur J Cancer 1993;29A: 1111–1114.

30. Tilanus-Linthorst MMA, Bartels CCM, Obdeijn AIM, Kuenen-Boumeester V, Klijn JGM, Oudkerk M. The effectiveness of surveillance for women with a family history of breast cancer; a retrospective study. Ned Tijdschr Geneeskd, 1995;139:445–449.

31. Salmon RJ, Vilcoq JR. Breast cancer after preventive subcutaneous mastectomy. Presse Med 1995; 24:1167–1168.

32. Seachrist L. Restating the risks of tamoxifen. Science 1994;263:910–911.

33. Leeuwen van LE, Benraadt J, Coebergh JWW, Kiemeney LALM, Gimbrère CHF, Otter R, Schouten LJ, Damhuis RAM, Bontenbal M, Diepenhorst FW, Belt vd-Dusebout, AW, Tinteren van H. Risk of endometrial cancer after tamoxifen treatment of breast cancer. Lancet 1994;343:448–452.

34. Jordan VC, Morrow M. Should clinicians be concerned about the carcinogenic potential of tamoxifen? Eur J Cancer 1994;30A:1714–1721.

35. Klijn JGM, Berns PMJJ, Bontenbal M, Alexieva-Figusch J, Foekens JA. Clinical breast cancer, new developments in selection and endocrine treatment of patients. J Steroid Biochem Molec Biol 1992; 43:211–221.

36. Klijn JGM, Setyono-Han B, Bontenbal M, Seynaeve C, Foekens JA. Novel endocrine therapies in breast cancer. Acta Oncol 1996;(In press).

37. Klijn JGM, Devilee P, van Geel AN, Tilanus-Linthorst MMA, Dudok-de Wit C, Meijers-Heijboer EJ. First Dutch experiences with presymptomatic DNA-testing in hereditary breast/ovarian cancer syndrome. Ned Tijdschr Geneeskd 1995;139:439–445.

38. Dudok de Wit AC, Meijers-Heijboer EJ, Tibben A, Frets PG, Klijn JGM, Devilee P, Niermeijer MF. Effect on a Dutch family of predictive DNA-testing for hereditary breast and ovarian cancer. Lancet 1994;344:197.

39. Cornelis R, Vasen H, Meijers-Heijboer H, Ford D, Van Vliet M, Van Tilborg A, Cleton F, Klijn J, Menko F, Meera Khan P, Cornelisse C, Devilee P. Age at diagnosis as an indicator of eligibility for BRCA1 DNA-testing in familial breast cancer. Hum Genet 1995;95:539–544.

40. Hogervorst F, Cornelis R, Bout M, Van Vliet M, Oosterwijk J, Olmer R, Bakker B, Klijn J, Vasen H, Meijers-Heijboer H, Menko F, Cornelisse C, Den Dunnen J, Devilee P, Van Ommen G. Rapid detection of BRCA1 mutations by the Protein Truncation Test. Nature Genet 1995;10:208–212.

41. Klijn JGM, Meijers-Heijboer EJ, Tilanus-Linthorst MMA, Bartels CCM, Van Geel AN, Logmans A, Niermeijer MF. Clinical Genetic and Oncological Aspects of Familial Breast Cancer: Implications for Risk, Screening and Prevention. 6th EORTC Breas Cancer Working Conference, Amsterdam, September 6–9, 1994.

42. Hille ETM, Klijn JGM, Meijers-Heijboer EJ, Cornelisse CJ, Rosendaal FR, Coebergh JWW, Vandenbroucke JB. Secular Trends in Mortality in Four Large Kindreds With Hereditary Breast-Ovarian Cancer. Abstract 7th EORTC Breast Cancer Working Conference (Bordeaux, 10–14 September), 1996.

43. Verhoog LC, van Geel AN, Henzen-Logmans SC, Seynaeve C, Tilanus-Linthorst M, Bartels CCM, Meijers-Heijboer M, Devilee P, Klijn JGM. Histologic Findings in Prophylactic Mastectomy Specimens From Women With Hereditary Risk Factors. Abstract 7th EORTC Breast Cancer Working Conference (Bordeaux, 10–14 September), 1996.

44. Seynaeve C, Logmans A, Meijers-Heijber EJ, Verhoog LC, Klijn JGM, Henzen-Logmans SC. Histologic Findings in Prophylactically Removed Ovaries From Women in Hereditary Breast/Ovarian Cancer (HBOC) Families, Including Follow-up Data. 21st Congress of the European Society of Medical Oncology (Wien, November 2–5, 1996).

45. Piver MS, Jiski MF, Tsukada Y, Nava G. Primary peritoneal carcinoma after prophylactic oophorectomy in women with a family history of ovarian cancer. Cancer 1993;71:2751–2755.

Identification of women at high risk of breast cancer due to inherited susceptibility

David E. Goldgar

International Agency for Research on Cancer, Lyon, France

Key words: BRCA1, BRCA2, breast cancer, genes.

Introduction

Breast cancer is one of the most common cancers affecting women in developed countries, and there is a trend of increasing incidence in developing countries as Western-style lifestyles are becoming more prevalent. Because metastatic breast cancer is an incurable disease, efforts to decrease breast cancer mortality have focused on early detection and improved treatment. Identification of women at particularly high risk of developing the disease provides not only a group on whom expensive and rigorous screening programs are cost-effective, but provides a cohort of women who may benefit from trials of chemopreventive agents. One of the strongest predictors of a woman's risk of breast cancer is the presence of the disease in her immediate family. Consequently, one of the most promising approaches for understanding the cause of breast cancer and creating an effective cancer control program is by identifying women who are genetically predisposed to have this disease. The discovery through genetic linkage studies and positional cloning of at least two genes, which when altered, confer markedly increased susceptibility to breast cancer, should facilitate the identification of a cohort of individuals with a particularly high risk of this disease.

Familiality of breast cancer

Evidence that women with a positive family history of breast cancer are at increased risk for developing breast cancer has been accumulating for over 50 years; nearly every study which examines this question has found significantly elevated relative risks to female relatives of breast cancer patients. Most studies have found relative risks between two and three for first degree relatives of breast cancer patients selected without regard to age at diagnosis or laterality.

In one of the first studies of familial breast cancer in a population-based series,

---

Address for correspondence: Dr David E. Goldgar, Chief Unit of Genetic Epidemiology, International Agency for Research on Cancer, 150 Cours Albert Thomas, 69372 Lyon Cedex 08, France. Tel.: +33-72-73-83-18. Fax: +33-72-73-85-75. E-mail: goldgar@iarc.fr

Ottman et al. [1] examined the risk of breast cancer regarding both age of onset as well as laterality. Their results demonstrated that risk was substantially increased for sisters of bilateral patients diagnosed at the age of 50 or younger (RR = 5.5); for sisters of bilateral cases at the age of 40 or younger the risk doubled to 10.5. Unilateral breast cancer cases diagnosed at the age of 50 or younger did not show significantly increased risk, however, sisters of unilateral patients diagnosed at the age of 40 or younger did appear to have an increased risk (RR = 2.4). For all age ranges, this study shows bilaterality of disease increasing risk by 4–5-fold.

The age at onset as an indicator of familial risk was analyzed by Claus et al. [2] in perhaps the largest population-based case-control study of familial breast cancer. Utilizing data from the Cancer and Steroid Hormone (CASH) case-control study of 4,730 probands with breast cancer diagnosed between the ages of 20 and 54, they estimated age-specific risks as a function of the age at diagnosis of the proband and the number of affected relatives. The risk to a mother of a case with breast cancer diagnosed at 50 years of age was 1.7, compared with 2.7 and 4.3 for cases diagnosed at ages 40 and 30 respectively. According to this analysis, a woman with a sister affected at the age of 50 has an estimated lifetime risk of 3.6 (95% CI 2.1–6.1), while a woman at the age of 50 with a mother and a sister affected has an estimated lifetime risk of 17.1 (95% CI 9.4–31.3). Data on laterality were unavailable in the CASH data set. Houlston et al. [3] showed a 6.4-fold increase in risk of breast cancer for first degree relatives of patients with bilateral breast cancer.

More recently, in a comprehensive population-based study of familial cancer, Goldgar et al. [4] studied the incidence of breast and other cancers among 49,202 first degree relatives of 5,559 breast cancer probands diagnosed before the age of 80. This study estimated a relative risk of 1.8 in relatives of these breast cancer probands. When the age criteria was reduced to early onset cancer (diagnosed before the age of 50), the relative risk of breast cancer among first-degree relatives increased to 2.6 and the risk for early onset breast cancer among these relatives was 3.7 (95% CI 2.8–4.6). Similarly, when the risk to subsequent relatives in families with two affected sisters was considered, the risk increased to 2.7 with a particularly high risk of 4.9 to breast cancers diagnosed before the age of 50. These studies, as well as complex segregation studies of families ascertained through population based resources [5,6], and simply the presence of remarkable high-risk families, strongly indicated the presence of genes which conferred a high lifetime risk of breast cancer. These findings paved the way for the genetic linkage studies and positional cloning efforts that followed and resulted in the identification of a number of breast cancer susceptibility genes.

Implications of major genes in breast cancer etiology

Over the past 5 years a number of genes responsible for inherited predisposition to breast and/or ovarian cancer have been identified or localized. In particular, BRCA1, BRCA2, the p53 gene, the ataxia-telangiectasia gene and the androgen receptor have been implicated in increased susceptibility to breast cancer. These genes differ in terms of the risks of cancer which they confer, the cancer phenotypes with which they are associated, and their gene frequencies. Because of their importance in familial breast cancer, the markedly increased risks they confer and their relatively high frequency in the population, this paper will focus on BRCA1 and BRCA2, with only brief descriptions of other genes known to confer increased susceptibility to breast cancer.

P53

The first gene to have been implicated in the genesis of breast cancer is the p53 gene on chromosome 17p [7]. Germline p53 mutations are most often associated with the Li-Fraumeni syndrome in which families typically exhibit multiple affected members with childhood cancers, primarily sarcomas and brain tumors [8]. Another hallmark of this syndrome is the presence in the family of cases of very early onset breast cancer, with the age at onset usually before the age of 30. It has been estimated that 60% of Li-Fraumeni families are due to germline p53 mutations. Overall, it is thought, however, that germline p53 mutations account for only a small (<5%) proportion of familial early onset breast cancer and a negligible fraction of familial breast cancer in general.

BRCA1

The existence of a specific gene, referred to as BRCA1, conferring increased susceptibility to breast cancer, was confirmed in late 1990 with the finding of a linkage between early onset breast cancer and a specific marker on the long arm of chromosome 17 [9]. Shortly thereafter it was recognized that families with inherited susceptibility to ovarian cancer as well as breast cancer were due to this gene [10]. A large study conducted by the Breast Cancer Linkage Consortium (BCLC) analyzed data from 214 families collected in Europe and North America. Based on genotypings at a series of marker loci surrounding the BRCA1 locus, the BCLC estimated that 45% of families with a high risk of breast cancer alone, and approximately 80% of breast cancer families who have one or more cases of ovarian cancer, are linked to the 17q site [11]. After an intensive and competitive 3-year hunt by many research groups from Europe and North America, the BRCA1 gene was isolated in 1994 through positional cloning by a collaborative effort led by Mark Skolnick at the University of Utah and Myriad Genetics [12]. Since that time, over 100 distinct mutations in over 200 high-risk families have been described in the BRCA1 gene [13,14].

Risks of cancer in BRCA1 mutation carriers

Now that BRCA1 has been cloned, precise estimates of the penetrance can be obtained from prospective population-based studies of mutations. However, even without these data it has been possible to obtain information regarding risks of cancer due to BRCA1 mutations from studies of high-risk families and from assessment of mutations in selected groups of early onset cases of relative pairs. Initially, we could only determine an individual woman's inherited risk in the context of a BRCA1-linked family from linkage studies through use of genetic markers that are tightly linked to the gene. The family must be sufficiently informative for linkage study, and several affected living family members who are closely related to the person whose risk is being evaluated must participate. However, given these limitations, it is possible to identify gene carriers in these families with a reasonable degree of confidence. Easton et al. [11], in the original analysis of the BCLC data, estimated an 85% lifetime risk of developing breast and/or ovarian cancer, an overall risk for breast and ovarian cancer of 59% by the age of 50, with more than 50% of the breast cancers occurring before the age of 50. At the few research centers where such testing may be done, the risks in BRCA1 linked families will most likely vary from these figures within the context of the pedigree analyzed.

More recently, Easton et al. [15] report an analysis of a subset of families submitted to the BCLC; these 33 families contained at least four cases of breast or ovarian cancer diagnosed before the age of 60 with evidence of linkage to the BRCA1 region of chromosome 17q. The estimated cancer risk for breast cancer conferred by BRCA1 in these families was 54% by the age of 60 (95% CI 27–71%). For ovarian cancer, the estimate was 30% by the age of 60 (8–47%). The age-specific incidence of breast cancer in BRCA1 mutation carriers follows a very different pattern from that seen in the general population: relative risks decline significantly with age from over 200-fold in the age group under 40 years to 15-fold in the 60–69 year age group [15].

One caveat in interpreting the risks of BRCA1 carriers is that the families participating in the BCLC consortium data were selected because multiple relatives developed breast cancer. Other families with breast cancer linked to less severe mutations in BRCA1 most likely exist. Women carrying less severe BRCA1 mutations might be at increased risk, but perhaps not so dramatically high as is seen in the BCLC families. With the cloning of BRCA1 it has been possible to search for mutations in a series of cases selected only for early age at diagnosis, without regard to family history. The results of such studies [16–18] have found the same pattern of mutations as in the high-risk families. Moreover, the frequency of BRCA1 mutations found in these series is consistent with the risks of cancer estimated from the linkage data on high-risk families.

BRCA2

Based on genotypings at a series of marker loci surrounding the BRCA1 locus, the BCLC estimated that 45% of families with a high risk of breast cancer alone, and approximately 80% of breast cancer families who have at least one case of ovarian cancer, are due to BRCA1. Interestingly, in a study by Stratton et al. [19], it was noted that the vast majority of families which contained a case of breast cancer in a male were unlinked to genetic markers in the BRCA1 region. This led to a collaborative effort between the University of Utah and the Institute of Cancer Research in London, to embark on a genome-wide search for high-risk predisposition loci for breast cancer other than BRCA1. This effort culminated in the late summer of 1994 with the localization of a second breast cancer gene, BRCA2, to the long arm of chromosome 13 [20]. This gene was identified by positional cloning in late 1995 [21] and its full sequence elucidated shortly thereafter [22]. A total of 15 mutations in high-risk families which showed evidence of linkage to chromosome 13q were reported in these two initial papers. A series of papers detailing additional mutations in family series have been recently published [23,24].

Although there is not a tremendous amount of information yet available, preliminary indications are that the risk of breast cancer conferred by BRCA2 mutations is similar to the risks due to BRCA1, while the risks of ovarian cancer in BRCA2 are less than those for BRCA1 but still considerably elevated over population figures [25]. Conversely, BRCA2 appears to confer about a 100-fold increased risk of male breast cancer, which due to the rarity of this condition, results in a fairly low (~6%) lifetime absolute risk [25].

Screening for BRCA1/2 mutations

Of course knowing that these genes exist and even knowing their complete sequence, is only the first step in the identification of high-risk mutations in individual breast cancer cases and their relatives. Because these genes are large genes (5.5 an 10.2 kb of coding sequence for BRCA1 and BRCA2, respectively) and more importantly, because there is a broad mutation spectrum with many distinct mutations spread across the entire gene, identifying the mutation in an individual sample with a high level of sensitivity and accuracy is a very labor-intensive and expensive process. Thus, when deciding who should be eligible for such screening, there will likely be some eligibility criteria imposed based on age at diagnosis and number of relatives affected. Once the mutation is identified in a given family, however, subsequent testing for other members of that family can be performed on a mutation-specific basis, with greatly reduced laboratory effort and cost.

For certain populations, however, the task of identifying mutation carriers is simplified by the presence of a single mutation in high frequency in that population. The most notable example is the BRCA1 185delAG mutation in individuals of Ashkenazi Jewish origin. It has been estimated that 1% of Ashkenazi Jews are carriers of this deleterious BRCA1 mutation [26]. When two series of young Jewish breast cancer patients diagnosed under 40 and 42 respectively, were examined [16,27], 24 of the 119 women examined (20%) were carriers of this mutation. In addition, in the second study [27], eight of 27 (30%) women diagnosed between the ages of 42 and 50 with an affected first degree relative were 185delAG-positive. Recently, a mutation in BRCA2, 6174delT has been identified in Ashkenazi Jewish breast cancer families and in six (7.5%) of the 80 cases diagnosed before the age of 42 [28]. Similarly, a BRCA2 mutation 999 del 5 has been observed in high frequency in Iceland, accounting for much of the familial breast cancer and an estimated 30%

of all cases of male breast cancer diagnosed in that country in the last 40 years [29]. The identification of common mutations in certain populations facilitates the task of carrier identification in these populations, although individuals who are negative for the most common mutations must still be screened for the entire BRCA1 and BRCA2 genes.

Other genes which may increase breast cancer risk

Although great excitement has been generated over the cloning of the BRCA1 and BRCA2 genes, it is clear that these genes account for only a minority of the familial risk observed for breast cancer. It is likely that other genes exist which may be more common in the population but which confer only moderately increased risk (3—5-fold) of breast cancer. An example of a gene which may be of this type is provided by the ataxia-telangiectasia (A-T) gene.

A-T is a progressive neurological disorder which appears to be inherited in an autosomal recessive fashion. It is associated with a high incidence of cancer (>61-fold), particularly lymphomas and leukemias, but also primary carcinomas of other organs, including the breast [30]. Patients with the disease are homozygous for a mutant gene, the A-T gene, assigned to the chromosomal region 11q23 [31]. It has been suggested that the high incidence of cancers with this disorder may be due to "fragile" chromosomes; the chromosomes of affected individuals seem particularly susceptible to damage from ionizing radiation, as well as specific cytotoxic drugs. It has been reported that about 1% of the population carry the A-T gene and that individuals who carry one abnormal copy of the A-T gene are also at an increased risk of cancer of any type, approximately twice that of the population at large [32]. The heterozygote relative risk for breast cancer in women carriers was estimated to be significantly higher, with a relative risk of 6.8 [30]. It should be noted that this paper generated a great deal of controversy; the results were questioned on the basis of methodological issues of control groups, as well as the radiation exposure assessment, which could reduce the risk reported [33—35]. However, if this result is true and the A-T gene frequency is as high as some estimates have indicated, this locus could account for a substantial proportion of the observed familial relative risk. However, in an examination of a number of early onset non-BRCA1-linked breast cancer families, no evidence of linkage to the A-T region of chromosome 11 was found [36]. More recently, the gene responsible for ataxia telangiectasia (ATM) was isolated [37]. This will enable in the near future direct assessment of the attributable fraction of breast cancer due to ATM and the risks conferred by mutations in this gene. If in fact ATM does confer increased susceptibility to breast cancer through increased radiosensitivity, this will have important implications for therapy, and perhaps for screening of women with or at risk of breast cancer.

Are there other high risk genes?

Evidence from linkage and mutation studies of a series of high risk families indicate that there may yet be one or more genes which convey a relatively high risk of breast cancer which remains to be identified ([23,24] unpublished data from Breast Cancer Linkage Consortium; Serova et al. (personal communication)). At this point a collaboration has been organized to gather informative families which show evidence against linkage to BRCA1 and BRCA2 and for which no mutations in these genes have been identified after screening of the complete coding sequence. These families will be used in a genome-wide search to try and identify other breast cancer susceptibility loci. Possible candidates based on somewhat tentative previous linkage reports are the Estrogen Receptor locus [38] and a region on chromosome 8p.

Summary

It is relatively well-established that a positive family history is the strongest epidemiologic risk factor known for breast cancer, stronger than any known reproductive, hormonal, or dietary factors. Although correlated family environment could account for some portion of the observed familiality, there is substantial evidence that the majority of this familial effect is due to the action of a number of specific genes. This evidence comes from several sources: the observation that there is an increased risk to more distant relatives of breast cancer probands who do not share common environments; the results of segregation analyses which show that the pattern of familiality is consistent with the actions of dominant high penetrant susceptibility loci; and, of course, most convincingly, the isolation of two such susceptibility genes, BRCA1 and BRCA2. Female carriers of BRCA1 or BRCA2 mutations, which may jointly comprise one in every 500 caucasian individuals, if unaffected at the age of 30, have a risk of approximately 3% per year of developing breast cancer in the following 20 years. This makes this group important to follow clinically and also could provide a cohort for more costly screening techniques or chemopreventive agents.

However, it is becoming increasingly clear that BRCA1 and BRCA2 do not account for the majority of the observed familial clustering of breast cancer. In fact, these genes together probably only account for about half of all families with three to five cases of breast cancer under the age of 60 and no evidence of ovarian cancer. It is likely that in the near future, at least one other high penetrant susceptibility locus for breast cancer will be identified through genetic linkage studies, and that the role of specific known genes such as ATM which seem to be associated with increased breast cancer risk will be clarified. It is also clear that in the near future, a large number of women who have a high-risk of developing breast cancer at a relatively young age will be identified through mutation testing of women with positive family histories. These women will need careful management in terms of screening, prevention, and psychosocial counselling.

References

1. Ottman R, Pike M, King MC, Casagrande JT, Henderson BE. Familial breast cancer in a population-based series. Am J Epidemiol 1986;123:15–21.

192

2. Claus EB, Risch N, Thompson WD. Age of onset as an indicator of familial risk in breast cancer. Am J Epidemiol 1990;131:961–972.

3. Houlston RS, McCarter E, Parbhoo S et al. Family history and risk of breast cancer. J Med Genet 1992;29:154–157.

4. Goldgar DE, Easton DF, Cannon-Albright LA, Skolnick MH. A systematic population-based assessment of cancer risk in first degree relative of cancer probands. J Natl Cancer Inst 1994;86: 1600–1608.

5. Newman B, Austin M, Lee M, King MC. Inheritance of human breast cancer: evidence for autosomal dominant transmission in high risk families. Proc Natl Acad Sci USA 1988;85:1–5.

6. Claus EB, Risch N, Thompson WD. Genetic analysis of breast cancer in the cancer and steroid hormone study. Am J Hum Genet 1991;48:232–242.

7. Malkin D, Li FP, Strong LC et al. Germ line p53 mutations in a familial syndrome of breast cancer, sarcomas, and other neoplasms. Science 1990;250:1234–1238.

8. Li FP, Fraumeni JF. Soft tissue sarcomas, breast cancer and other neoplasms: a familial syndrome? Ann Int Med 1969;71:747–760.

9. Hall JM, Lee MK, Newman B et al. Linkage of early-onset familial breast cancer to chromosome 17q21. Science 1990;250:1684–1689.

10. Narod SA, Feunteun J, Lynch HT et al. Familial breast-ovarian cancer locus on chromosome 17q12-q23. Lancet 1991;338:82–83.

11. Easton DF, Bishop DT, Ford D, Crockford GP. Genetic linkage analysis in familial breast and ovarian cancer: Results from 214 Families. Am J Hum Genet 1993;52:678–701.

12. Miki Y, Swensen J, Shattuck-Eidens D, Futreal PA et al. A strong candidate for the 17q-linked breast and ovarian cancer susceptibility gene BRCA1. Science 1994;266:66–71.

13. Shattuck-Eidens D, McClure M, Simard J et al. A collaborative survey of 80 mutations in the BRCA1 breast and ovarian cancer susceptibility gene: Implications for presymptomatic testing and screening. JAMA 1995;273:535–541.

14. Couch FJ, Weber BL, Breast Cancer Information Core (BIC). Mutations and polymorphisms in the familial early onset breast cancer (BRCA1) gene. Human Mutat 1996;(In press).

15. Easton DF, Ford D, Bishop DT, Breast Cancer Linkage Consortium. Breast and ovarian cancer incidence in BRCA1 mutation carriers. Am J Hum Genet 1995;56:265–271.

16. Fitzgerald MG, MacDonald DJ, Kranier M et al. Germline BRCA1 mutations in Jewish and non-Jewish women with early-onset breast cancer. N Engl J Med 1996;334:143–149.

17. Langston AA, Malone KE, Thomson JD, Daling JR, Ostrander EA. BRCA1 mutations in a population-based sample of young women with breast cancer. N Engl J Med 1996;334:137–142.

18. Ithier G, Girard M, Stoppa-Lyonnet DL. Correspondence. N Engl J Med 1996;334:1198–1199.

19. Stratton MR, Ford D, Seal S et al. Familial male breast cancer is not linked to the BRCA1 locus on chromosome 17q. Nature Genet 1994;7:103–107.

20. Wooster R, Neuhausen S, Mangion J et al. Localization of a breast cancer susceptibility gene, (BRCA2), to chromosome 13q12-13. Science 1994;265:2088–2090.

21. Wooster R et al. Identification of the breast cancer susceptibility gene BRCA2. Nature 1995;378: 789–791.

22. Tavtigian SV, Simard J, Rommens J et al. The complete BRCA2 gene and mutations in chromosome 13q-linked kindreds. Nature Genet 1996;12:333–337.

23. Phelan CM, Lancaster J, Tonin P et al. Mutation analysis of the BRCA2 gene in 49 site-specific breast cancer families. Nature Genet 1996;13:120–122.

24. Couch FJ, Farid L, Deshano M et al. BRCA2 germline mutations in male breast cancer cases and breast cancer families. Nature Genet 1996;13:123–125.

25. Easton DF, Steele L, Fields P, Daly PA, Ormiston W, Neuhausen SL, Ford D, Wooster R, Cannon-Albright LA, Stratton MR, Goldgar DE. Cancer risks in two large breast cancer families linked to BRCA2 on chromosome 13q12-13. Am J Hum Genet 1996;(In press).

26. Struewing JP et al. The carrier frequency of the BRCA1 185delAG mutation is approximately 1 percent in Ashkenazi Jewish individuals. Nature Genet 1995;11:1–5.

27. Offit K, Gilewski T, McGuire P, Schluger A, Brown K, Neuhausen S, Skolnick M, Norton L, Goldgar D. Germline BRCA1 185delAG mutations in Jewish women affected by breast cancer. Lancet 1996;(In press).

28. Neuhausen S, Gilewski T, Notton L et al. Recurrent BRCA2 6174delT mutations in Ashkenazi Jewish women affected by breast cancer. Nature Genet 1996;13:126–128.

29. Thorlacius S, Olafsdottir G, Tryggvadottir L et al. A single mutation in the BRCA2 gene in male and female breast cancer families with varied cancer phenotypes. Nature Genet 1996;13:117–119.

30. Swift M, Reitnauer PJ, Morrell D, Chase CL. Incidence of cancer in 161 families affected by ataxia telangiectasia. N Eng I Med 1991;325:1831–1836.

31. Gatti RA, Berkel I, Boder E et al. Localization of the ataxia telangiectasia gene to chromosome 11q22-23. Nature 1988;336:577–580.

32. Swift M, Reitnauer PJ, Morrell D, Chase CL. Breast and other cancers in families with ataxia telangiectasia. N Engl J Med 1987;316:1289–1294.

33. Hall CE, Geard CR, Brenner DJ. Correspondence: risk of breast cancer in ataxia telangiectasia. N Engl J Med 1992;326:1359–1360.

34. Land CE. Correspondence: risk of breast cancer in ataxia telangiectasia. N Engl J Med 1992; 326:1359–1360.

35. Wagner LK. Correspondence: risk of breast cancer in ataxia telangiectasia. N Engl J Med 1992;326:1359–1360.

36. Savitsky K, Bar-Shira A, Gilad S et al. A single ataxia telangiectasia gene with a product similar to PI-3 kinase. Science 1995;268:1749–1753.

37. Zuppan P, Hall JM, Lee MK, Ponglikitmongko M, King MC. Possible linkage of the estrogen receptor gene to breast cancer in a family with late-onset disease. Am J Hum Genet 1991;48: 1065–1068.

38. Keranguevan F, Essioux L, Dib A et al. Loss of heterozygosity and linkage analysis in breast carcinoma: indications for a putative third susceptibility gene on the short arm of chromosome 8. Oncogene 1995;10:1023–1026.

Available results on chemopreventative effects of tamoxifen and other drugs on mammary cancer

The Scientific Bases of Cancer Chemoprevention.
C. Maltoni, M. Soffritti and W. Davis, editors.

Experimental results on the chemopreventive and side effects of tamoxifen using a human-equivalent animal model

Cesare Maltoni, Franco Minardi, Fiorella Belpoggi, Carmine Pinto, Angela Lenzi and Federica Filippini
Cancer Research Centre, European Ramazzini Foundation of Oncology and Environmental Sciences, Bologna, Italy

Abstract. *Background.* The reported experiments were performed to obtain more precise information on the chemopreventive effects of tamoxifen on mammary cancer and other tumours, as well as data to assess its carcinogenic potential.

Materials and Methods. Tamoxifen was tested on female Sprague-Dawley rats, which develop spontaneous tumours, that must be considered equivalent to the human counterpart.

— Experiment 1: tamoxifen was administered to groups of 100 8-week-old female rats at the daily doses of 3.3 (group I) and 0 (group II) mg/kg b.w. (10 times the dose delivered to women given 20 mg daily), in water suspension, by stomach tube, once daily, six times weekly, for the life-span.

— Experiment 2: tamoxifen was administered to groups of 139 56-week-old female rats, at the daily doses of 3.3 (group I) and 0 (group II) mg/kg b.w., in water suspension, by stomach tube, once daily, six times weekly, for 40 weeks, after which the animals were kept alive until spontaneous death.

— Experiment 3: tamoxifen was administered to groups of 139–151 56-week-old female rats, at the daily doses of 3.3 (group I), 1 (group II), 0.33 (group III), 0.10 (group IV), 0 (group V) mg/kg b.w., in water suspension, by stomach tube, once daily, six times weekly, for 40 weeks, after which the animals were sacrificed.

Results. In the tested conditions, tamoxifen shows a strong chemopreventive effect on mammary cancer. The number of mammary cancers/100 animals and the Protection Index (PI) in the various groups of the three experiments, resulted as follows:

— Experiment 1: 13.0 in the control group and 0 in group I (PI = 100.00).

— Experiment 2: 10.8 in the control group and 2.8 in group I (PI = 74.1).

— Experiment 3: 12.7 in the control group; 0.7 in group IV (PI = 94.5); 0 in group III (PI = 100.0); 0.7 in group II (PI = 94.5); 0 in group I (PI = 100.0).

The chemopreventive effect was shown also at a dose much lower than that used in the clinical practice. Tamoxifen also lowers the incidence of benign mammary tumours, pituitary gland adenomas, and uterine polyps. When administered at 3.3 mg/kg b.w. for the life-span, it causes only a borderline increase of liver tumours and of uterus-vagina tumours.

Conclusion. The experiments suggest a large gap between the dose of tamoxifen which causes cancer risk and the dose of the drug still effective for tumour chemoprevention. Further research is needed to more precisely assess the lowest doses still effective in chemoprevention.

Key words: carcinogenesis, chemoprevention, mammary cancer, rat, tamoxifen.

Address for correspondence: Cesare Maltoni, Cancer Research Centre, European Ramazzini Foundation of Oncology and Environmental Sciences, Castle of Bentivoglio, 40010 Bentivoglio, Bologna, Italy.

Introduction

Tamoxifen is a drug which is widely used in medical oncology as an antioestrogen. This effect is due to its competitive action on oestrogen receptors, but other mechanisms can be implied. Most likely, tamoxifen may also act via the hypophysis by lowering the production of ovarian oestrogens.

The use of tamoxifen in oncology started in 1971 [1] and it has been progressively and gradually expanding. Up to the present day it seems that over 5 million women have undergone treatment with this drug. Ordinarily, tamoxifen is administered at the daily dose of 20 mg, but sometimes 30 or 40 mg are also prescribed.

Tamoxifen has been found efficacious, and is, therefore, used in primary hormonotherapy for female and male mammary carcinoma and for endometrial cancer. Its use has also been proposed in other tumours, mainly melanomas. Its therapeutical effect on mammary cancer has also been proved with experimental animal models [2].

Nowadays, tamoxifen is widely used in postsurgical adjuvant therapy for mammary carcinoma in women. There are at present 14 clinical trials on this use [3–18], and the updated results seem to show an advantageous effect of the drug on disease-free survival time and on the overall survival.

Tamoxifen has been shown to have chemopreventive effects on mammary cancers experimentally induced in rats, or arisen in a strain of mice which develop mammary tumours spontaneously at a high incidence [2,19–25], and on the spontaneous mammary cancers of the colony of Sprague-Dawley rats, used in our laboratory [26–38]. The results obtained on spontaneous mammary carcinomas in female Sprague-Dawley rats show a strong chemopreventive effect of tamoxifen, and they are particularly relevant for clinical extrapolation since this animal model must be considered human-equivalent, due to the histological pattern, biological behaviour, global incidence and age-equivalent distribution of these tumours.

The chemopreventive effect of tamoxifen on mammary carcinoma is also supported by a protective effect of tamoxifen in the controlateral mammary tumours observed in the trials evaluating the effect of the drug in adjuvant therapy. Of a total of 30,000 women included in these trials (180,000 woman years), 379 cases of controlateral mammary carcinomas have been observed up to present in the control group, vs. 276 cases of these tumours in the tamoxifen-treated group, with an odds reduction of 35% (2P = 0.00001) (personal communication).

These experimental and clinical observations prompted three chemopreventive clinical trials, one in the USA on 16,000 women [39–41], one in Italy on 20,000 women [42] and one in the UK on 15,000 women [43,44]. The daily dose employed in these trials is 20 mg/die. The Italian clinical trial is performed on hysterectomized women.

Much is known about the short- and middle-term, wanted and unwanted effects of tamoxifen in treated women [33,45–51].

It is also known that the drug has a carcinogenic potential. Information on the carcinogenic effects of tamoxifen is of primary importance, because of the use of tamoxifen in adjuvant therapy, involving large groups of women who must be considered already cured by surgery alone, and because of the chemopreventive trials which are now ongoing and whose results may eventually open the door to the adoption of tamoxifen treatment for chemoprevention of mammary cancer on large groups of women all over the world.

Pioneering observations in the Swedish adjuvant trial showed, even in 1989, an increase in endometrial carcinomas in women treated with tamoxifen at 40 mg daily [52]. The effect has now been confirmed also in women treated with the daily dose of 20 mg [53].Among the total 30,000 control and treated women of the ongoing adjuvant trials, 78 cases of endometrial carcinoma have been observed up to present in treated women, vs. 21 in the control group (2p < 0.00001) (personal communication).

Five experimental studies in rats of different strains were performed to evaluate the carcinogenic effect of tamoxifen on liver. The results, summarized in Table 1, indicate that tamoxifen is indeed a hepatocarcinogen at very high doses. The still effective lower dose is 5 mg/kg b.w., which corresponds to 15 times the current clinical dose (in the case of a woman weighing 60 kg, the current daily dose of 20 mg corresponds to 0.33 mg/kg b.w.). It must be pointed out, on the other hand, that the maximum duration of these experimental hepatocarcinogenicity studies was 24 months.

In this context three sets of information are needed:
1. Data on the full carcinogenic potential of tamoxifen based upon life-span experiments.
2. Data on the duration of the protective effect of tamoxifen, after the drug administration is stopped.
3. Data on the minimum doses still efficacious for chemoprevention, in order to lower as far as possible the risk of unwanted carcinogenic effects.

Within the framework of an experimental research project on the chemopreventive and carcinogenic effect of tamoxifen, which includes 14 studies and was started in 1986, three experiments were planned to obtain some of this needed information.

— Experiment 1: was planned to study the full chemopreventive and carcinogenic potential of tamoxifen, by exposing the animals to a high dose from an early age to death.
— Experiment 2: was planned to study the chemopreventive and carcinogenic potential of tamoxifen following a limited treatment and, furthermore, the duration of the protective effect of the drug by allowing the animals to live until spontaneous death.
— Experiment 3: was planned to assess the chemopreventive potential of a range of doses of tamoxifen, including one lower than that ordinarily used in clinical practice (20 mg/die).

The results of these experiments are herein presented.

Table 1. Incidence of hepatocarcinomas in various rat strains submitted to long-term treatment with tamoxifen.

Strain of rats	Daily dose (mg/kg b.w.)	No. of animals		Duration of the experiment (months)	Hepatocarcinoma (bearing animals) (%)	References
		At start	Corrected			
Sprague-Dawley	2.8	57	22	15	0	[54]
	11.3	57	11	15	45	
	45.2	55	4	12	75	
Wistar	5.0	52	51	24	16	[55]
	20.0	52	51	24	64	
	35.0	52	51	24	64	
Sprague-Dawley	11.3	84	36	12	44	[56]
	22.6	75	24	12	100	
Sprague-Dawley	11.3	5	5	15	60	[57]
	45.0	8	6	15	83	
Fischer F344	12.5	20	8	15	0	[58]

Plan of experiments, Materials and Methods

The plan of the experiments, which were started in 1988 (BT 5T) and in 1991 (BT 11T and BT 12T), is shown in Table 2.

The tamoxifen tested is the one marketed by Zeneca, under the commercial name of ®Nolvadex.

The tested animals were female Sprague-Dawley rats of the colony which has been used for 30 years in the laboratories of the CRC/BT, for which there is extensive information on expected nonneoplastic and neoplastic pathology, available for about 10,000 control animals.

In this strain, the incidence of mammary tumours is of the same order as that observed in women in industrial countries: within the years in which the experiments herein presented were performed, usually mammary cancer arises in about 10% of the females (range 7—12%), and the number of mammary cancers per 100 animals ranges from nine to 13 (since the same animal can bear more than one mammary malignancy). The distribution by equivalent ages in this animal model and in women overlaps. The mammary cancers show all the various morphological patterns which characterize the human types and subtypes.

The animals were weaned at 5 weeks of age, identified by ear punch and randomized in order to have no more than one animal of each litter in the same group. From weaning, the animals received feed and water ad libitum. The animals were housed five per cage, in makrolon cages with a solid top of stainless steel. A shallow layer of white wood shavings served as bedding. The animals were kept in a temperature-controlled laboratory at 19°—20° C, with 12-h light-dark intermittence.

Tamoxifen was administered by stomach tube in 1 ml of water suspension, once daily, 6 days weekly, while water alone was administered to the control animals.

The animals were submitted daily to observation; feed and water consumption and body weight were measured periodically (weekly within the first 13 weeks of experiment, and then every 2 weeks). The gross lesions, with particular regard to the mammary lumps, were described and recorded every 2 weeks.

At death, all animals were submitted to systematic necropsy. Specimens for histopathology include mammary glands, mammary tumours, brain, pituitary gland, Zymbal glands, salivary glands, Harderian glands, head (five sections) (with oral and nasal cavities and external and internal ear ducts), tongue, thyroid and parathyroids, pharynx, larynx, thymus and mediastinal lymph nodes, trachea, lung, heart, diaphragm, liver, spleen, pancreas, kidneys and adrenal glands, oesophagus, stomach, intestine (four levels), bladder, uterus, vagina, ovaries, interscapular fat pad, subcutaneous and mesenteric lymph nodes, femur, and any other organs and tissues with pathological lesions. The histological slides were examined independently by two pathologists, and then reviewed by a third pathologist.

The experiments were performed in compliance with the Good Laboratory Practices (GLP).

Table 2. Plan of the three experiments on the chemopreventive effects of tamoxifen on female Sprague-Dawley rats (Exp. BT 5T, BT 11T, BT 12T).

Experiment	Group	Daily dose (mg/kg b.w.)[a]	Animals no.	Age at start (weeks)	Duration of the treatment (weeks)	Duration of the experiment (weeks)
1 (BT 5T)	I	3.3	100	8	life-span	life-span (167)
	II	0	100	8	life-span	life-span
2 (BT 12T)	I	3.3	139	56	40	life-span (143)
	II	0	139	56	40	life-span
3 (BT 11T, BT 12T)	I	3.3	139	56	40	96
	II	1.0	145	56	40	96
	III	0.33	151	56	40	96
	IV	0.1	151	56	40	96
	V	0	149	56	40	96

[a]The tested four doses, 3.3, 1.0, 0.33, 0.1 mg/kg b.w., correspond, respectively, to the daily clinical doses of 200, 66, 20, 6.6 mg, in a woman weighing 60 kg.

Results

Feed and water consumption

In the first experiment the treated animals showed a reduced drinking water intake, while the feed consumption was affected to a minimal extent. In the second and third experiments the treated animals still showed a reduction in drinking water intake, even if minimal; no differences were observed in feed consumption.

Body weight

In tamoxifen-treated animals a reduction in body weight was observed, which parallels the length and intensity of treatment. Such a reduction, which was marked in the first experiment, is due to a reduction of body size as a whole.

Survival

In all three experiments, a slight increase of survival was observed in tamoxifen-treated groups with respect to control groups.

Nononcological changes

No evident behavioural changes were found in tamoxifen-treated animals. In female rats, atrophic changes in cervical mucosa were observed at the histological examination, following continuous treatment with tamoxifen when started at a young age.

Carcinogenic and anticarcinogenic (chemopreventive) effects

— Experiment 1 (BT5T). In the tamoxifen-treated group there was a decreased incidence of total benign tumours (Table 3), and a borderline decrease in the incidence of total malignant tumours (Table 4). With respect to specific types of tumours, tamoxifen was found: 1) to completely inhibit the onset of benign and malignant mammary tumours (Tables 5 and 6); 2) to decrease the pituitary gland tumours (Table 7), and polyps of the uterus (Table 8); and 3) to slightly increase tumours and correlated oncological lesions of the liver (Table 9), and tumours of the uterus and vagina (Table 10).
— Experiment 2 (BT12T). In the tamoxifen-treated group there was again a decreased incidence of total benign tumours (Table 11) and a slight decrease of total malignant tumours (Table 12). In the tamoxifen-treated group a reduction in benign mammary tumours (Table 13) was observed. As far as mammary cancer is concerned, at the end of the treatment there was a complete inhibition, and, on a life-span basis, a protection index of 74.1 was still found (Table 14). A reduction of the polyps of the uterus (Table 15) was also found. No carcinogenic effect of tamoxifen was found on the liver (Table 16) and the uterus and vagina

Table 3. Results of experiment 1 (BT 5T): incidence of total benign tumours.

| Group | Daily dose (mg/kg b.w.) | Animals | | Benign tumours | | | |
| | | Sex | No. | Animals with tumours | | Tumours | |
				No.	%	No.[a]	Per 100 animals
I	3.3	F	100	26	26.0	28	28.0
II	0	F	100	57	57.0	110	110.0

[a]One animal can bear more than one tumour.

Table 4. Results of experiment 1 (BT 5T): incidence of total malignant tumours.

| Group | Daily dose (mg/kg b.w.) | Animals | | Malignant tumours | | | |
| | | Sex | No. | Animals with tumours | | Tumours | |
				No.	%	No.[a]	Per 100 animals
I	3.3	F	100	31	31.0	34	34.0
II	0	F	100	27	27.0	37	37.0

[a]One animal can bear more than one tumour.

Table 5. Results of experiment 1 (BT 5T): incidence of benign mammary tumours.

Group	Daily dose (mg/kg b.w.)	Animals		Benign mammary tumours				
		Sex	No.	Animals with tumours		Tumours		Protection index[b]
				No.	%	No.[a]	Per 100 animals	
I	3.3	F	100	0	—	0	—	100.0
II	0	F	100	36	36.0	55[c]	55.0	

[a]One animal can bear more than one tumour; [b]percent decrease of tumour incidence (referred to tumours per 100 animals); [c]fibromas and fibroadenomas.

Table 6. Results of experiment 1 (BT 5T): incidence of malignant mammary tumours

Group	Daily dose (mg/kg b.w.)	Animals		Malignant mammary tumours				
		Sex	No.	Animals with tumours		Tumours		Protection index[b]
				No.	%	No.[a]	Per 100 animals	
I	3.3	F	100	0	—	0	—	100.0
II	0	F	100	9	9.0	13[c]	13.0	

[a]One animal can bear more than one tumour; [b]percent decrease of tumour incidence (referred to tumours per 100 animals); [c]12 adenocarcinomas, 1 fibrosarcoma.

Table 7. Results of experiment 1 (BT 5T): incidence of pituitary gland tumours.

Group	Daily dose (mg/kg b.w.)	Animals		Animals with tumours	
		Sex	No.	No.	%
I	3.3	F	100	2	2.0
II	0	F	100	16	16.0

Table 8. Results of experiment 1 (BT 5T): incidence of polyps of the uterus.

Group	Daily dose (mg/kg b.w.)	Animals		Animals with tumours	
		Sex	No.	No.	%
I	3.3	F	100	0	—
II	0	F	100	13	13.0

Table 9. Results of experiment 1 (BT 5T): incidence of tumours and other lesions on oncological interest of the liver.

Group	Daily dose (mg/kg b.w.)	Animals		Animals with liver changes							
		Sex	No.	Nodular hyperplasias		Nodular dysplasias		Hepato-adenomas		Hepato-carcinomas[a]	
				No.	%	No.	%	No.	%	No.	%
I	3.3	F	100	6	6.0	1	1.0	1	1.0	3	3.0
II	0	F	100	6	6.0	0	–	0	–	0	–

[a] All with small deviation.

Table 10. Results of experiment 1 (BT 5T): incidence of malignant tumours of the uterus and vagina

Group	Daily dose (mg/kg b.w.)	Animals		Animals with tumours											
		Sex	No.	Uterus				Vagina				Total			
				Carcinomas		Sarcomas		Carcinomas		Sarcomas		Carcinomas		Sarcomas	
				No.	%	No.	%	No.	%	No.	%	No.	%	No.	%
I	3.3	F	100	1	1.0	3	3.0	1	1.0	0	–	2	2.0	3	3.0
II	0	F	100	0	1.0	2	2.0	0	–	0	–	1	1.0	2	2.0

208

Table 11. Results of experiment 2 (BT 12T): incidence of total benign tumours.

Group	Daily dose (mg/kg b.w.)	Animals		Benign tumours			
		Sex	No.	Animals with tumours		Tumours	
				No.	%	No.[a]	Per 100 animals
I	3.3	F	139	69	49.6	128	92.1
II	0	F	139	92	66.2	199	143.2

[a] One animal can bear more than one tumour.

Table 12. Results of experiment 2 (BT 12T): incidence of total malignant tumours.

Group	Daily dose (mg/kg b.w.)	Animals		Malignant tumours			
		Sex	No.	Animals with tumours		Tumours	
				No.	%	No.[a]	Per 100 animals
I	3.3	F	139	45	32.4	53	38.1
II	0	F	139	43	30.9	59	42.4

[a] One animal can bear more than one tumour.

Table 13. Results of experiment 2 (BT 12T): incidence of benign mammary tumours.

Group	Daily dose (mg/kg b.w.)	Animals		Benign mammary tumours				
		Sex	No.	Animals without tumours		Tumours		
				No.	%	No.[a]	Per 100 animals	Protection index[b]
I	3.3	F	139	48	35.2	65[c]	46.8	34.9
II	0	F	139	65	46.8	100[c]	71.9	

[a]One animal can bear more than one tumour; [b]percent decrease of tumour incidence (referred to tumours per 100 animals); [c]fibromas and fibroadenomas.

Table 14. Results of experiment 2 (BT 12T): incidence of malignant mammary tumours.

Group	Daily dose (mg/ kg b.w.)	Animals		Malignant mammary tumours				
		Sex	No.	Animals with tumours		Tumours		
				No.	%	No.[a]	Per 100 animals	Protection index[b]
I	3.3	F	139	4	2.8	4[c]	2.8	74.1
II	0	F	139	12	8.6	15[d]	10.8	

[a]One animal can bear more than one tumour; [b]percent decrease of tumour incidence (referred to tumours per 100 animals); [c]two adenocarcinomas, two fibrosarcomas; [d]13 adenocarcinomas, one fibrosarcoma, one liposarcoma.

Table 15. Results of experiment 2 (BT 12T): incidence of polyps of the uterus.

Group	Daily dose (mg/kg b.w.)	Animals		Animals with tumours	
		Sex	No.	No.	%
I	3.3	F	139	7	5.0
II	0	F	139	14	10.1

Table 16. Results of experiment 2 (BT 12T): incidence of tumours and other lesions of oncological interest of the liver.

Group	Daily dose (mg/kg b.w.)	Animals		Animals with liver changes									
		Sex	No.	Nodular hyperplasias		Nodular dysplasias		Hepato-adenomas		Hepato-carcinomas		
				No.	%	No.	%	No.	%	No.	%	
I	3.3	F	139	8	5.7	0	–	0	–	0	–	
II	0	F	139	8	5.7	0	–	0	–	0	–	

(Table 17).

— Experiment 3 (BT11T, BT12T). The four tested doses produced a sharp reduction of benign mammary tumours (Table 18) and a near complete protection from mammary cancer (Table 19). In the range of the tested doses, with a ratio of 30:1, there are practically no differences in the protective effect. In these experimental conditions, no carcinogenic effect has been detected.

Conclusion and Discussion

Under the tested conditions, the results of the three experiments show that:

1. Tamoxifen has a strong inhibiting (chemopreventive) effect on spontaneous mammary tumour in female rats, more pronounced in the case of malignant tumours than in that of benign lumps.
2. Such chemopreventive effect lasts when the treatment is stopped.
3. Tamoxifen reduces the incidence of other tumours (including pituitary tumours and polyps of the uterus).
4. When given at the dose of 3.3 mg/kg b.w., 10 times the ordinary dose in women, continuously for the life-span, tamoxifen causes a slight increase in liver tumours and a borderline increase in malignancies of the uterus and vagina.
5. When the drug was given at the same dose, continuously but for a limited period of time (40 weeks), in adult female rats, no carcinogenic effect on the liver and uterus was detected. It must be pointed out that in this experiment, not only is the dose 10 times higher than the current clinical dose, but the period of treatment with respect to the life-span of the animal tested is much longer than that considered in adjuvant therapy and in the chemoprevention of mammary cancer, with respect to the average life-span of women.
6. When the drug was given at the doses of 3.3, 1, 0.33 and 0.10 mg/kg b.w. (corresponding to the daily dose of 200, 66, 20 and 6.6 mg in a woman of 60 kg), it completely or nearly completely inhibited the onset of mammary cancer.

On the basis of our data and of the experimental and clinical information from the scientific literature, the carcinogenic effects of tamoxifen on the liver and uterus appear to be related to the total dose. Such a dose relationship is clearly demonstrated for liver carcinogenesis in rats and also, to some extent, for uterine carcinogenesis in women: in fact, it is not by chance that the first evidence of endometrial cancer was detected in the Swedish adjuvant therapy trial, in which tamoxifen was administered at the dose of 40 mg/die.

The chemopreventive effect of tamoxifen on mammary carcinoma is specifically effective in the control of breast cancer. However, even the carcinogenic side effects cannot be underestimated. As very often occurs in medical practice, the problem now is to assess whether there is a dose of the drug which is effective for chemoprevention but which does not entail serious carcinogenic risks. There are two facts which support the expectation that such a dose may exist. Our data show that a life-span treatment with tamoxifen at a dose 10 times higher than that ordinarily employed in medical practice, entails only marginal carcinogenic effects (Experiment 1), which on

Table 17. Results of experiment 2 (BT 12T): incidence of malignant tumours of the uterus and vagina.

Group	Daily dose (mg/kg b.w.)	Animals		Animals with tumours											
				Uterus				Vagina				Total			
				Carcinomas		Sarcomas		Carcinomas		Sarcomas		Carcinomas		Sarcomas	
		Sex	No.	No.	%	No.	%	No.	%	No.	%	No.	%	No.	%
I	3.3	F	139	5	3.6	5	3.6	0	—	0	—	5	3.6	5	3.6
II	0	F	139	3	1.2	6	4.3	1	0.7	0	—	4	2.9	6	4.3

Table 18. Results of experiment 3 (BT 11T, BT 12T): incidence of benign mammary tumours.

Group	Daily dose (mg/kg b.w.)	Animals		Benign mammary tumours			Per 100 animals	Protection index[b]
		Sex	No.	Animals with tumours		Tumours		
				No.	%	No.[a]		
I	3.3	F	139	21	15.1	28[c]	20.1	68.8
II	1.0	F	145	13	9.0	14[c]	9.6	85.1
III	0.33	F	151	25	16.5	25[c]	16.5	74.4
IV	0.1	F	151	22	14.6	23[c]	15.2	76.4
V	0	F	149	66	44.3	96[c]	64.4	—

[a]One animal can bear more than one tumour; [b]% decrease of tumour incidence (referred to tumours per 100 animals); [c]fibromas and fibroadenomas.

Table 19. Results of experiment 3 (BT 11T, BT 12T): incidence of malignant mammary tumours.

Group	Daily dose (mg/ kg b.w.)	Animals		Malignant mammary tumours				
		Sex	No.	Animals with tumours		Tumours		Protection index[b]
				No.	%	No.[a]	Per 100 animals	
I	3.3	F	139	0	–	0	–	100.0
II	1.0	F	145	1	0.7	1[c]	0.7	94.5
III	0.33	F	151	0	–	0	–	100.0
IV	0.1	F	151	1	0.7	1[d]	0.7	94.5
V	0	F	149	18	12.1	19[d]	12.7	–

[a]One animal can bear more than one tumour; [b]% decrease of tumour incidence (referred to as tumours per 100 animals); [c]fibrosarcoma; [d]adenocarcinomas.

214

the other hand do not emerge in the experiment where the drug was given for a limited, although not short, period, and still at a high dose (Experiment 2). On the other hand, Experiment 3 of the project demonstrated that 0.1 mg/kg b.w. of tamoxifen, corresponding to 6.6 mg daily in women, still completely inhibited the onset of spontaneous mammary cancer in our colony of rats, therefore, indicating that doses much lower than 20 mg daily may still be effective in the treatment for chemoprevention (and for adjuvant therapy). The time has come to review tamoxifen posology, in order to continue to benefit from its chemopreventive/therapeutic effects, without creating risk situations.

References

1. Cole MP, Jones CTA, Todd IDH. A new anti-oestrogenic agent in late breast cancer. An early clinical appraisal of ICI 46474. Br J Cancer 1971;25:270–275.
2. Jordan VC. Effect of tamoxifen (ICI 46,474) on initiation and growth of DMBA-induced rat mammary carcinomata. Eur J Cancer 1976;12:419–424.
3. Ludwig Breast Cancer Studt Group. Randomized trial of chemo-endocrine therapy and mastectomy alone in postmenopausal patients with operable breast cancer and axillary node metastases. Lancet 1984;1:1256–1260.
4. Senanayake F. Adjuvant hormonal chemotherapy in early breast cancer: early results from a controlled trial. Lancet 1984;2:1148–1149.
5. Cummings FJ, Gray R, Davis TE, Tormey DC, Harris JE, Falkson G, Arsenau. Adjuvant tamoxifen treatment of elderly women with stage II breast cancer. A double blind comparison with placebo. Ann Intern Med 1985;324–329.
6. Palshof T, Carstenson B, Mouridsen HT, Dombernowsky P. Adjuvant endocrine therapy in pre- and postmenopausal women with operable breast cancer. Rev Endocrine Rel Cancer 1985;17(Suppl): 43–50.
7. Rose C, Thorpe SM, Andersen KW, Pedersen BV, Mouridsen HT, Blicher-Toft M, Rasmussen B. Beneficial effect of adjuvant tamoxifen therapy in primary breast cancer patients with high estrogen receptor values. Lancet 1985;1:16–19.
8. Breast Cancer Trials Committee, Scottish Cancer Trials Office. Adjuvant tamoxifen in the management of operable breast cancer: The Scottish trial. Lancet 1987;2:171–175.
9. Delozier T, Julien JP, Juret P, Veyret C, Couette JE, Grai Y, Olliver JM, de Ranieri E. Adjuvant tamoxifen in postmenopausal breast cancer: preliminary results of a randomized trial. Breast Cancer Res Treat 1987;7:105–110.
10. Ptirchard K, Meakin JW, Boyd NF et al. Adjuvant tamoxifen in postmenopausal women with axillary node positive breast cancer: an update. In: Salmon SE (ed) Adjuvant Therapy of Cancer. Orlando: Grune and Stratton, 1987;391–400.
11. Rudqvist IE, Cedermark B, Glas U, Johansson H, Nordenskjöold B, Skoog L, Somell A, Theve T, Friberg S, Askergren J. The Stockholm trial on adjuvant tamoxifen in early breast cancer. Breast Cancer Res Treat 1987;10:255–266.
12. Biance AR, Gallo C, Marinelli D, d'Istria M, de Placido S, Tagliarulo C, Petrella G, Del Rio G. Adjuvant therapy with tamoxifen in operable breast cancer: 10 years results of the Naples (GUN) study. Lancet 1988;2:1095–1099.
13. CRC Adjuvant Breast Trial Working Party. Cyclophosphamide and tamoxifen as adjuvant therapies in the management of breast cancer. Br J Cancer 1988;57:604–607.
14. Nolvadex Adjuvant Trial Organization. Contolled trial of Tamoxifen as a single adjuvant agent in the management of early breast cancer. Br J Cancer 1988;57:608–611.
15. Ribeiro G, Swindell R. The Christie Hospital adjuvant tamoxifen trial. Status at 10 years. Br J Cancer 1988;57:601–603.

16. Fisher B, Constantino J, Redmond C, Poisson R, Bowman D, Couture J, Dimitrov NV, Wolmark N, Wickerham DL, Fisher ER, Margolese R, Robidoux A, Shibata H, Terz J, Paterson AHG, Feldman MI, Farrar W, Evans J, Lickley HL, Ketner M, and others. A randomized clinical trial evaluating tamoxifen in the treatment of patients with node-negative breast cancer who have estrogen-receptor-positive tumors. N Engl J Med 1989;320:479–484.

17. Cummings FJ, Gray R, Tormey DC, Davis TE, Volk H, Harris J, Falkson G, Bennett JM. Adjuvant tamoxifen versus placebo in elderly women with node-positive breast cancer: long-term follow-up and causes of death. J Clin Oncol 1993;11:29–35.

18. Fisher B, Constantino J, Wickerham L, and others. Adjuvant therapy for node-negative breast cancer: an update of NSABP findings. Proc Am Soc Clin Oncol 1993;12:79.

19. Jordan VC, Allen KE, Dix CJ. Pharmocology of tamoxifen in laboratory animals. Cancer Treat Rep 1980;64:745–759.

20. Pento JT, Magarian RA, King MM. A comparison of the efficacy for antitumor activity of the non-steroidal antiestrogenss analog II and tamoxifen in 7,12-dimethylbenz[a]anthracene-induced rat mammary tumors. Cancer Lett 1982;15:261–269.

21. McCormick DL, Moon RC. Retinoid-tamoxifen interaction in mammary cancer chemoprevention. Carcinogenesis 1986;7:193–196.

22. Gottardis MM, Jordan VC. Antitumor actions of keokifene and tamoxifen in the N-nitrosomethylurea-induced rat mammary carcinoma model. Cancer Res 1987;47:4020–4024.

23. Teelmann K, Bollag W. Therapeutic effects of the arotenoid Ro 15-0778 on chemically induced rat mammary carcinoma. Eur J Cancer Clin Oncol. 1988;24:1205–1209.

24. Ratko TA, Detrisac CJ, Dinger NM, Thomas CF, Kelloff GJ, Moon RG. Chemopreventive efficacy of combined retinoid and tamoxifen treatment following surgical excision of a primary mammary cancer in female rats. Cancer Res 1989;49:4472–4476.

25. Jordan VC, Lababidi MK, Mirecki DM. Anti-oestrogenic and anti-tumour properties of prolonged tamoxifen therapy in C3H/OUJ mice. Eur J Cancer 1990;26:718–721.

26. Maltoni C, Pinto C, Paladini G. Project of experimental bioassays on chemoprevention agents performed at the Bologna Institute of Oncology: report on tamoxifen control of spontaneous mammary tumors on Sprague-Dawley rats. Cancer Invest 1988;6:643–658.

27. Maltoni C, Soffriti M, Pinto C, e Mobiglia A. Il contributo sperimentale alla chemioprevenzione. In: Morino F, Caldarola A, Mussa P, Calderini D, Carretti, Maltoni C (eds) Atti XIV Congresso Nazionale di Oncologia, Il Ruolo della Terapia Chirirgica in Oncologia, 2. Bologna: Monduzzi, 1988; 1073–1100.

28. Maltoni C, Pinto C, Mobiglia A, Soffritti M. La chemioprevenzione dei tumori: bilanci, richerche in corso e prospettive. In: Rasà G, Maltoni C, Amato S, Castiglione G, Grasso G, Palmeri ML, Cuva F. Aggiornamenti in Oncologia Medica. Bologna: Monduzzi, 1989;3–89.

29. Maltoni C, Pinto C, Soffritti M, Mobiglia A. La chemioprevenzione dei tumori della mammella: acquisizione disponibili, con particolare riguardo ai dati sperimentali. In: Maltoni C, Marrano D, Rubini S, Rivelli DF, Patella V (eds) I tumori della mammella. Bologna: Monduzzi, 1989;305–359.

30. Maltoni C, Minardi F, Pinto C, Soffritti M, Mobiglia A. Long-term Bioassays on the Toxic, Carcinogenic and Tumour Chemopreventive Effects (Particularly on Mammary Carcinomas) of Tamoxifen on Sprague-Dawley Rats: Ongoing Studies and Early Results. Acta Oncol 1990;11: 289–305.

31. Maltoni C, Pinto C, Mobiglia A, Soffritti M, Belli A. La chemioprevenzione dei tumori: lo stato attuale delle conoscenze ad il progetto di ricerca dell'Istituto di Oncologia di Bologna. In: Battelli T (ed) Aggiornamenti in Oncologia Medica. Bologna: Monduzzi, 1990;111–169.

32. Maltoni C, Pinto C, Soffritti M, Mobiglia A. Chemioprevenzione dei tumori della mammella. Argomenti di Oncologia 1990;11:1–22.

33. Maltoni C, Minardi F, Pinto C. Il tamoxifen come potenziale agente chemioprevenzione nel carcinoma mammario nella donna: scenario, presupposti scientifici, recenti acquisizione sperimentali e studi clinici disponibili e in programmazione. In: Robustelli della Cuna G, Pannuti F (eds) Progresi in Oncologia Clinica, Tamoxifene, 1. Pavia: Edizione Medico Scientifiche, 1991;117–138.

34. Maltoni C, Minardi F, Pinto C, Soffritti M, Belli A. Un nuovo approccio al controllo del carcinoma mammario nella donna: la chemioprevenzione. Adria Medica 1991;2:11–50.

35. Maltoni C, Minardi F, Pinto C, Soffritti M, Mobiglia A, Belli A. La chemioprevenzione del carcinoma mammario: bilancio delle conoscenze e prospettive. Atti delle Giornate Medico-Chirurgiche Internazionali in onore de Achille Mario Dogliotti, 1. Torino: Minerva Medica, 1991; 91–172.

36. Maltoni C, Minardi F, Pinto C, Soffritti M. La chemioprevenzione del carcinoma mammario: basi scientifiche e orientamenti. In: Batteli T, Manocchi P, Mattioli A, Pilone S, Delpret S, Rossini G, De Signoribus G, Silva RR, Carretti D, Maltoni C (eds) Atti del XVIII Conresso Nazionale di Oncologia, Il Cancro della Mammelle alle Soglie del Duemila, 1. Bologna: Monduzzi, 1992;127–142.

37. Maltoni C, Minardi F, Soffritti M, Pinto C, Paladini G. La prevenzione del carcinoma mammario: presupposti scientifici e programmi. Acta Oncol 1992;13:523–530.

38. Maltoni C, Minardi F, Soffritti M, Pinto C, Belpoggi F. The role of experimental research in cancer chemoprevention using human-equivalent animal models: a project on tamoxifen. In: Motta M, Serio M (eds) Sex Hormones and Antihormones in Endocrine Dependent Pathology: Basic and Clinical Aspects. Elsevier: Amsterdam, 1994;319–329.

39. Fisher B. The evolution of paradigms for the management of breast cancer: a personal perspective. Cancer Res 1992;52:2371–2383.

40. Love RR. The National Surgical Adjuvant Breast Project (NSABP) Breast cancer prevention trial revisited. Cancer Epidemiol Biomarker Prev 1993;2:403–407.

41. Lippman SM, Benner SE, Hong WK. Cancer chemoprevention. J Clin Oncol 1994;12:851–873.

42. Veronesi U, Maltoni C. Protocollo di chemioprevenzione del carcinoma mammario con tamoxifen.

43. Cuzick J. Protocol for the UKCCCR National Multicentre Tamoxifen Breast Cancer Prevention Trial, 1992.

44. Powles TJ, Jones AL, Ashley SE, O'Brien MER, Tidy VA, Treleaven JG, Cosgrove D, Nash AG, Sacks N, Baum M, McKinna JA, Davey JB. The Royal Marsden Hospital pilot tamoxifen chemoprevention trial. Breast Cancer Res Treat 1994;31:73:82.

45. Blackburn AM, Amiel SA, Millis RR, Rubens RD. Tamoxifen and liver damage. Br Med J 1984; 289:288.

46. Clarysse A. Hormone-induced tumor flare. Eur J Cancer Clin Oncol 1985;21:545–547.

47. Diver JM, Jackson IM, Fitzgerald JD. Letter to the editor, Tamoxifen and nonmalignant indication. Lancet 1986;1:733.

48. Smith I. Adjuvant tamoxifen for early breast cancer. Br J Cancer 1988;57:527–528.

49. Love RR. Prospects for antiestrogen chemoprevention of breast cancer. J Natl Cancer Inst 1989;82: 18–21.

50. Powles TJ, Hardy JR, Ashley SE, Cosgrove D, Davey JB, Dowsett M, McKinna A, Nash AG, Rundle SK, Sinnett HD, Tillyer CR, Treleaven JG. Chemoprevention of breast cancer. Breast Cancer Res Treat 1989;14:23–31.

51. Powles TJ, Hardy JR, Ashley SE, Farrington GM, Cosgrove D, Davey JB, Dowsett M, McKinna JA, Nash AG, Sinnett HD, Tillyer CR, Treleaven JG, A pilot trial to evaluate the acute toxicity and feasability of tamoxifen for prevention of breast cancer. Br J Cancer 1989;60:126–131.

52. Fornander T, RutQvist LE, Cedermark B, Glas U, Mattsson A, Silfversward C, Skoog A, Somell A, Theve T, Wilking N, Askergren J, Hjalmar ML. Adjuvant tamoxifen in early breast cancer: occurrence of new primary cancer. Lancet 1989;1:117–120.

53. Fisher B, Constantino JP, Redmond CK, Fisher ER, Wickerham DL, Cronin WM, and other NSABP Contributors. Endometrial cancer in tamoxifen-treated breast cancer patients: findings from the National Surgical Adjuvant Breast and Bowel Project (NSABP) B-14. J Natl Cancer Inst 1994;86: 527–537.

54. Williams GM, Iatropoulos MJ, Djordjevic MV, Kaltenberg OP. The triphenylethylene drug tamoxifen is a strong liver carcinogen in the rat. Carcinogenesis 1993;14:315–317.

55. Greaves P, Goonetilleke R, Nunn G, Topham J, Orton T. Two-year carcinogenicity study of tamoxifen in Alderly Park Wistar-derived rats. Cancer Res 1993;53:3919–3924.

56. Hard GC, Iatropoulos MJ, Jordan K, Radi L, Kaltenberg OP, Imondi AR, Williams GM. Major difference in the hepatocarcinogenicity and DNA adduct forming ability between toremifene and tamoxifen in female Crl: CD (BR) rats. Cancer Res 1993;53:4534—4541.

57. Hirsimäki P, Hirsimäki Y, Nieminen L, Payne BJ. Tamoxifen induces hepatocellular carcinoma in rat liver: a 1-year study with two antiestrogens. Arch Toxicol 1993;67:49—54.

58. Dragany YP, Fahey S, Street K, Vaughan J, Jordan VC, Pitot HC. Studies of tamoxifen in female Fischer F344 rats. Breast Cancer Res Treat 1994;31:11—25.

Psychological implications of tamoxifen treatment in women at high risk to breast cancer

Lesley Fallowfield

Communication and Counselling Research Centre, Department of Oncology, University College Hospitals Medical School, London, UK

Abstract. The epidemiological and experimental data suggesting the importance of oestrogen in the promotion of breast cancer and indications that antioestrogenic intervention with tamoxifen might prevent or delay expression of the disease in women at high genetic risk, has led to multicentre, randomised, prevention trials worldwide. Although early work with tamoxifen has suggested that physical toxicity is minimal, there have to date been no publications from controlled studies of the psychological or sexual impact of the long-term use of the drug in pre- and postmenopausal women. Such research is extremely important, if chemoprevention does produce unwanted psychosexual side effects, we need to be able to provide women with appropriate information about them and to design and offer ameliorative interventions. Failure to conduct this kind of research might well compromise compliance and undermine the first really major breakthrough in preventing breast cancer in an "at risk" population.

In this paper some early data are presented from British women participating in the International Breast Cancer Intervention Study (IBIS). This placebo-controlled double-blind randomised trial has provided us with a unique opportunity to conduct a parallel psychological study on a large cohort of women at increased risk to breast cancer.

Key words: anxiety, breast cancer, family history clinics, genetic counselling, screening, sexual activity.

Introduction

There have been many reports published showing that the diagnosis and treatment of breast cancer provokes considerable psychological, social and sexual difficulties for a significant minority of women [1]. The past 2 decades have seen increasing worldwide media attention being paid to both the physical and psychosocial sequelae of breast cancer and large numbers of articles have appeared in the lay press. This explosion of interest in the topic is due, in part, to the prevalence of the disease. In the Western world, the lifetime risk of a woman developing breast cancer is high and for reasons that are not clearly understood, the incidence rates appear to have been increasing by approximately 1% per annum over the last 20 years [2]. Breast cancer is clearly a major public health issue and more recently there has been a heightened awareness of the fact that some women may have an inherited predisposition to breast cancer that places them potentially at increased risk. The fears and anxiety women

---

Address for correspondence: Lesley Fallowfield, Communication and Counselling Research Centre, Department of Oncology, University College Hospitals Medical School, 48 Riding House Street, London W1P 7PL, UK.

have about the disease have been fuelled further by the publicity given to the identification of the BRCA 1 and 2 genes. Although the percentage of women who develop breast cancer because of their genetic predisposition is small (<5%) [3], the prevalence of the disease means that this still represents a large number of women. As well as considering the psychological effects, the increasing availability of genetic testing raises many difficult moral, ethical and legal issues that need more debate.

A vast literature now exists containing data on the psychosocial impact of treatment for breast cancer. Some of this research has been used to help develop effective ameliorative interventions such as counselling or support groups [4] or to change medical practice in ways that may prevent psychological trauma [5]. Unfortunately there is still a dearth of literature dealing with psychosocial factors in women who are at increased risk of breast cancer because of their family histories [6].

We have an urgent need to conduct more systematic psychosocial studies that would provide us with the information that we require when: 1) discussing personal risk factors with women, 2) recommending different surveillance and screening strategies, 3) encouraging participation in and adherence to early detection programmes, 4) helping women with decisions about prevention strategies, and 5) developing appropriate counselling and other supportive interventions for probands and their relatives who may be affected by the knowledge that they are at increased risk.

The International Breast Cancer Intervention Study (IBIS)

Clinicians in the UK have been participating in IBIS, a multicentre randomised trial of tamoxifen vs. placebo in women at high familial risk of breast cancer. This trial has provided us with a unique opportunity to address some of the behavioural consequences and important psychosocial issues that arise when dealing with women whose family histories place them at increased risk. The eligibility criteria for the main trial require that women are between 45 and 65 years old, and that they have a greater than 2-fold risk of breast cancer. Some younger women with an even higher risk may also be eligible. The primary aim of the parallel psychological study is to monitor the quality of life of women recruited to the tamoxifen trial. Particular attention is being paid to the impact that hormonal influences may have on vasomotor changes which in turn may affect libido and mood state. The way in which knowledge that one is at increased risk affects anxiety and behaviour, is also being investigated. The data collected will enable recommendations to be made about the specific communication and counselling needs of women at high risk to breast cancer. The results are vital if balanced information, support and reassurance are to be provided that will encourage and motivate asymptomatic women to take medication or accept surveillance over a long-term period.

To date 550 women have been recruited to the psychological arm of the study. We are also monitoring women who though eligible for the main trial decline an opportunity to participate. Until the code is broken revealing which study participants have been taking active drug and which placebo, results from data concerning many of the aims listed above cannot be reported. However, there are a few other interesting observations made already that will be discussed in this paper. These observations concern three main topics: 1) how women's estimates of the population risk of breast cancer influence their willingness to join a prevention trial [7], 2) the anxiety found in women at increased genetic risk of developing breast cancer who attend family history clinics compared with those who do not [8], and 3) the sexual activity of high risk women participating in the prevention study compared with that of other groups [9].

Risk perception

Women often have inaccurate perceptions about both their own personal risk and the general population risk of developing breast cancer, e.g., in a study of 242 women attending for routine mammographic screening as part of the UK National Breast Screening Programme, merely 14% knew the general population risk to be approximately one in 12 [10]. Among attenders of a family history clinic only 33% of 200 women correctly understood the general population risk and only 41% knew their own risk despite careful counselling [11].

Knowledge about the general population risk of developing breast cancer could be used as a reference point against which women could evaluate their own personal risk and this could then influence behaviour, e.g., women contemplating bilateral prophylactic mastectomy, mammographic surveillance or long-term chemoprevention, may base their decisions to decline or take part in such programmes, on a comparison of the perceived threat of breast cancer to women in general with their own personal perceived risk. We have investigated the relationship between knowledge of breast cancer risk in the general population and willingness to participate in the tamoxifen prevention trial.

A total of 149 women attending a breast cancer family history clinic, who were eligible to join the prevention trial, were asked to estimate whether the approximate chances of a woman in the UK getting breast cancer were less than one in 100, about one in 55 or one in 12. Data analysis showed that agreement to participate in the prevention trial was related to an individual's perception of risk in the general population. Of the 74 women who consented to join the trial, 51 (66%) correctly identified the general population risk to be one in 12. Significantly more, 63 (83%) of the 74 women who declined entry into the trial, knew the general population risk (p < 0.008) [7].

These results have some potentially important implications for the manner in which information is given to high risk women and highlights the necessity to check what an individual has understood. This is especially relevant when getting informed consent from asymptomatic women for treatment of uncertain efficacy and/or their participation in clinical trials. Perhaps estimates of personal risk should always be given in the context of general population risk. We have evidence suggesting that a high risk woman who believes the population risk to be one in 55 or one in 100, may well become alarmed and make inappropriate or uninformed decisions when told that her own risk is one in four. In contrast a woman who recognises that breast cancer risk is already high in the general population may decide against a prevention policy in which the long-term side effects and consequences are still unknown.

Relative risks are sometimes difficult to understand and odds ratios are very hard for lay people to comprehend and interpret appropriately. We can illustrate this problem with an hypothetical example of a woman with three sisters. This woman may well have sought advice at a family history clinic as she had a mother who died at an early age from breast cancer. She might well be told that her family history has increased her risk to one in four. If one of her sisters then develops breast cancer, she may correctly recognise that having two close relatives now with breast cancer places her at even higher risk. Unfortunately another woman might interpret this scenario entirely differently and reason that her own risk must now be diminished as her sister was the unlucky one in four who developed the disease! Another potential difficulty and confusion arises through individuals within the same family having different risks as odds ratios apply to the "average" woman with a family history not to an individual woman.

It is obvious that specialist counselling is necessary for women at high genetic risk and we could do with some innovative research aimed at helping geneticists and others to convey information to women in ways that are easier to understand and permit more appropriate decision making.

Anxiety

It is difficult to pick up a newspaper or magazine these days without encountering an article about breast cancer. Likewise there have been many television and radio programmes devoted to the topic. Not all of the information provided by the media is useful to women and it can exacerbate anxiety about the disease. It is hardly surprising that the prospect of developing breast cancer creates fear in many women even if they do not have a family history that puts them at much greater risk. There have been at least two reports in the US literature suggesting that women with a high familial risk attending family history clinics are especially anxious [12,13] but there are few published data concerning the anxiety of women who have a family history that places them at risk but who do not attend family history clinics. In the absence of such data it is possible, if one considers the US results, to assume that family history clinics either see a population of the most anxious women or that attendance creates or exacerbates anxiety.

In the UK, the risk perceptions and anxiety of 99 women participating in the tamoxifen prevention trial were compared with those of 87 women with and 86 women without a family history of breast cancer, who were attending for mammographic screening as part of the National Breast Screening Programme (NBSP) [8]. All subjects completed a questionnaire concerning knowledge about breast cancer and estimations of risk in the general population, together with a standardised anxiety inventory by Spielberger [14].

Results showed that the tamoxifen trial participants had a significantly more accurate view of the general population risk of breast cancer in comparison to the NBSP women (p = 0.004). Out of a total of 99, 47 of the trial participants recognised the risk to be approximately one in 12, in comparison to 44 of 173 women in the screening programme. Awareness of population risk did not differ between those women in the NBSP with a family history and those without. As far as anxiety was concerned, the least anxious women were the following: all the tamoxifen trial participants, all the NBSP women without a family history and the NBSP women with a family history who were also unaware of the risk in the general population. The most anxious women were those from the NBSP sample who did have a familial risk and who correctly recognised the general population risk. This group's mean Spielberger score of 45.5 (SD 9.5) was higher than a normal sample of women aged 50–69 without breast cancer, mean 31.79 (SD 7.78), and higher than that reported in women with breast cancer 34.86 (SD 9.95) [15].

These data can be interpreted in different ways. It could be that attending a family history clinic improves understanding about risk and that this, with the surveillance offered, reduces overall anxiety. Another explanation for the findings is that women with accurate risk perceptions who are also highly anxious, avoid such clinics. The results contradict the US findings of high anxiety in women attending clinics. The lowered anxiety in the UK sample might reflect cultural differences or differences in the counselling offered. The US data were from women attending clinics with a family history but who were not participating in a prevention programme. Despite the often hostile publicity surrounding the tamoxifen prevention trial, it could be that this participation in itself, rather than mere attendance at the clinic reduces anxiety.

Sexual activity

Hormonal therapy may exacerbate menopausal symptoms or induce an early menopause in younger women. Symptoms such as hot flushes, sweats, weight gain and emotional lability can significantly impair a woman's quality of life. Oestrogen deficiency may also reduce vaginal lubrication and this dryness can make intercourse less enjoyable, thus the menopause often affects sexual activity. Various studies of women undergoing a natural menopause report a decline in both sexual desire and sexual activity [16,17]. Women who experience a premature menopause in association with hormonal treatment for cancer, seem to suffer more sexual dysfunction, greater psychological distress and report more troubling menopausal symptoms in comparison with a healthy sample of women [18].

If tamoxifen does reduce breast cancer in women at high risk, then it is important that we have information available about the possible side effects of treatment including the impact that the drug may have on sexual activity. This would then allow asymptomatic women an opportunity to make some cost-benefit analysis before opting to take the drug. Furthermore a systematic study of unwanted effects may identify areas of difficulty that are potentially amenable to some intervention and highlight other problems that require the development of further ameliorative interventions.

The Sexual Activity Questionnaire (SAQ) was developed especially for use in the tamoxifen prevention trial [9]. It was felt that as most of the available standardised instruments had been developed for use in sexual dysfunction clinics they were either too lengthy or deemed unnecessarily explicit for the purposes of this study. The SAQ is a short 14 item self-report questionnaire with three scales that assess: 1) pleasure from sexual intercourse, i.e., desire, enjoyment and satisfaction, 2) discomfort, i.e., dryness and pain, and 3) habit, i.e., how usual was the reported sexual activity. For data, we have only baseline data from the study available. They show that the sexual functioning of our sample of high risk women is, not surprisingly, very similar to that of a normal population of women of similar age (35–65) years.

A total of 527 women completed the questionnaire and of these 108 (20.5%) were sexually inactive. The most frequently cited reason for celibacy was lack of a partner. Among the women who were sexually active, younger women reported higher frequencies of sex and there was a significant difference in the reported monthly frequency of sexual activity between menopausal categories. Premenopausal women were more sexually active than postmenopausal women including those taking HRT ($p = 0.0001$). Older women also indicated that sexual activity was less pleasurable for them than younger women ($p = 0.008$), although there was no interaction between hormonal status and pleasure scores. Older women in the sample also reported more discomfort from sexual activity. This was related to hormonal status with greatest discomfort in the postmenopausal, slightly less in those on HRT and lowest discomfort found in the premenopausal women ($p = 0.0001$).

The SAQ appears to be a reliable and sensitive measure of sexual activity that should provide us with the information that we need about the impact that tamoxifen has over a 5-year period in pre- and postmenopausal women in the chemoprevention trial.

Conclusions

The prevalence of breast cancer and the unpleasant sequelae of treatment makes the disease a worrying prospect for any woman. Recognition of the extra psychological burden imposed by the knowledge that a family history may place one at even greater risk is an increasingly important area of research. We need to increase our own knowledge about the effects that disclosure of genetic risk have on both individuals and their families, and to consider how information about risk is best conveyed. We also have to develop means of helping women who have an elevated risk, to make rational choices between such things as long-term surveillance, chemoprevention and prophylactic surgery.

Acknowledgements

The author wishes to thank the Cancer Research Campaign for their financial support of the research being conducted in the chemoprevention trial. She would also like to acknowledge the help of the study coordinators Dr Kathryn Thirlaway and Janice Osgood and clinical collaborators especially Drs Jack Cuzick, Trevor Powles, Anthony Howell and Gareth Evans.

References

1. Fallowfield LJ, Hall A. Psychosocial and sexual impact of diagnosis and treatment of breast cancer. Br Med Bull 1991;47:388–399.
2. American Cancer Society. Cancer Facts and Figures – 1992. A.C.S. Atlanta, USA 1991.
3. Evans DGR, Fentiman IS, Macpherson K et al. Familial breast cancer. Br Med J 1993;308:183–197.
4. Fallowfield LJ. Psychosocial interventions in cancer. Br Med J 1996;311:1316–1317.
5. Fallowfield LJ. Has psychosocial oncology helped in the management of women with breast cancer? Breast 1996;2(1):107–113.
6. Lynch HT, Lynch J, Conway T, Severin M. Psychological aspects of monitoring high risk women for breast cancer. Cancer 1994;74(Suppl 3):1184–1192.
7. Thirlaway K, Fallowfield LJ, Evans G, Howell A. Entry into the tamoxifen prevention trial depends on women's estimates of the population risk of breast cancer. Breast 1995;4:203–204.
8. Thirlaway K, Fallowfield L, Nunnerly H, Powles T. Anxiety in women "at risk" of developing breast cancer. Br J Cancer 1996;73:(In press).
9. Thirlaway K, Fallowfield L, Cuzick J. The sexual activity questionnaire: A measure of women's sexual functioning. Qual Life Res 1996;5:81–90.
10. Fallowfield LJ, Rodway A, Baum M. What are the psychological factors influencing attendance and re-attendance at a breast screening centre? J R Soc Med 1990;83:547–551.
11. Evans DGR, Blair V, Greenhalgh R, Hopwood P, Howell A. The impact of genetic counselling on risk perception in women with a family history of breast cancer. Br J Cancer 1994;70:934–938.
12. Kash KM, Weinberg GB, Small A, Hendon MS. Breast cancer screening among relatives of women with breast cancer. Am J Pub Health 1992;81:1174–1179.
13. Lerman C, Croyle R. Psychological issues in genetic screening for breast cancer susceptibility. Arch Int Med 1994;154:609–616.
14. Spielberger C. Manual for the State-Trait Anxiety Inventory. Consulting Psychologists Press, Palo Alto, CA. 1983.
15. Fallowfield LJ, Hall A, Maguire GP, Baum M. Psychological outcomes of different treatment policies in women with early breast cancer outside a clinical trial. Br Med J 1990;301:575–580.
16. Hunter M, Battersby R, Whitehead M. Relationships between psychological symptoms, somatic complaints and menopausal status. Maturitas 1986;8:217–218.
17. McCoy NL, Davidson JM. A longitudinal study of the effects of the menopause on sexuality. Maturitas 1985;87:203–210.
18. Moadel A, Ostroff JS, Lesko LM, Bajoronas DR. Psychosexual adjustment among women receiving hormone replacement therapy for premature menopause following cancer treatment. Psycho-oncology 1995;4:273–282.

Ongoing trials on the chemoprevention of breast cancer with tamoxifen

Alberto Costa, Virgilio Sacchini, Bernardo Bonanni, Peter Boyle, Umberto Veronesi and the Italian Tamoxifen Units

European Institute of Oncology, Milan, Italy

Abstract. Inhibition or reversal of breast carcinogenesis with Tamoxifen currently appears to be the most potentially successful chemopreventive strategy against breast cancer. To verify its efficacy, three major studies have been designed, in the UK, the USA and Italy. The design of the Italian study is similar to the US and the UK studies: it is a double-blind, randomized study with placebo vs. tamoxifen (20 mg/day), in healthy women aged 35 to 70. The main difference is in the target population, which is hysterectomised women only. The Italian study is showing the feasibility to run these chemoprevention trials in hysterectomized women, thus avoiding the risk of endometrial cancer, which is the major side effect of tamoxifen.

Drugs interfering with the initiation and promotion of breast cancer have recently allowed for the development of a new strategy for the reduction of the incidence of this disease. Experimental studies on the possibility of chemical tumor prevention with tamoxifen [1—7] and the clinical results relating to adjuvant tamoxifen in breast cancer patients over the past years [8—12] have emphasized that tamoxifen is the drug which best meets the requirements of effectiveness and tolerability in potentially preventing breast cancer. Myocardial infarction and bone fractures are less frequent in women treated with this drug [9], which also seems to have a beneficial effect on bone density [13—16], and in the prevention of cardiovascular illnesses [17—19]. Such observations have led to tamoxifen being considered as a possible agent to prevent or delay the development of breast cancer together with an increased control of cardiovascular diseases and osteoporosis in postmenopausal women.

In this framework, chemoprevention of breast cancer with tamoxifen represents a major effort involving the participation of some 12,000 women without breast cancer in long-term randomized trials, which commit them taking either tamoxifen or a placebo for 5 years [9—12,20]. Three of such studies (one in the UK, one in the USA, and a third one in Italy) are currently being conducted by randomizing healthy subjects, in a double-blind trial.

The major endpoint of the Italian trial is the reduction of incidence and mortality from breast cancer. Secondary endpoints are the effects on bone metabolism and related fractures [13—16], the effects on the cardiovascular system and the thrombo-

Address for correspondence: Virgilio Sacchini MD, European Institute of Oncology, via Ripamonti 435 20141 Milan, Italy. Tel.: +39-2-57489-719. Fax: +39-2-57489-725.

embolic events [17—20].

Since 1973, tamoxifen has been administered to more than 1 million women with breast cancer and to over 20,000 women in controlled studies for periods of 1 to 3 years without major long-term side effects [9—12,20]. Some minor side effects (gastrointestinal intolerance, fluid retention, anorexia, headache, depression, giddiness) were noted in a small percentage of cases (2—4%). However, the same effects were also seen in patients treated with placebo in the NATO study [11]. Some rare cases of thromboembolism (one/800 patients) have been observed during treatment with tamoxifen [20]. The incidence of deep venous thrombosis in the NSABP protocol B-14 on the evaluation of adjuvant tamoxifen in breast cancer patients was 1.3% for women taking tamoxifen vs. 0.2% for those taking placebo. However, a previous history of thrombophlebitis may be determinant in increasing this side effect, and the exclusion of such patients drastically reduces the incidence of thrombophlebitis in women taking tamoxifen. Macular degeneration has been reported as a side effect of tamoxifen in a Greek study [21]. There are no adequate data linking tamoxifen to ocular problems in controlled clinical trials. Menopausal symptoms (hot flushes, vaginal dryness and vaginal discharge) are often reported, but apart from a small number of cases, these symptoms are rather well-tolerated by most patients. This is because the above side effects usually occur only in the first few months of treatment, after which their intensity decreases. The cancers most frequently associated with tamoxifen treatment include endometrial carcinoma, hepatocellular carcinoma and gastrointestinal cancer.

Special attention was always devoted to the endometrial cancer issue. The increased incidence of endometrial cancer in patients treated with adjuvant tamoxifen which had appeared in a few articles [22—24] was the argument that convinced us to limit our trial to hysterectomized women only since the beginning. Although the role of tamoxifen in promoting endometrial cancer is still controversial, we have to consider the recent statement of the International Agency for Research on Cancer [25] that, "there is sufficient evidence in humans of the carcinogenicity of tamoxifen in increasing the risk of endometrial cancer".

These conclusions are actually no more than a confirmation of well-known studies and do not question the wider benefits of the drug in the treatment of hormone-dependent breast cancers which result in prolonging the survival and lowering the risk of a recurrence and of a second contralateral primary cancer [26—29]. Moreover, the risk of an endometrial cancer in patients taking tamoxifen as adjuvant treatment could well be assessed by a regular schedule of ultrasound monitoring of the uterus with transvaginal probe [30]. The risk of endometrial cancer in healthy women receiving tamoxifen in the frame of a chemoprevention trial is, of course, a different matter.

The investigators who had the major role in the conception of the Italian trial (U. Veronesi and C. Maltoni) never overlooked the risk on the endometrium and thus decided to design a trial addressed to hysterectomised women only to avoid any such risk [31]. This can well be considered a certainly safe decision, after the recent papers [29,32] published 3 years into the study.

Indeed, the NSABP-B14 trial in 2661 women with stage I breast cancer who received tamoxifen for 5 years as adjuvant treatment has shown a risk of contracting endometrial cancer approximately 7 times greater than that of randomized placebo subjects and more than 2 times greater than that of population-based rates. More importantly, a trend toward a higher mortality risk has also been observed, thus prompting the National Cancer Institute to instruct clinicians conducting the American study to re-write consent forms and ask all participants to re-sign [29].

Concerns about the development of hepatocellular carcinoma with tamoxifen are based solely upon laboratory experiments [33]. It has been reported that very large doses of tamoxifen produce liver tumors in rats [34—37] and DNA adducts in rat liver [38,39], while protein adducts have been noted in vitro. Adduct formation has not been demonstrated from patients taking tamoxifen and there are no reports of primary liver cancer in patients receiving tamoxifen 20 mg daily, while there have been such reports in two cases given 40 mg [23]. In the western world hepatocellular carcinoma is, however, a very rare disease (5/100.000 per year), and women taking oral contraceptives for 5—8 years have a 10-fold increased relative risk of developing this disease, an increase which is considered insignificant by epidemiologists.

A report on the data obtained from the Swedish tamoxifen study [40], known as the Stockholm Trial, seems to show more clearly an almost 6-fold increased risk of endometrial cancer and no increased risk of liver cancer in women taking 40 mg tamoxifen daily for 2 to 5 years (the increase of endometrial cancer was 3-fold in patients taking 20 mg tamoxifen daily for at least 5 years in the NSABP B-14 study). Additionally [41], they noted a trend towards an increased risk of stomach and colorectal cancers, although further research should be carried out to confirm this risk [40]. To further analyze their data, Rutqvist and his colleagues pooled information from the Stockholm trial with surveys of second cancers in two other studies, the Danish Breast Cancer Group Trial and the South Swedish Trial, in which women with breast cancer were randomised to receive postoperative radiotherapy with or without 30 mg tamoxifen daily for 1 year. The pooled analysis of risk for second cancers, on a total of 4914 subjects, showed a 3-fold increased risk of endometrial cancer, no increased risk of liver cancer, and a less than 2-fold increased risk of colorectal cancer (the NSABP B-14 trial has not reported any increased risk for gastrointestinal cancers). This analysis and the findings on colorectal cancers have been questioned [42,43], because of the differences in dose and treatment duration among the pooled studies and the variable risk factors from country to country. It has been suggested that the increased gastrointestinal risk might be limited to patients exposed to other treatments, like chemotherapy and radiotherapy; the combination of such treatments with tamoxifen may produce a synergistic effect for carcinogenesis. There has also been criticism on the usefulness and weaknesses of the pooled analysis of risk [43].

There are also new data suggesting that colorectal cancer risk is reduced by hormone replacement therapy in postmenopausal women [44—45].

Update of the Italian study

In October 1992, the coordinating center in Milan started randomization of eligible subjects. There are currently 48 units regularly randomizing. As of 31 December 1995, 4,320 women have been randomized in the study. The mean age is 51 years, with 77.5% of them belonging to the 45–64 age group. Of the 4,320 women, 45% contacted the centers spontaneously due to information programs, while 55% of these randomized women found in hospital record charts were contacted through letters or telephone calls.

Of the randomized women in the study, 21% have at least one first-degree relative with breast cancer, 96% of the participants have had a total hysterectomy, 3.7% a subtotal hysterectomy and 33% have had a hysterectomy without any ovarian surgery. Bilateral oophorectomy is associated with 47% of the women and monolateral oophorectomy with 20%.

Of all the randomized subjects, 16% were using estrogen replacement therapy (HRT) at the time of randomization; this is not an exclusion criterion in our trial. In every eligible subject we always assess the cardiovascular risk, based on the presence of one or more main or secondary risk factors. The results define a tentative cardiovascular score. Another baseline evaluation regards the menopausal symptomatology.

Preliminary data show a median time of exposure to the trial agents of 15.1 months. A total of 64% of the women reported complaints. The most frequent are menopausal disturbances, such as hot flushes (38.9%), vaginal dryness (12.3%), vaginal discharge (12.3%), gastrointestinal symptoms, especially nausea (6.8%), and urinary symptoms (6.8%).

Among the cardiovascular events, in the follow-up period observed, we registered mainly 28 venous vascular events divided into: one pulmonary embolism (PE), four deep vein thrombosis (DVT) of the lower limbs, 23 superficial thrombophlebitis (SPT) of the lower limbs. Five out of these 28 women were at least 60 years old (one PE and four SPT); no fatal outcome has been observed. PE and DVT were defined as major events and were diagnosed by an instrumental method, while SPT were defined as minor events and were diagnosed clinically; when SPT occurred an instrumental test (B mode venous ecoscan) was performed to exclude the presence of DVT.

Discussion

Chemoprevention is a new fascinating area of cancer control which aims at inhibiting the carcinogenic process and preventing cancer occurrence. Many compounds are under study for this purpose, and randomised clinical trials are ongoing to evaluate the effectiveness of potentially preventive agents and their long-term side effects.

From the biochemical point of view, breast cancer is an important model in which the carcinogenic process is influenced by hormonal reactions: the possible role of tamoxifen in preventing breast cancer might be due to its competitive binding to the estrogenic nuclear receptor, contrasting the promotion of estrogens in carcinogenesis. Other mechanisms under study hypothesize interaction with growth factors. To evaluate the effectiveness of tamoxifen in preventing breast cancer in healthy women, and to assess the risk-benefit ratio, three studies are in progress in the USA, UK and Italy. While the US and the UK trials are enrolling high-risk women only, the Italian study involves only hysterectomised women in order to avoid the endometrial risk of tamoxifen. Thus, the trial enrolls any healthy women between 35 and 70 years of age [31]. Statistical information on the Italian population revealed a prevalence of 500,000 hysterectomized women which was a base consideration for the feasibility of the study [46].

Menopausal symptoms are the major complaints reported during the study. In our series 17% out of 36% of hot flushes were already present at the baseline, but in contrast vaginal discharge or dryness, was present only in 5.4% at the baseline, vs. 22.3% reported at the follow-up. Hormone replacement therapy or estrogenic vaginal cream administered for a short period may reduce these menopausal symptoms, allowing the women to continue taking the pill (tamoxifen or placebo). Sixteen percent of the randomized women are taking estrogen replacement therapy plus tamoxifen or placebo since the beginning and this subgroup of women is carefully evaluated regarding possible side effects, alteration of hemocoagulatory parameters, liver function, lipid profile, bone density, in order to be alert to possible increased toxicity of this combination of drugs or synergistic action on bone or cardiovascular protection, compared to the group with only hormone replacement therapy and placebo.

Polls in a pilot clinical trial using tamoxifen and placebo, did not find a significant difference between these two groups regarding menopausal symptoms. The same finding was found by Fisher [47]. Although our trial may appear restrictive, being addressed to hysterectomized women only, the decision to protect the healthy participants appeared to be a priority at the time of the study design.

Identification of women at high risk for endometrial cancer due to tamoxifen may be achieved by means of intravaginal ultrasound or endometrial flow cytometry [48] and this may permit the trial being extended to general population. Moreover, better definition of high risk breast cancer patients by means of genetic markers [49] or serum hormonal levels [50] can justify the increased risk due to tamoxifen administration.

Acknowledgements

This work is supported by the Italian League against Cancer (Milan), the Italian Association for Cancer Research (Milan), the American-Italian Cancer Foundation (New York), the Italian Foundation for Cancer Research (Milan), the Foundation for the Training in Oncology (Milan), the National Research Council (Rome), the ASSILS (Rome) and the Italian Diagnostic Center (Milan).

Alberto Costa and Bernardo Bonanni work on a chemoprevention program supported by the Italian Foundation for Cancer Research (FIRC)

The authors would like to thank Aliana Guerrieri Gonzaga, MSc., for her assistance in the preparation of the manuscript.

232

References

1. Jordan VC et al. Suppression of mouse mammary tumorigenesis by long-term tamoxifen therapy. J Natl Cancer Inst 1991;83:492–496.
2. Jordan VC. Antitumour activity of the antioestrogen tamoxifen (ICI 46,474) in the dimethylbenzanthracene (DMBA) induced rat mammary carcinoma model. J Steroid Biochem 1974;5:354.
3. Sporn MB. Carcinogenesis and cancer: different perspectives on the same disease. Cancer Res 1991;51:6215–6218.
4. Maltoni C et al. Project of experimental bioessays on chemoprevention agents performed at the Bologna Institute of Oncology: report on tamoxifen control of spontaneous mammary tumours on Sprague-Dawley rats. Cancer Invest 1988;6:643–658.
5. Turcot-LeMay L, Kelley PA. Characterization of estradiol, progesterone and prolactin receptors in N-nitrosomethylurea-induced mammary tumours and effects of antioestrogen treatment on the development and growth of these tumours. Cancer Res 1980;40:3232–3240.
6. Jordan VC. Effect of tamoxifen (ICI 46,474) on initiation and growth of DMBA-rat mammary carcinomata. Eur J Cancer 1976;12:419–424.
7. Gottardis MM, Jordan VC. The antitumour actions of keoxifene and tamoxifen in the N-nitrosomethylurea-induced rat mammary carcinoma model. Cancer Res 1987;47:4020–4024.
8. Kedar RP et al. Effects of tamoxifen on uterus and ovaries of postmenopausal women in a randomised breast cancer prevention trial. Lancet 1994;343:1318–1321.
9. Stewart HJ et al. Scottish adjuvant tamoxifen trial at 10 years. International Congress on long-term antihormonal therapy for breast cancer. Lake Buena Vista, Florida, July 2, 1991;12.
10. Early Breast Cancer Trialists Collaborative Group. Systemic treatment of early breast cancer by hormonal, cytotoxic or immune therapy. Lancet 1992;339:1–15.
11. Nolvadex Adjuvant Trial Organisation (NATO). Controlled trial of tamoxifen as a single adjuvant agent in the management of early breast cancer. Lancet 1985;1:836–840.
12. Cancer Research Campaign Breast Cancer Trials Group. The effect of adjuvant tamoxifen: the latest results from the Cancer Research Adjunct Breast Trial. Eur J Oncol 1992;28A:904–907.
13. Love RR et al. Effect of tamoxifen on bone mineral density in postmenopausal women with breast cancer. N Engl J Med 1992;326:852–856.
14. Zylberberg B et al. Breast cancer: effect of tamoxifen on the mineral density of bone. Eur J Obstet Gynec Reprod Biol 1993;52:147–148.
15. Ward RL et al. Tamoxifen reduces bone turnover and prevents lumbar spine and proximal femoral bone loss in early postmenopausal women. Bone Miner 1993;22:87–94.
16. Kristensen B et al. Tamoxifen and bone metabolism in postmenopausal low risk breast cancer patients: a randomized study. J Clin Oncol 1994;12:992–997.
17. Love RR et al. Effects of tamoxifen on cardiovascular risk factors in postmenopausal women. Ann Int Med 1991;115:860–864.
18. Rutqvist LE, Mattson A. Cardiac and Thromboembolic morbidity among postmenopausal women with early-stage cancer in a randomized trial of adjuvant tamoxifen. J Natl Cancer Inst 1993;85:1398–1406.
19. McDonald CC, Stewart HJ. Fatal myocardial infarction in Scottish adjuvant tamoxifen trial. Br Med J 1991;303:435–437.
20. Saphner T et al. Venous and arterial thrombosis in patients who received adjuvant therapy for breast cancer. J Clin Oncol 1991;9:286–291.
21. Pavlidis NA et al. Clear evidence that long-term, low dose tamoxifen treatment can induce ocular toxicity. Cancer 1992;69:2961–2964.
22. Gottardis MM et al. Contrasting actions of tamoxifen in endometrial and breast tumor growth in the athymic mouse. Cancer Res 1988;44:4006–4010.
23. Fornander T et al. Adjuvant tamoxifen in early breast cancer: occurrence of new primary cancers. Lancet 1989;1:117–120.
24. Horwitz RI, Feintstein AR. Estrogens and endometrial cancer: responses to arguments and current

status of and epidemiological controversy. Am J Med 1986;81:503—507.

25. IARC Monographs on the evaluation of carcinogenic risks to humans, vol 66, (In press).

26. Fornander T et al. Descriptive clinicopathologic study of 17 patients with endometrial cancer during or after adjuvant tamoxifen in early breast cancer. J Natl Cancer Inst 1993;85:1850—1855.

27. van Leuwen FE et al. Risk of endometrial cancer after tamoxifen treatment of breast cancer. Lancet 1994;343:448—452.

28. Magriples U et al. High grade endometrial carcinoma in tamoxifen treated breast cancer patients. J Clin Oncol 1993;11:485—490.

29 Fisher B et al. Endometrial cancer in tamoxifen treated breast cancer patients: findings from the National Surgical Adjuvant Breast and Bowel Project(NSABP) B14. J Natl Cancer Inst 1994;86: 527—537.

30. Kedar RP et al. Effects of tamoxifen on uterus and ovaries of postmenopausal women in a randomized breast cancer prevention trial. Lancet 1994;343:1318—1321.

31. Veronesi U: for the Italian Tamoxifen Prevention Study (ITAMPS). Prevention of breast cancer with tamoxifen: the Italian study in hysterectomized women. Breast 1995;4:267—272.

32. Cuzick J. Methodologic aspects of prevention trials. In: Stoll BA (ed) Approaches to Breast Cancer Prevention. Amsterdam: Kluwer Academic Press, 1991;181—190.

33. Jordan VC. Tamoxifen for breast cancer prevention. Proc Soc Exp Biol Med 1995;208:144—149.

34. Wiliams GM et al. The triphenylethylene drug tamoxifen is a strong liver carcinogen in the rat. Carcinogenesis 1993;14:315—317.

35. Greaves P et al. Two year carcinogenicity study of tamoxifen in Alderley Park Wistar-derived rats. Cancer Res 1993;53:3919—3924.

36. Hard GC et al. Major differences in the hepatocarcinogenicity and DNA adduct forming ability between toremifene and tamoxifen in female CrL: CD (BR) rats. Cancer Res 1993;53:4534—4541.

37. Dragan YP et al. Tumor promotion as a target for oestrogen/antioestrogen effects in rat hepatocarcinogenesis. Prev Med 1991;20:15—26.

38. Han X, Liehr JG. Induction of covalent DNA adducts in rodents by tamoxifen. Cancer Res 1992;52:1360—1363.

39. White INH et al. Genotoxic potential of tamoxifen and analogues in female Fischer 344/n rats, DBA/2 and C557BL/6 mice and in human MCL-5 cells. Carcinogenesis 1992;13:2197—2203.

40. Furner SE et al. A case control study of large bowel cancer and hormone exposure in women. Cancer Res 1989;49:4936—4940.

41. Rutqvist LE et al. Adjuvant tamoxifen therapy for early stage breast cancer and second primary malignancies. J Natl Cancer Inst 1995;87:645—651.

42. Jordan VC. Tamoxifen tumourgenicity: a predictable concern. J Natl Cancer Inst 1995;87:623—626.

43. Simon R. Discovering the truth about tamoxifen: problems of multiplicity in statistical evaluation of biomedical data. J Natl Cancer Inst 1995;87:627—629.

44. Chute CG et al. A prospective study of reproductive history and exogenous estrogens on the risk of colorectal cancer in women. Epidemiology 1991;2:201—207.

45. Gerhard SS et al. Reproductive factors exogenous female hormones and colorectal cancer by subsite. Cancer Causes Control 1992;3:355—360.

46. Berrino F et al. Incidenza dei tumori e cause di morte in Lombardia. Notizie Sanitarie 10/85 Regione Lombardia March 1986;11—95.

47. Fisher B et al. A randomized clinical trial evaluating tamoxifen in the treatment of patients with node-negative breast cancer who have estrogen-receptor-positive tumors. N Engl J Med 1989;320: 479—484.

48. Decensi A et al. Effect of tamoxifen on endometrial proliferation. J Clin Oncol 1996;14:434—439.

49. Easton DF et al. Breast and ovarian incidence in BRCA1 mutation carriers. Am J Hum Genet 1995;56:265—271.

50. Berrino F et al. Serum sex hormone levels after menopause and subsequent breast cancer. J Natl Cancer Inst 1996;88:291—296.

Experimental studies on the chemopreventive effects of medroxyprogesterone acetate (MPA) on mammary cancer, using a human-equivalent animal model

Franco Minardi, Luciano Bua, Alberto Santi, Loretta Menarini, Silva Rossi and Cesare Maltoni

Cancer Research Centre, European Ramazzini Foundation of Oncology and Environmental Sciences, Bologna, Italy

Abstract. *Background.* Because of the maturative effect of progestins on mammary gland cells, and of some evidence of therapeutical effects of these hormones on advanced mammary cancer, medroxyprogesterone acetate (MPA), the major progestin drug used in oncology, has been submitted to an experimental bioassay to evaluate its chemopreventive effects on mammary carcinogenesis in rats.

Material and Methods. MPA was tested on female Sprague-Dawley rats, which develop spontaneous tumours that must be considered equivalent to the human counterpart. MPA was administered to groups of 139–144 56-week-old female rats, at the daily doses of 83.3 (group I), 33.3 (group II), 1.7 (group III), 0 (group IV) mg/kg b.w., in water suspension, by stomach tube, once daily, 6 times weekly, for 40 weeks, after which the animals were sacrificed.

Results. The number of mammary cancers/100 animals, and the Protection Index (PI) in the various groups of the experiment, resulted as follows: 7.2 in the control group, 0.7 in group III (PI = 90.3), 0 in group II (PI = 100) and 1.4 in group I (PI = 80.5).

Conclusions. In the tested conditions MPA shows a strong chemopreventive effect on mammary cancer. Further experimental studies are now ongoing to assess such chemopreventive potential more extensively, and to obtain information on side effects.

Key words: chemoprevention, rat, mammary cancer, medroxyprogesterone acetate.

Introduction

Progestins are considered maturative hormones for the mammary gland and endometrium. Because of the antagonism between proliferation and maturation, theoretically progestins can be assumed as drugs eligible to be tested for the chemoprevention of mammary and endometrial cancers. Moreover, one of the most used progestins in clinical oncology, medroxyprogesterone acetate (MPA) has been shown to have an antitumour effect on DMBA-induced mammary cancer in female rats, which is similar to the one of ovariectomy, at the dose of 100 mg/kg b.w. [1]. When administered at doses ≥500 mg, MPA induces a temporary partial remission of advanced mammary cancer in postmenopausal women [2].

Address for correspondence: Dr Franco Minardi, Cancer Research Centre, European Ramazzini Foundation of Oncology and Environmental Sciences, Castle of Bentivoglio, 40010 Bentivoglio, Bologna, Italy.

For these reasons MPA has been included in the list of drugs to be tested for their eligibility for mammary cancer chemoprevention, in the framework of a project of experimental studies of tumour chemoprevention ongoing in our laboratory.

As all the other compounds studied in the project, MPA has been tested on spontaneous mammary carcinogenesis in female Sprague-Dawley rats of the colony of CRC/BT. Spontaneous mammary tumours in the females of this colony of rats are very similar to the ones in women for incidence, age-equivalent time of onset, biological behaviour and morphology, to such an extent that they may be considered human equivalent.

This report deals with the results of this bioassay. To our knowledge these results are the first dealing with the chemopreventive effects of the progestins on mammary cancer.

Plan of the experiment, materials and methods

The plan of the experiment, which was started in 1991, is shown in Table 1.

The MPA tested is the one marketed by Upjohn, under the commercial name of Depo-Provera.

The tested animals were female Sprague-Dawley rats of the colony which has been used for 30 years in the laboratories of the CRC/BT, for which there is extensive information on expected non-neoplastic and neoplastic pathology, available for about 10,000 control animals.

In this strain, the incidence of mammary tumours is of the same order as that observed in women in industrial countries. Within the years in which the experiment herein presented was performed, usually mammary cancer arises in about 10% of the females (range 7–12%), and the number of mammary cancers per 100 animals ranges from nine to 13 (since the same animal can bear more than one mammary malignancy). The distribution by equivalent ages in this animal model and in woman overlaps. The mammary cancers show all the various morphological patterns which characterise the human types and subtypes.

The animals were weaned at 5 weeks of age, identified by ear punch and randomized in order to have no more than one animal of each litter in the same group. From weaning, the animals received feed and water ad libitum. The animals were housed five per cage, in makrolon cages with a solid top of stainless steel. A

Table 1. Plan of the experiment on the chemopreventive effect of MPA on the incidence of spontaneous mammary cancer in female Sprague-Dawley rats (Exp. BT 12T).

Group	Daily dose/mg/kg b.w.	Animals	
		Age at start/weeks	No.
I	83.3	56	139
II	33.3	56	134
III	1.7	56	141
IV	0	56	139

shallow layer of white wood shavings served as bedding. The animals were kept in a temperature-controlled laboratory at 19–20°C, with 12-h light-dark intermittence.

MPA was administered, by stomach tube, in 1 ml of water suspension once daily, 6 times weekly, at the doses of 83.3, 33.3, 1.7 mg/kg b.w., corresponding to 5,000, 2,000, 100 mg in a woman of 60 kg, while water alone was administered to the control group. The animals were treated from 56 weeks of age, and kept under continuous treatment and control for 40 weeks, and then sacrificed at 96 weeks of age (since between 56 and 96 weeks of age the highest onset of mammary cancer in the untreated animals is observed).

The animals were submitted daily to observation, and feed and water consumption and body weight were measured periodically (weekly within the first 13 weeks of experiment, and then every 2 weeks). The gross lesions, with particular regard to the mammary lumps, were described and recorded every 2 weeks.

At death, all animals were submitted to systematic necropsy. Specimens for histopathology include mammary glands, mammary tumours, brain, pituitary gland, Zymbal glands, salivary glands, Harderian glands, head (five sections) (with oral and nasal cavities, and external and internal ear ducts), tongue, thyroid and parathyroids, pharynx, larynx, thymus and mediastinal lymph nodes, trachea, lung, heart, diaphragm, liver, spleen, pancreas, kidneys and adrenal glands, oesophagus, stomach, intestine (four levels), bladder, uterus, vagina, ovaries, interscapular fat pad, sub-cutaneous and mesenteric lymph nodes, femur, and any other organs and tissues with pathological lesions. The histological slides were examined independently by two pathologists, and then reviewed by a third pathologist.

The experiment was performed in compliance with the Good Laboratory Practices (GLP).

Results

Feed and water consumption

No differences in feed and water consumption were observed among the groups.

Body weight

In all the groups treated with MPA there was a slight increase of mean body weight, which was not dose related (Fig. 1).

Survival

MPA treatment, at the three tested doses, does not affect the survival (Fig. 2).

Nononcological changes

No evident behavioural changes were found in MPA-treated animals.

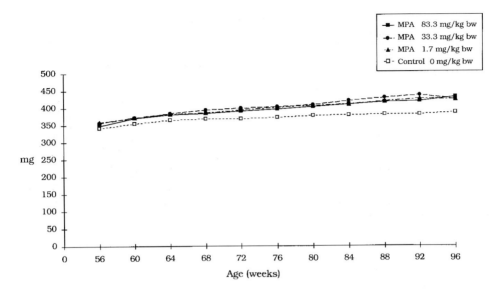

Fig. 1. Mean body weight of female Sprague-Dawley rats treated with different levels of MPA.

Carcinogenic and anticarcinogenic (chemopreventive) effects

The incidence of mammary cancer is reported in Table 2. There was a sharp decrease of mammary cancer in all the MPA-treated groups. No difference in the morphology of tumours was found.

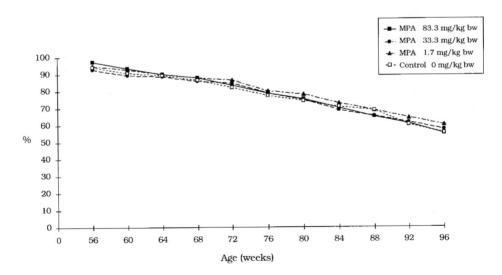

Fig. 2. Survival of female Sprague-Dawley rats treated with different levels of MPA.

Table 2. Incidence of mammary cancer in female Sprague-Dawley rats following treatment with MPA delivered at different doses (Exp. BT 12T).

Group	Animals No.	Daily dose/ mg/kg b.w.	Malignant mammary tumours				
			Animals with tumours		Tumours		
			No.	%	No.[a]	Per 100 animals	Protection index[b]
I	139	83.3	2	1.4	2[c]	1.4	80.5
II	134	33.3	0	—	0	—	100.0
III	141	1.7	1	0.7	1[c]	0.7	90.3
IV	139	0	8	5.7	10[d]	7.2	—

[a]One animal can bear more than one tumour; [b]percentage decrease of tumour incidence (referred to tumours/100 animals; [c]adenocarcinomas; [d]nine adenocarcinomas and one liposarcoma.

Discussion and Conclusion

The present results show that MPA, in the tested experimental conditions, has a strong chemopreventive effect on mammary cancer, very similar to that observed with tamoxifen in the same animal model [3,4].

The fact that the average protection index due to the drug is about 90 means that the onset of the majority of the carcinogenic foci is blocked by progestins.

These observations call for further studies to assess whether and how progestins in general, and MPA in particular, alone or in association, can be used for mammary cancer chemoprevention. A study has been undertaken at the CRC/BT to assess the chemopreventive effects on mammary carcinogenesis of very low doses of MPA associated with very low doses of tamoxifen and leuprolide.

The strong inhibitory effect of MPA on the early stages of carcinogenesis, as demonstrated by the results herein presented, suggests a different approach in the use of MPA in cancer hormonotherapy. To date this drug has been used as a second line drug, when the tumours are far advanced and in general less hormone (progestin)-dependent. Clinical trials should now be planned to assess the effect of MPA as a drug for adjuvant therapy and for the therapy of mammary cancer at early recurrences.

However, before extending the use of MPA to chemoprevention and to adjuvant therapy, further scientific information is needed to know the long-term effects of this drug. A life-span bioassay of MPA, aimed at assessing its side effects, is in the list of priorities of the CRC/BT.

References

1. Danguy A, Legros N, Devleeshoumer N, Heuson-Stennon JA, Heuson JC. Effects of medroxyprogesterone acetate (MPA) on growth of DMBA-induced rat mammary tumors: histopathological and endocrine studies. In: Jacobelli S, Di Marco A (eds) Role of Medroxyprogesterone in Endocrine-Related Tumors. New York: Raven Press, 1980;21–28.

2. Pannuti F, Martoni A, Zamagni C, Melotti B. Progestins I: medroxyprogesterone acetate. In: Powles TJ, Smith IE (eds) Medical Management of Breast Cancer. London: Martin Dunitz, 1991;95—103.
3. Maltoni C, Pinto C, Paladini G. Project of experimental bioassays on chemoprevention agents performed at the Bologna Institute of Oncology: report on tamoxifen control of spontaneous mammary tumours in Sprague-Dawley rats. Cancer Invest 1988;6:643—658.
4. Maltoni C, Minardi F, Soffritti M, Pinto C, Belpoggi F. The role of experimental research in cancer chemoprevention using human-equivalent animal models: a project on tamoxifen. In: Motta M, Serio M (eds) Sex Hormones and Antihormones in Endocrine Dependent Pathology: Basic and Clinical Aspects. Amsterdam: Elsevier, 1994;319—329.

Results of experimental bioassays on the chemopreventive effects of vitamin A and N-(4-hydroxyphenyl)-retinamide (HPR) on mammary cancer

Morando Soffritti, Alberto Mobiglia, Carmine Pinto, Lucia Bortoluzzi, Giuseppe Lefemine and Cesare Maltoni

Cancer Research Centre, European Ramazzini Foundation of Oncology and Environmental Sciences, Bologna, Italy

Abstract. *Background.* The reported experiments were conducted to assess the chemopreventive effects, on mammary cancer in rats, of vitamin A and 4-(N-hydroxyphenyl)-retinamide (HPR), which have been considered eligible for the chemoprevention of breast cancer in women without adequate experimental bases.

Materials and methods. Vitamin A (retinol acetate and palmitate) and HPR were tested on female Sprague-Dawley rats, which develop spontaneous tumours, that must be considered equivalent to their human counterpart. Vitamin A was administered in the diet to groups of 200 6-week-old female rats, at the dose levels of 3,900 (group I), 16,900 (group II), 75,000 (group III), 150,000 (group IV) IU per kg of feed, for the life-span. HPR was administered to groups of 107—108 56-week-old female rats, at the dose levels of 0 (group I) and 33 (group II) mg/kg b.w., by stomach tube, in water suspension, once daily, six times weekly, for 38 weeks, after which the animals were sacrificed at 94 weeks of age.

Results. The number of mammary cancers/100 animals in the vitamin A experiment resulted as follows: 7.5 in group I, 16.0 in group II, 16.0 in group III, 18.5 in group IV. The number of mammary cancers/100 animals in the HPR experiment was as follows: 19.4 in group I, 15.9 in group II.

Conclusion. In the tested animal system, vitamin A and HPR failed to show chemopreventive effects on mammary carcinogenesis. On the contrary vitamin A is associated with an increase of mammary cancer.

Key words: 4-(N-hydroxyphenyl)-retinamide, carcinogenesis, chemoprevention, mammary cancer, rat, vitamin A.

Introduction

Previous studies seemed to suggest that a high intake of vitamin A (retinol) and of correlated compounds (such as β-carotene and retinoids) might be associated with a reduced risk of cancer. In particular, some epidemiological studies have indicated that the intake of vegetables rich in β-carotene is associated with a decreased risk of malignancies, especially of lung cancer [1,2].

Several authors have also suggested that vitamin A and vitamin A analogs may inhibit the onset of mammary carcinomas [3—5], however, such hypotheses lack solid

Address for correspondence: Dott. Morando Soffritti, Cancer Research Centre, European Ramazzini Foundation of Oncology and Environmental Sciences, Castle of Bentivoglio, 40010 Bentivoglio, Bologna, Italy.

experimental, epidemiological and clinical bases.

The claim that vitamin A and its analogs, other vitamins, such as vitamin C and vitamin E, and other micronutrients may be inhibitors of carcinogenesis and may protect mankind from carcinogenic risk, has become a widespread belief. Such a belief has in turn generated widespread dietary fashions, an increased human intake of "protective" drugs, and to some extent a major readiness to accept exogenous carcinogenic risks, on the basis of the assumption that there are possible antidotes. Rarely in the history of modern medicine, has such a widespread phenomenon been based on so little scientific evidence.

In recent years, five major clinical trials have been conducted to investigate the tumour chemopreventive effects of vitamin A and its analogs. Two of these trials study the chemopreventive effects of vitamin A and β-carotene on lung cancer in high risk groups [6,7]. Two other trials deal with the cancer chemopreventive effects of β-carotene in males (physicians) and women [7]. A fifth study was planned to evaluate the chemopreventive effects of the retinoid HPR, on the onset of contra-lateral breast carcinoma in women who had undergone mastectomy for breast cancer [8].

It is surprising that these five trials, which recruited about 82,500 apparently healthy people, which involved many physicians and scientists, and which required a huge economical commitment, were performed without any scientific evidence or on the basis of equivocal data, and more specifically without any adequate experimental support.

In 1986 a large systematic and integrated project, which included 14 experiments, was started, aimed at evaluating the cancer chemopreventive effects of vitamin A (retinyl palmitate and acetate) and of HPR on the various spontaneous tumours of male and female Sprague-Dawley rats, of the colony which has been used and studied in our laboratory, for nearly 30 years. This project has been performed on a large number of animals and has required, to present, near 9,000 animals.

This report refers the results of two experiments on the effects of vitamin A and HPR, respectively, on the incidence of malignant mammary tumours in female rats.

Plan of the experiments, Materials and Methods

The plans of the experiments, which were started in 1986 (BT 8001) and 1988 (BT 4T), are shown in Tables 1 and 2.

Vitamin A (retinol acetate and palmitate) was supplied by Roche SpA. HPR was supplied by McNeil Pharmaceuticals (through the National Tumour Institute of Milan).

The tested animal were female Sprague-Dawley rats of the colony which has been used for 30 years in the laboratories of the CRC/BT, for which there is extensive information on expected nonneoplastic and neoplastic pathology, available for about 10,000 control animals.

In this strain, the incidence of mammary tumours is of the same order as that observed in women in industrial countries. The distribution by equivalent ages in this

Table 1. Plan of the experiment of the chemopreventive effect of vitamin A in the diet on the incidence of spontaneous malignant mammary tumours in female Sprague-Dawley rats (Exp. BT 8001).

Group	Vitamin A levels (IU/kg of diet)	Animals	
		Age at start (weeks)	No.
I	3900	6	200
II	16900	6	200
III	75000	6	200
IV	150000	6	200

animal model and in woman overlaps. The mammary cancers show all the various morphological patterns which characterise the human types and subtypes.

Vitamin A was added to the standard diet, without any vitamin supplement (the lower tested level), in accordance with the different experimental regimens required. HPR was supplied in water, and 1 ml of the suspension was administered by stomach tube, once daily, six times weekly; 1 ml of water was administered to the control animals in the same way.

The animals were weaned at 5 weeks of age, identified by ear punch and randomized in order to have no more than one animal of each litter in the same group of each experiment. From weaning, the animals received feed and water ad libitum. The animals were housed five per cage, in makrolon cages with a solid top of stainless steel. A shallow layer of white wood shavings served as bedding. The animals were kept in a temperature-controlled laboratory at 19–20°C, with 12-h light-dark intermittence.

In the experiment on vitamin A (Table 1) the animals were treated from 6 weeks of age, and kept under continuous treatment with various regimens of vitamin A and under observation for the life-span. In the experiment with HPR (Table 2) the animals were treated from 56 weeks of age, kept under continuous treatment and control for 38 weeks, and then sacrificed at 94 weeks of age (since between 56 and 94 weeks of age the higher onset of mammary cancer in the untreated animals was observed).

The animals were submitted daily to observation; feed and water consumption and body weight were measured periodically (weekly within the first 13 weeks of experiment, and then every 2 weeks). The gross lesions, with particular regard to the mammary lumps, were described and recorded every 2 weeks.

At death, all animals were submitted to systematic necropsy. Specimens for

Table 2. Plan of the experiment on the chemopreventive effect of HPR by gavage on the incidence of spontaneous malignant mammary tumours in female Sprague-Dawley rats (Exp. BT 4T).

Group	Daily dose (mg/kg b.w.)	Animals	
		Age at start (weeks)	No.
I	0	56	108
II	33	56	107

histopathology include mammary glands, mammary tumours, brain, pituitary gland, Zymbal glands, salivary glands, Harderian glands, head (five sections) (with oral and nasal cavities and external and internal ear ducts), tongue, thyroid and parathyroids, pharynx, larynx, thymus and mediastinal lymph nodes, trachea, lung, heart, diaphragm, liver, spleen, pancreas, kidneys and adrenal glands, oesophagus, stomach, intestine (four levels), bladder, uterus, vagina, ovaries, interscapular fat pad, subcutaneous and mesenteric lymph nodes, femur, and any other organs and tissues with pathological lesions. The histological slides were examined independently by two pathologists, and then reviewed by a third pathologist.

The experiments were performed in compliance with the Good Laboratory Practices (GLP).

Results

Experiment on vitamin A

— Feed and water consumption: no differences in feed and water consumption were observed in the different groups.
— Body weight: among the groups no difference in mean body weight was observed (Fig. 1).
— Survival: no difference was observed in survival of the different groups (Fig. 2).
— Nononcological changes. No evident behavioural changes were found among the four groups of animals.
— Carcinogenic and anticarcinogenic (chemopreventive) effects: the incidence of

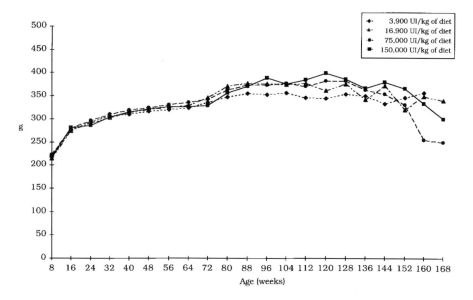

Fig. 1. Mean body weight of female Sprague-Dawley rats treated with different levels of vitamin A (Exp. BT 8001).

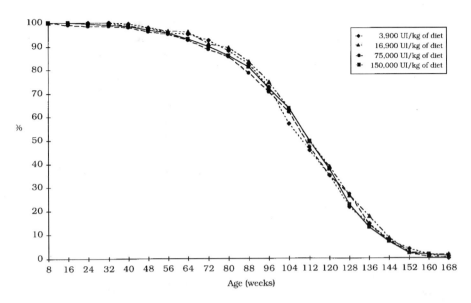

Fig. 2. Survival of female Sprague-Dawley rats treated with different levels of vitamin A (Exp. BT 8001).

malignant mammary tumours is reported in Table 3. In the three groups with the highest levels of vitamin A in their diet, there is a higher onset of mammary malignancies, without, however, a defined dose-response relationship.

Experiment on HPR

— Feed and water consumption: no differences were found in feed consumption between the control and the HPR-treated animals. A slight decrease of drinking water consumption was noticed in the treated group (Fig. 3).
— Body weight: the HPR-treated animals showed a slight decrease of body weight (Fig. 4).

Table 3. Incidence of malignant mammary tumours in female Sprague-Dawley rats treated with different levels of vitamin A (Exp. BT 8001).

Group	Vitamin A levels (IU/ kg of diet)	Animals (No.)	Malignant mammary tumours			
			Animals with tumours		Tumours	
			No.	%	No.[a]	Per 100 animals
I	3900	200	11	5.5	15[b,c]	7.5
II	16900	200	27	13.5	32[b]	16.0
III	75000	200	26	13.0	32[b,c]	16.0
IV	150000	200	30	15.0	37[b]	18.5

[a]One animal can bear more than one carcinoma; [b]adenocarcinomas; [c]one with sarcomatous component.

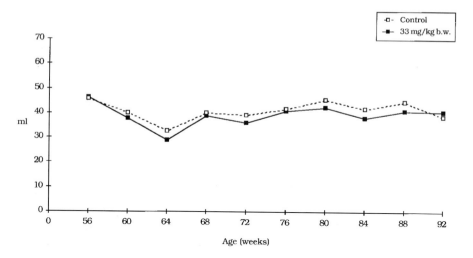

Fig. 3. Water consumption of female Sprague-Dawley rats, untreated (control) and treated with HPR (Exp. BT 4T).

— Survival: no difference in survival rates in the two groups was observed (Fig. 5).
— Nononcological changes: no evident behavioural changes were found among the two groups of animals.
— Carcinogenic and anticarcinogenic (chemopreventive) effects: practically no differences were observed in the incidence of malignant mammary tumours between the animals in the control and treated groups (Table 4).

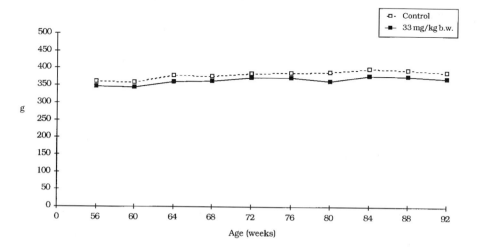

Fig. 4. Body weight of female Sprague-Dawley rats, untreated (control) and treated with HPR (Exp. BT 4T).

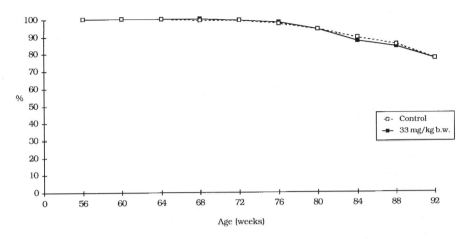

Fig. 5. Survival of female Sprague-Dawley rats, untreated (control) and treated with HPR (Exp. BT 4T).

Conclusion and Discussion

In the experimental conditions described above, a higher incidence of mammary cancer has been observed in the three groups of females whose diet was supplemented with vitamin A. In these three groups the incidence of mammary cancer is more than doubled when compared to that found in the animals whose diet contained the lowest level of vitamin A.

The increased incidence of malignant mammary tumours observed in the three groups with the highest levels of vitamin A intake, does not parallel the increased intake of vitamin A; this may be due to metabolic saturation.

Our results do not prove that vitamin A has any protective effect on mammary cancer, but rather show that vitamin A increases the onset of this malignancy.

On the basis of our data, this effect cannot be explained by the variation in body weight of the various groups, nor can it be biased by the variation in mortality between the groups.

No chemopreventive effects of HPR on mammary carcinogenesis have been demonstrated by the reported experiment.

Table 4. Incidence of malignant mammary tumours in female Sprague-Dawley rats untreated (control) and treated with HPR (Exp. BT 4T).

Group	Daily dose (mg/kg b.w.)	Animals (No.)	Malignant mammary tumours			
			Animals with tumours		Tumours	
			No.	%	No.[a]	Per 100 animals
I	108	0	10	9.3	21[b]	19.4
II	107	33	9	8.4	17[b]	15.8

[a]One animal can bear more than one carcinoma; [b]adenocarcinomas.

All together the presented data do not support the claim that vitamin A and HPR can prevent mammary cancer, but rather show that an excess of vitamin A may entail a carcinogenic risk. The far-reaching implications of these results should be given adequate consideration in order to avoid the risk of cancers derived from an excess intake of retinol.

From a more general point of view, the reported data indicate that any hypothesis in medicine must be scientifically proved before being presented as a fact, and before being used as a basis for public health policy.

The time has come to design scientific protocols to establish the eligibility of drugs for cancer chemoprevention, on the basis of defined advantages and possible disadvantages. In such a protocol, bioassays on animal systems represent a mathematically precise tool (less cancers, same cancers, more cancers) which must not be eluded.

Such a protocol appears to be still more urgently needed if one considers the recent disappointing results of three of the major five trials on vitamin A, β-carotene and HPR [1,2,6,7], stated and conducted before acquiring experimental proofs of the benefits of such treatments. The available results of the two trials on the chemopreventive effects of vitamin A and β-carotene on lung cancer in high risk groups show a higher incidence of cancers in participants taking the two compounds [6,7]. In the trial on physicians, after more than 12 years of treatment, no significant benefit of β-carotene on cancer was found.

Acknowledgements

The experimental project has been partially supported by the "Associazione Italiana per la Ricerca sul Cancro" (AIRC) (Italian Association for the Research on Cancer), Milan.

References

1. Peto R, Doll R, Buckley JD, Sporn MB. Can dietary beta-carotene materially reduce human cancer rates? Nature 1981;290:201–208.
2. National Research Council. Diet, nutrition, and cancer. Washington DC: National Academy Press, 1982.
3. Sporn MB, Dunlop NM, Newton DL, Smith JM. Prevention of chemical carcinogenesis by vitamin A and its synthetic analogs (retinoids). Fed Proc 1976;35:1332–1338.
4. Moon RC, Grubbs CJ, Sporn MB, Goodman DG. Retinyl acetate inhibits mammary carcinogenesis induced by N-methyl-N-nitrosourea. Nature 1977;267:620–621.
5. Moon RC, McCormick DL, Mehta RG. Inhibition of carcinogenesis induced by retinoids. Cancer Res 1983;43(Suppl):2469–2475.
6. The Alpha-Tocopherol, Beta-Carotene Cancer Prevention Study Group. The effect of vitamin E and beta carotene on the incidence of lung cancer and other cancers in male smokers. N Engl J Med 1994;330:1029–1035.
7. National Institutes of Health, US Department of Health and Human Services. Beta-carotene and vitamin A halted in lung cancer prevention trial. Embargoes for release, January 18, 1996.
8. Costa A, Formelli F, Chiesa F, Decensi A, De Palo G, Veronesi U. Prospects of chemoprevention of human cancers with the synthetic retinoid fenretinide. Cancer Res 1994;54(Suppl):2032–2037.

Ongoing clinical chemoprevention study of breast cancer with fenretinide

G. De Palo[1], T. Camerini[1], E. Marubini[1], F. Formelli[1], R. Miceli[1], L. Mariani[1], A. Costa[2], U. Veronesi[2], C. Maltoni[3], M. Rosselli Del Turco[4], A. Decensi[5], F. Boccardo[5] and G. D'Aiuto[6]

[1]Istituto Nazionale Tumori, Milan; [2]European Institute of Oncology, Milan; [3]Istituto di Oncologia "F. Addarii", Bologna; [4]Centro per lo Studio e la Prevenzione Oncologica, Florence; [5]Istituto Scientifico Tumori, Genoa; and [6]Istituto Tumori "Fondazione Pascale", Naples, Italy

Abstract. The aim of the study was to test the efficacy of fenretinide (4-HPR) in the prevention of contralateral primary in women already treated for breast cancer. Patients operated on for T1/T2 N-breast cancer who have not received any kind of adjuvant therapy and without relapse of the disease were randomized, after an informative written consent, into two groups: 4-HPR at the dose of 200 mg p.o. daily vs. no treatment (control (CTR) group). The duration of treatment was 5 years plus 2 years of follow-up. Treated and untreated patients had the same clinical and laboratory follow-up. The study started in March 1987 and accrual was closed on 31 July 1993. A total of 2,848 patients (1,421 in the 4-HPR group and 1,427 in the CTR group) are available. The groups are well-balanced for age, menopausal status, tumour size, type of surgery and histology. The status of study at February 12, 1996 is the following: 560 patients are ongoing, 1,345 patients have completed the first 5 years and 943 patients have interrupted the study for: complaints (62 in the 4-HPR group, 26 in the CTR group), refusals (175 in the 4-HPR group, 75 in the CTR group), intercurrent events not related to the disease (82 in the 4-HPR group, 45 in the CTR group), unfavourable events (213 in the 4-HPR group, 255 in the CTR group) and other causes (four in the 4-HPR group, six in the CTR group). At this time no differences are seen in the rate of contralateral breast cancer. Follow-up is ongoing.

Key words: breast cancer, chemoprevention, fenretinide.

Introduction

There is experimental evidence for the efficacy of the synthetic retinoid fenretinide (N-(4-hydroxyphenyl)retinamide) (4-HPR) in the prevention of breast cancer. The inhibition of chemically induced mammary carcinoma in rats by 4-HPR was first described by Moon et al. [1]. In vivo evaluations showed that 4-HPR significantly reduced the overall incidence of mammary tumours and the latency of tumour development in carcinogen-treated rats and in nulliparous mice [1]. It also inhibited the appearance of subsequent mammary tumours following removal of the first palpable tumour in carcinogen-treated rats [2]. 4-HPR inhibition of carcinogenesis was enhanced by oophorectomy in rats with nitrosomethylurea-induced mammary

---

Address for correspondence: Prof G. De Palo, Istituto Nazionale Tumori, via Venezian 1, 20133 Milan, Italy.

cancer [3]. When 4-HPR was administered in the diet of rats whose first tumours were surgically removed, these animals had fewer recurrences and delayed latency compared with the control group. When the first tumour was not removed, 4-HPR induced a regression of the lumps to a nonpalpable stage [4]. 4-HPR has been shown to work synergistically with the antioestrogen drug tamoxifen in inhibiting the induction of mammary tumours in carcinogen-treated rats. Furthermore, the combination of 4-HPR and tamoxifen was shown to be more effective than treatment with either agent alone in blocking the progression of mammary tumours following removal of the first palpable mammary tumour [5]. A study in humans has shown that 4-HPR decreases circulating serum levels of insulin-like growth factor 1 (IGF-1), which is a potent mitogen for human breast cancer cells in vitro [6].

4-HPR appears to be better tolerated than other retinoids with lower toxicity and teratogenicity [7,8]. However, 4-HPR causes dermatological side effects, although its dermatological tolerability is good even after more than 3 years of administration. The major adverse effect of 4-HPR is impaired dark adaptation (nictalopia). Impaired dark adaptation is the result of decreased retinol serum levels together with a proportional decrease in RBP levels, with consequent interference with retinal function. Impaired dark adaptation is dose-related, reversible upon drug interruption, and the incidence is low with a daily dose of 200 mg (reviewed in [9—11]).

Breast cancer is the most common malignant tumour in women of western countries, with a continuously rising incidence. The incidence curve rises suddenly at 45 years and at 70 years. Breast cancer is the primary cause of cancer death in women 35—55 years old. Early diagnosis and improved treatment are known to increase the survival rate, but reducing incidence would be even better, and chemoprevention appears promising.

The high incidence of breast cancer and the above-mentioned characteristics of 4-HPR led one of us (U. Veronesi) to the idea of using this compound to prevent contralateral primaries in women already treated for breast cancer, whose risk is 0.8% per year within 10 years from primary treatment. The final objective is obvious. If 4-HPR can succeed in preventing second primaries in breast cancer patients, it could possibly be useful for a wider group of subjects with high breast cancer risk. The study was supported by a grant from the NIH-NCI of Bethesda.

Material and Methods

The randomized study was planned according to a design with two arms: intervention vs. no treatment. Patients in the intervention group were treated with 4-HPR at 200 mg p.o. daily, a dosage that results in minimal adverse effects based on data of the phase I study. Since 4-HPR lowers plasma retinol levels, and vitamin A deficiency is associated with impaired dark adaptation, a 3-day drug holiday at the end of each month was planned to allow a recovery of retinol concentration (reviewed in [9—11]). Furthermore, it was recommended that 4-HPR be taken after a meal when absorption is higher [12].

Treatment duration was 5 years. The 5-year treatment duration was based on the assumption that the possible efficacy of 4-HPR to halve the risk of contralateral breast cancer may be expected from the 3rd year onwards (3-year lag time).

Study participants were breast cancer patients aged 30–70 years, treated with ablative or conservative (plus radiotherapy) surgery for T1 tumour (less than 2 cm) or T2 tumour (less than 5 cm), all infiltrating types without nodal metastases. In order to be eligible, patients had to have no evidence of local recurrences and/or distant metastases, and no previous treatment with adjuvant chemotherapy and/or hormone therapy. They had to have normal metabolic and liver function tests, and avoid pregnancy during the study. Ineligibility criteria were concomitant or previous neoplastic disease (with the exception of basal cell carcinoma of the skin and cervical intraepithelial neoplasia), lobular carcinoma in situ (LCIS) or Paget's disease, geographic inaccessibility or neuropsychiatric difficulties and those who are related to the physicians or participating in another study. The same applied to patients with ocular or other concomitant diseases. Patients with intraductal carcinoma were considered as protocol deviation and were admitted to the study. Patients were able to enter the study through one of the two mechanisms: those identified as potentially eligible through a review of the medical records, and those operated on after 1 March 1987 and proven eligible.

The following tests were performed at baseline: general objective examination, dermatologic examination, ocular questionnaire, laboratory findings (HB, HT, WBC, PLTS, SGOT, SGPT, BIL, AP, total proteins, BUN, creatinine, blood sugar, cholesterol, triglycerides, retinol blood levels), pregnancy test (for those of childbearing age), mammography, chest X-ray, bone scan, liver echography. The ocular questionnaire was designed to assess dark adaptation, low-light vision and recovery after dazzling. The ocular questionnaire was considered positive if at least two out of three items were positive, doubtful if one out of three was positive, and negative when no item was positive. If by this test the visual function was judged normal, the subject was considered eligible. The ocular questionnaire was performed at each control visit. Both groups, intervention and control, were followed with the same tests: physical examination and laboratory determination every 6 months, mammography, chest X-ray and liver echography every year, bone scan at 18, 36 and 60 months, and 4-HPR and retinol levels each year in all treated patients.

The sample size was calculated as follows: assuming a 3-year lag time needed to obtain full intervention efficacy, a 50% reduction of the incidence rate of contralateral breast cancer, a 2-year follow-up of all patients after the end of intervention, and a 10% drop-out rate [13], by using the procedure described by Wu et al. [14], the total sample size was established at 3,500 subjects, so as to yield a 90% power for a two-sided test.

Complaints were subdivided in four categories: general, dermatologic, ophthalmologic and visual. General complaints were nausea/vomiting, diarrhea, dyspeptic syndrome, dizziness, etc. Dermatologic complaints included dryness of skin and mucosae, itching, desquamation, etc. Ophthalmologic complaints were conjunctivitis, ocular dryness, etc. Visual complaints consisted in a positive or doubtful ophthalmologic questionnaire with positive, doubtful or negative electroretinogram. With the exception of visual complaints, the severity of the symptom was left to the physician's estimation for definition. The criteria used for establishing the side effect in laboratory values have been previously reported [15].

All the records and flow sheets were regularly reviewed. Protocol violations, complaints, intercurrent and unfavourable events were discussed in a collegiate manner. Intercurrent events were all the events not related to the disease which occur during follow-up (e.g., hepatitis, cardiomyopathy, pregnancy, etc.). Unfavourable events were relapses (local, regional, distant), second new primaries, contralateral breast cancer. They were considered at the time they were cytologically histologically radiologically documented. Intraductal carcinoma was considered as an unfavourable event, while lobular in situ carcinoma was not considered as an unfavourable event.

Results

The study started in March 1987 and accrual closed on 31 July 1993. At this time 2,848 patients (1,421 in the 4-HPR group and 1,427 in the control group) were available. The two groups are well-balanced for age, menopausal status, primary tumour treatment, histology, tumour size and number of years from primary surgery to randomization.

The compliance to 4-HPR treatment was evaluated by pill count. Compliance is high: 90.2% of patients who are still ongoing and 90.5% of patients who completed treatment have a compliance rate between 90–100%.

By February 1996, out of 2,848 available patients, 1,345 completed the first 5 years, 560 are still ongoing, and 943 patients had interrupted the study for: complaints (62 in the 4-HPR group, 26 in the CTR group), refusals (175 in the 4-HPR group, 75 in the CTR group), intercurrent events (82 in the 4-HPR group, 45 in the CTR group), unfavourable events (213 in the 4-HPR group, 255 in the CTR group) and other causes (four in the 4-HPR group, six in the CTR group) (Table 1). The total number of first unfavourable events (local, regional or distant relapse, new primary in other sites and contralateral breast cancer) is 622 (Table 2). The number of unfavourable events is reported according to the total number of available patients, based on the concept of "intention to treat" (randomized therefore analyzed), i.e.

Table 1. 4-HPR breast cancer study, status of study at 12 February 1996.

	4-HPR	CTR	Total
Evaluable patients	1421	1427	2848
Ongoing	254	306	560
Completed the first 5 years	631	714	1345
Discontinued	**536 (38%)**	**407 (28.5%)**	**943**
Complaints	62	26	88
Refusals	175	75	250
Intercurrent events	82	45	127
Unfavourable events	213	255	468
Lost	4	6	10

Table 2. 4-HPR breast cancer study, total number of first unfavourable events at 12 February 1996.

	4-HRP	CTR	Total
Evaluable patients	1421	1427	2848
With unfavourable event	313[a]	309[b]	622
Local relapse	88	103	191
Regional relapse	27	11	38
Distant relapse	120	118	238
Contralateral breast cancer	47	51	98
New primary	31	26	57

[a]After treatment discontinuation in 60 patients and after treatment completion in 40 patients; [b]after discontinuation in 54 patients.

including patients with treatment discontinuation for refusal, intercurrent events or complaints. The CTR group shows 309 first unfavourable events of which 255 occurred within the first 5 years. In the 4-HPR group there are 313 first unfavourable events, of which 60 occurred after treatment discontinuation for other causes (refusal, complaints, intercurrent events) and 40 after completion of the 5-year treatment. At this time no differences are seen in the rate on contralateral breast cancer in the two groups, although it is worthy of note that considering the incidence of contralateral breast cancer according to menopausal status at randomization, there is a trend in favour of premenopausal patients of the 4-HPR group. The study is ongoing and the 5-year intervention plan will end in December 1997.

Conclusion

It is well-known that cancer chemoprevention trials are difficult to implement since they require a large number of participants, a long follow-up period, and a high compliance rate. This is particularly true when healthy subjects are considered, and the endpoint of the study tumour incidence. But it is also true when the population under study is represented by patients in which the endpoint is the prevention of a new tumour. In this type of study, the eligible subjects are often not willing to enter the trial so that the accrual period tends to be prolonged. The long follow-up period, required to observe a sufficient number of events, has as consequence the risk of a high drop-out rate.

Our study started on March 1987 and accrual was closed at July 1993. Although the approach to eligible subjects has been difficult (data not yet published), the accrual was completed in 77 months and the drop-out rate, estimated at 10%, was 9%. The planned 5-year period is not yet completed in 560 patients and the estimated end of the first 5-year intervention plan is at December 1997. Since the incidence of contralateral breast cancer is defined as the occurrence of a new cancer in the opposite breast at any time during the whole period of observation (intervention: 5 years; and follow-up: 2 years), the analysis will be a comparison between the curves for the cumulative incidence of a contralateral breast cancer over time when all patients will have been followed for 7 years. Therefore the results of the efficacy of 4-HPR in the prevention of contralateral breast cancer are not yet available.

References

1. Moon RC, Thompson HJ, Becci JP, Grubbs JC, Gander RJ, Newton DL, Smith JM, Phillips SL, Henderson WR, Mullen TT, Brown CC, Sporn MB. N-(4-hydroxyphenyl) retinamide. A new retinoid for prevention of breast cancer in rat. Cancer Res 1979;39:1339–1346.
2. Moon RC, Pritchard JF, Mehta RG, Nomides CT, Thomas CF, Dinger NM. Suppression of rat mammary cancer development by N-(4-hydroxyphenyl)retinamide (4-HPR) following surgical removal of first palpable tumor. Carcinogenesis 1989;10:1645–1649.
3. McCormick DL, Mehta RG, Thompson CA. Enhanced inhibition of mammary carcinogenesis by combined treatment with N-(4-hydroxyphenyl)retinamide and ovariectomy. Cancer Res 1982;42:508–512.
4. Dowlatshahi K, Mehta RG, Thomas CF, Dinger NM, Moon RC. Therapeutic effect of N-(4-hydroxyphenyl)retinamide on N-methyl-N-nitrosourea-induced rat mammary cancer. Cancer Lett 1989;47:187–192.
5. Ratko TA, Detrisac DJ, Dinger NM, Thomas CF, Kelloff GJ, Moon RC. Chemopreventive efficacy of combined retinoid and tamoxifen treatment following surgical excision of a primary mammary cancer in female rats. Cancer Res 1989;49:4472–4476.
6. Torrisi R, Pensa F, Orengo MA, Catsafados E, Ponzani P, Boccardo F, Costa A, Decensi A. The synthetic retinoid fenretinide lowers plasma insulin-like growth factor I levels in breast cancer patients. Cancer Res 1993;53:4769–4771.
7. Paulson JD, Oldham JW, Preston RF. Lack of genotoxicity of the cancer chemopreventive agent N-(4-hydroxyphenyl) retinamide. Fundam Appl Toxicol 1985;5:144–149.
8. Kenel MF, Krayer JH, Merz EA. Teratogenicity of N-(4-hydroxyphenyl)-all-trans-retinamide in rats and rabbits. Teratog Carcinog Mutag 1988;8:1–11.
9. Costa A, Formelli F, Chiesa F, Decensi A, De Palo G, Veronesi U. Prospects of chemoprevention of human cancers with the synthetic retinoid fenretinide. Cancer Res 1994;54:2032s–2037s.
10. Decensi A, Formelli F, Torrisi R, De Palo G, Costa A. Fenretinide in breast cancer chemoprevention (review). Oncology Reports 1994;1:817–824.
11. De Palo G, Veronesi U, Marubini E, Camerini T, Chiesa F, Nava M, Formelli F, Del Vecchio M, Costa A, Boracchi P, Mariani L. Controlled clinical trials with fenretinide in breast cancer, basal cell carcinoma and oral leukoplakia. J Cell Biochem 1995;22(Suppl):11–17.
12. Doose DR, Minn FL, Stellar S, Nayak RK. Effects of meals and meal composition on the bioavailability of fenretinide. J Clin Pharm 1992;32:1089–1095.
13. Veronesi U, De Palo G, Costa A, Formelli F, Marubini E, Del Vecchio M. Chemoprevention of breast cancer with retinoids. JNCI Monogr 1992;12:93–97.
14. Wu M, Fisher M, De Mets D. Sample size for long-term medical trial with time-dependent dropout and event rates. Contr Clin Trials 1980;1:109–111.
15. Veronesi U, De Palo G, Costa A, Del Vecchio M, Marubini E, Coopmans de Yoldi GF, Attili A, Mascotti G, Moglia D, Magni A, Cerrotta A, Delle Grottaglie M, Crippa A, Palvarini M, Maltoni C, Rosselli Del Turco M, Saccani G, Boccardo F. Controlled clinical trial with fenretinide in the prevention of contralateral breast cancer. Rationale, design, methodological approach and accrual. In: De Palo G, Sporn M, Veronesi U (eds) Progress and Perspectives in Chemoprevention of Cancer, vol 79. Serono Symposia: Raven Press, 1992;243–259.

Chemoprevention — where we are

The Scientific Bases of Cancer Chemoprevention.
C. Maltoni, M. Soffritti and W. Davis, editors.

257

An overview of recent results of chemoprevention trials

Eva Buiatti

Epidemiology Unit, Centre for Cancer Study and Prevention, Florence, Italy

Abstract. *Background.* Results from four large and well-designed chemoprevention trials on β-carotene, other micronutrients and cancer risk have become recently available: the ATBC, CARET, Linxian and Physicians Health Study (PHS). These results, although preliminary, originated a wide discussion on methodological issues and public health concerns.

Methods. This paper compares the four studies in terms of population involved, smoking habits, baseline levels of β-carotene, doses and duration of treatment and outcomes.

Results. Two studies were negative for lung cancer (PHS and Linxian, though the second suggested a nonsignificant protective effect) the other two showed a significant positive association between treatment with β-carotene and lung cancer risk. The Linxian study, but not the ATBC, also evidenced a protection of treatment on stomach cancer.

Conclusions. The two studies showing a positive association with lung cancer incidence/mortality are based on heavy smokers, treated with 20–30 mg/day of β-carotene after the age of 40 for 5 years. Interaction with smoking of β-carotene at high doses in the late stages of carcinogenesis is strongly suspected. These findings do not necessarily contradict previous results from observational studies, but they practically exclude β-carotene from possible chemopreventive agents on lung cancer. Its effect on other cancer sites in nonsmokers is still under question.

Key words: β-carotene, lung cancer, smoking.

Introduction

Measuring the effect of chemopreventive agents in human populations has become one of the main objectives in cancer research. While new potential chemopreventive agents are being developed through laboratory research and animal experiments, several of these are already being experimented in human subjects.

Randomised, double-blind chemoprevention trials are universally recognised as the gold standard design for evaluating chemopreventive action in humans [1]. In these, the main potential biases of observational studies, i.e., information and selection bias, are in principle excluded. In fact, according to a recent review [2], near to 100 chemoprevention trials on cancer of different sites are ongoing, testing a wide range of chemicals, and sometimes involving thousands of subjects.

Only a few of the largest and more promising trials have by now reached the state of publishing the first results. These, however, have been often controversial or unexpected.

Address for correspondence: Eva Buiatti, Epidemiology Unit, Centre for Cancer Study and Prevention, Health Unit 10, Via di San Salvi 12, 50136 Florence, Italy.

The aim of the present paper is to compare study design, how they were conducted and outcomes of the main trials for which by now results are available.

Chemopreventive trials: agents tested, dose ranges and cancer sites

In a review published in 1994, 91 cancer prevention trials published or ongoing during the 1990s were evaluated [2]. Out of these, 78 were testing one or more specific chemopreventive agents, 12 were aimed to evaluating the preventive potential of dietary changes, and one was a vaccination trial.

In Table 1 the distribution of the chemopreventive trials by agent(s) tested, cancer

Table 1. Summary of treatments used in prevention and chemoprevention trials by cancer site.

Treatment	Cancer site	Number of trials			Dose-range
		Published	On-going	Total	
Vitamin A	Oral	2	1	3	50–60 mg/week
	Lung	1	3	4	25–50,000 IU/d
	Skin	–	3	3	25000 IU/d
	Total	3	7	10	
Vitamin C	Colon	1	–	1	3 g/day
	Stomach	–	2	2	2 g/day
	Total	1	2	3	
Synthetic	Oral	2	1	3	0.25–2 mg/kg/d
retinoids	Cervix	–	1	1	topic
	Lung	–	1	1	
	Skin	2	3	5	5–70 mg/d
	Head and neck	1	2	3	50–100 mg/mc
	Breast	–	1	1	200 mg/d
	Total	5	9	14	
β-carotene	Colon	–	2	2	30 mg/d
	Oral	3	1	4	15/40 mg/d
	Cervix	–	1	1	18 mg/d
	Lung	1	5	6	20–50 mg/d
	Skin	1	1	2	50 mg/d
	Stomach	1	1	–	
	Total	6	11	15	
Other	Oral	–	1	1	
vitamins	Cervix	1	1	2	
	Lung	1	1	2	
	Total	2	3	5	
Combined	Colon	1	3	4	
vitamins	Oral	2	2	4	
	Oesoph.	1	1	2	
	Cervix	–	1	1	
	Lung	–	3	3	
	Stomach	–	2	2	
	Total	4	12	16	

site, and dose-range is presented. A majority of these trials (64%) involve vitamins, their precursors or derivatives tested on a wide variety of epithelial cancers (colon, oral, oesophagus, lung, cervical, skin, head and neck, breast, stomach). The more frequently represented agents, alone or in combination, are β-carotene (alone in 16, in combination in 10 trials), retinol (administered alone or in combination in 23 trials) synthetic retinoids (alone in 14, in combination in one trial), and calcium (tested in 13 trials on colon and oesophageal cancers).

The criteria for having chosen a certain dose are not always reported in detail. Quite wide variation is shown for the same chemical, even larger when the cumulative dose (dose × time of treatment) is considered because of the further variation of length of treatment. In some studies, the baseline level of the agent in the population is considered as determinant for the choice of the dose; in others, the dose is related with the expected pharmacological effect, based on experimental studies, independent of the baseline level.

The interest shown in the potentialities of vitamins, their precursors and derivatives for a chemopreventive effect on cancer is based on a large amount of evidence, especially with reference to β-carotene. Exposure to high levels of β-carotene, measured as estimates of intake and/or as plasma levels, has been inversely correlated with the risk of epithelial lung, oral cavity, oesophagus, colon and stomach cancers in numerous and consistent case-control and cohort studies [3,4]. In fact, such an amount of consistent evidence from observational epidemiological studies on exposures related with cancer occurrence has seldom been available. Animal studies have further contributed to identify this agent as a promising chemopreventive candidate [5,6].

The evidence on vitamin A, vitamin E and calcium is not as consistent in epidemiological studies, but their potential beneficial effect is strongly suggested by in vitro and animal studies [7].

Four major trials on β-carotene, other vitamins and microelements: comparison of early results

Four trials using β-carotene alone or in combination with other agents have now published or anticipated their early results: the Linxian study on oesophageal and stomach cancer [8]; the α-tocopherol, β-carotene cancer prevention study (ATBC) on lung cancer [9]; the β-carotene and retinol efficacy trial (CARET) on lung cancer [10,11] and the Physician Health Study (PHS) [12]. In Table 2 these are described in terms of the subjects involved, the area in which they were conducted and the target organ(s). The four studies differ widely in terms of characteristics of the population: while the ATBC and the CARET trial involve heavy smokers and subjects at very high risk for lung cancer (asbestos exposed who are or were heavy smokers), the Linxian study and the PHS refer to groups from the general population which have an exposure to cigarettes lower than the average, being in one case a Chinese population and in the other US physicians; further, the Linxian trial has been developed in an area with environmental, dietary, general health conditions typical

Table 2. Populations involved and primary target cancer sites of four large chemopreventive trials (Linxian [8], ATBC [9], CARET [10,11] and PHS [12]).

Study	Population	Area	Target organ
Linxian	General	China	Oesophagus, stomach
ATBC	Male Smokers	Finland	Lung
CARET	Smokers, ex-smokers[a], asbestos exp.[b]	USA	Lung
PHS	Male physicians	USA	Epithelial cancers

[a]Former smokers since less than 5 years; [b]exposed to asbestos (20% with positive X-rays, 46% with positive X-rays and positive occupational history, 34% with positive occupational history) who are currently smokers or former smokers since less than 5 years.

of third world, while the other studies refer to Western populations. In Table 3, the size of the trials, age groups, agents employed, dose and duration of treatment are compared.

Doses of β-carotene range from 15 mg/day in the Linxian study to 30 mg/day in the CARET trial. In the Linxian study doses are in the range of those used in

Table 3. Size, chemopreventive agents, dose and duration of treatment in the four chemoprevention trials (Linxian, ATBC, CARET and PHS) dealing with β-carotene, other antioxidants and trace elements as preventative agents.

Study	Population	Age	Agent[a]	Dose	Duration
Linxian	29584 (males + females)	40—69	1. ret + zinc 2. ribof + niac 3. VitC + molyb. 4. Bcar + VitE + selenium 5. placebo	5000 IU + 15 mg 3.2 mg + 40 mg 120 mg + 30 μg 15 mg + 30 mg + 50 μg	5 years
ATBC	29133 (male smokers)	50—69	1. VitE 2. Bcar 3. VitE + Bcar 4. placebo	50 mg 20 mg	5—8 years
CARET	14254 smokers or ex-smokers, 4060 asb. exp. and smokers or ex-smokers (males + females)	50—69	1. VitA + Bcar 2. placebo	25000 IU + 30 mg	stopped at 4 years
PHS (1987)	22071	40—84	1. Bcar 2. asp 3. Bcar + asp 4. placebo	50 mg/2 days 325 mg/2 days	13 years

[a]ret = retinol, ribof = riboflavin, niac = niacin, molyb = molybdenum, Bcar = β-carotene, asp = aspirin.

Table 4. Cigarette smoking in the four trials.

Study	Smokers	Average amount
Linxian	30% (males)	
ATBC	all	20 cigarettes/day × 36 years
CARET	66% (60% males and 40% females)	40–49 pack/year
	44% former smokers <5 years	
PHS	11% (51% former smokers)	

deprived populations for supplementation [8]. In the other trials, doses were chosen as those possibly assuring a high pharmacological activity [12].

The only study which involves a wide range of age groups is the PHS (40–84). The same also implies the longest duration of treatment (13 years).

In Table 4 the smoking habits of the subjects involved in the trials are described in more detail. The PHS participants are apparently those at the lowest exposure to cigarette smoking, although no information is given on the average amount of cigarettes/day of the 30% smokers in the Linxian population. Taking into account the very low recorded lung cancer death rates (see below), the use of cigarettes by these subjects must have been recent and sporadic.

Baseline levels of β-carotene are also different in the study groups (Tables 5 and 6), being very similar in Finnish and US smokers, while they are almost 3 times lower in Linxian. In this last case, the 5-year period of the trial corresponded with changes in food availability in the general population [13], with a doubling in vitamin levels in the placebo arm. Compared with average levels of β-carotene in Western populations, as expected, the Finnish smokers in the ATBC study and the CARET

Table 5. The ATBC study: baseline levels and effect of supplementation on β-carotene and α-tocopherol seric levels (mg/Lt).

Agent	Median	Ratio 2/1
α-tocopherol		
Treatment		
1. baseline	11.5	1.5
2. at 3 years	17.3	
Placebo		
1. baseline	11.4	
2. at 3 years	12.4	1.1
β-carotene		
Treatment		
1. baseline	0.17	
2. at 3 years	3.0	17.6
Placebo		
1. baseline	0.17	
2. at 3 years	0.18	1.1

From [9], modified

Table 6. The Linxian study: baseline levels (mean and SD) and effect of supplementation with β-carotene + selenium + vitE on β-carotene plasmatic levels (mg/Lt); (values adjusted for season). The CARET study: effect of β-carotene and retinol supplementation on β-carotene baseline levels.

Study	Mean	SD	Ratio 2/1
Linxian trial			
β-carotene			
1. baseline	0.059	0.052	14.5
2. at 5 years	0.855	0.785	
Placebo			
1. baseline	0.068	0.058	2.6
2. at 5 years	0.120	0.150	
CARET trial			
β-carotene			
1. baseline	0.17	12.3	
2. at 6 years	2.10—2.30		
Placebo			
1. baseline	0.17	1.0	
2. at 6 years	0.15—0.17		

From: [8,10,11], modified.

participants (smokers and ex-smokers) have somewhat lower values (a range from 0.22 mg/Lt to 0.29 mg/Lt has been reported for US males at the end of the 1980s in some transversal studies [14,15]). The relative increase of β-carotene in the three studies, however, is remarkably similar (12—17 times). The absolute levels after treatment are also similar in the ATBC and in the CARET study. In Linxian at the end of treatment the supplemented subjects reach levels which are 5 times (and not 12—17 times) higher than those at baseline in the other two studies, and only about 3 times higher than the average in US males.

Results for lung cancer in the four trials are summarized in Table 7 [8—10,16,17]. It should be noted that those reported are early results for the Linxian and for the ATBC study (short follow-up), and a preliminary report for the other two trials [17]. Further, the lung was not the target organ in the Linxian study; the power of the trial for this site is very low and multiple comparisons may explain the effects described.

Results, however, are far from consistent, they range from a suggested protective effect of β-carotene + vitamin E + selenium in the Linxian study (lung cancer mortality: OR = 0.5, n.s.), to no effect in the PHS trial and to a significant excess of lung cancer incidence in both CARET and ATBC studies, respectively related with β-carotene + vitamin A and with β-carotene alone (RR = 1.28 and 1.18, both significant).

In Table 8, results on stomach cancer incidence and mortality are given comparing the Linxian and the ATBC studies. Stomach cancer was the target organ, together with oesophageal cancer, in Linxian; the ATBC study produced information on stomach cancer mortality, but without testing for significance the differences between treatment and placebo. While no effect on stomach cancer risk is apparent in this last

Table 7. Results on lung cancer from Linxian, ATBC, CARET and PHS.

Study	Lung cancer incidence		Lung cancer mortality	
	Rate × 10,000py	RR	Rate × 10,000py	RR
Linxian				
β-car. + α-toc + selenium			1.5	0.55 (n.s.)
placebo			2.7	
ATBC				
α-toc	51.3 (n.s.)	0.98	33.6	1.02 (n.s.)
non-""	52.4		32.8	
β-car	56.3	1.18	35.6	1.15
non-""	47.5	(p = 0.01)	30.8	
CARET				
β-car + retinol		1.28 (sign.)		1.17
placebo				(sign.)
PHS		NO SIGNIFICANT EFFECT		
β-car.				
placebo				

trial, in Linxian a borderline significant protective effect is shown for β-carotene + vitamin E + selenium, consistently on incidence and on mortality.

Discussion

Early results from some large and well designed trials are now available, although far from conclusive, they have produced immensely valuable information for reorienting the future of cancer chemoprevention. In the interpretation of these results, several questions should be addressed:

Table 8. Results on stomach cancer incidence and mortality from the Linxian and the ATBC trials.

Study	Stomach cancer incidence		Stomach cancer mortality
	Rate × 10,000py	RR	RR
Linxian			
retinol + zinc		0.96 (0.81—1.14)	1.03 (0.83—1.28)
riboflavin + niac		1.04 (0.88—1.23)	1.00 (0.81—1.24)
vitC + molibd.		1.10 (0.92—1.30)	1.09 (0.88—1.36)
β-car + vitE + selen		0.84 (0.71—1.00)	0.79 (0.64—0.99)
placebo		1	1
ATBC			
α-toc	8.3	1.2	
non-""	6.6		
β-car	8.3	1.2	
non-""	6.3		

— Are these results clearly stating that treatment with β-carotene is not able to prevent lung cancer?
— Are they stating that β-carotene actually increases the risk of lung cancer?
— Do results apply to the general population? And, if not, which limitations should be considered?
— Is there evidence of an effect on other target organs?
— Are these results such to contradict those on diet and cancer risk deriving from observational epidemiology?

Relating with the first questions, the PHS is probably the study which is more informative: in fact, it is the only one which did recruit a population comprehensive of smokers and nonsmokers (although selected in the direction of nonsmokers) and in which treatment was given for a reasonably long period.

Taking into account the natural history of lung cancer, this second point may be crucial, as treatment lasting 3–5 years and beginning not before the age of 50 (such as in the ATBC and CARET study) may well be limited to the end of the promotion-progression phase of the disease (Table 9). β-carotene, on the contrary, is a candidate for interfering mostly with the early phases of carcinogenesis [7].

According to PHS results, however, β-carotene treatment is not associated at all with lung cancer. The question whether this study, based on a population at low cancer risk, had the power to evidence a possible small association, remains open.

The CARET and ATBC studies provide evidence of a positive association of β-carotene, given at doses of 20–30 mg/day to subjects who have been recently heavily exposed to cigarette smoking or are still exposed, if treatment is given in the late stages of carcinogenesis. This finding is relevant in terms of public health and for the understanding of interactions at a cellular level between carcinogens and antioxidants. In fact, the interaction of smoking with dietary levels of antioxidants is not well understood [18] and there is some suggestion that vitamins, even when taken inside natural products such as fruit and vegetables, could prevent lung cancer only or mostly in nonsmokers [19].

Some other interpretation of the CARET and ATBC results may also be suggested, including the remark that these two studies are also characterized by high doses (higher than in the Linxian and PHS study) and by high final plasmatic levels of β-carotene in the treated arm. If this possible dose-related effect has some meaning it is not known by now, as the populations involved in the four studies are strikingly different in terms of smoking.

From the point of view of public health, these findings practically exclude β-

Table 9. Lung cancer natural history in humans.

Age	Initiation		Promotion		Progression	
	20	30	40	50	60	70
	Onset of exposure				Treatment	

carotene from the list of possible preventive agents for lung cancer. Even if it were effective in nonsmokers, as suggested by the Linxian study, this would be of very limited general interest.

These results do not necessarily contradict observational epidemiology on diet and lung cancer: treatment with synthetic β-carotene for 4—13 years cannot be compared with a long-lasting diet rich in fresh fruit and vegetables, in terms of age at first exposure, duration, dose, molecules involved and complexity of exposure. In fact, in the control arm of the ATBC study, a protective effect of high intake of fruit and vegetables has been confirmed [9]. It could well be, however, that β-carotene is not the chemical which explains the protective effect seen in observational studies on lung cancer, but simply the one which is easier to measure [20].

Evidence on the effect of β-carotene on other cancer sites is still preliminary; more studies (in nonsmokers) will provide information on stomach cancer prevention potentialities [2].

References

1. Hennekens CH. Design Strategies in Epidemiologic Research In: Hennekens CH, Buring JE (eds) Epidemiology in Medicine. Boston: Little, Brown 1987;26—27.
2. Buiatti E. Intervention Trials of Cancer Prevention. Lyon: IARC Technical Report No. 18, 1994.
3. von Poppel G. Carotenoids and cancer: an update with emphasis on human intervention studies. Eur J Cancer 1993;29A(9):1335—1344.
4. Block G. Fruits, vegetables and cancer prevention: a review of the epidemiological evidence. Nutr Cancer 1992;18:1—29.
5. Malone WF. Studies evaluating antioxidants and beta-carotene as chemopreventives. Am J Clin Nutr 1991;53:305S—313S.
6. Peto R, Doll R, Buckley JD, Sporn MB. Can dietary beta-carotene materially reduce human cancer rates? Nature 1981;290:201—209.
7. DiGiovanni J. Inhibition of chemical carcinogenesis. In: Cooper CS, Grover PL (eds) Chemical Carcinogenesis and Mutagenesis II. Berlin: Springler Verlag, 1990;159—202.
8. Blot WJ, Li Jun-Yao, Taylor PR, Guo W, Dawsey S, Wang Guo-Qing, Yang CS, Zheng Su-Fang, Gail M, Li Guang-Yi, Yu Yu, Liu Buo-qi, Tangrea J, Sun Yu-hai, Liu F, Fraumeni J Jr, Zhang You-Hui, Li B. Nutrition intervention trials in Linxian, China: supplementation with specific vitamin/mineral combinations, cancer incidence, and disease-specific mortality in the general population. J Natl Cancer Inst 1993;85:1483—1492.
9. The Alpha-tocopherol, Beta-carotene Cancer Prevention Study Group. The effect of vitamin E and beta-carotene on the incidence of lung cancer and other cancers in male smokers. N Engl J Med 1994;330:1029—1035.
10. Goodman GE, Metch BJ, Omenn GS. The effect of long-term beta-carotene and vit. A administration on serum concentrations of alpha-tocopherol. Cancer Epiderm Biomark Prev 1994;3:429—432.
11. Omenn GS, Goodman G, Thornquist M, Grizzle J, Rosenstock L, Barnhart S, Balmes J, Cherniack MG, Cullen MR, Glass A, Keogh J, Meyskens F Jr, Valanis B, Williams J Jr. The beta-carotene and retinol efficacy trial (CARET) for chemoprevention of lung cancer in high risk populations: smokers and asbestos-exposed workers. Cancer Res 1994;54:2038s—2043s.
12. Hennekens CH. Issues in the design and conduct of clinical trials. J Natl Cancer Inst 1984;73: 1473—1476.
13. Day NE, Bingham SA. Re: Nutrition intervention trials in Linxian, China: Supplementation with specific vitamin/mineral combinations, cancer incidence and disease-specific mortality in the general population. (Letter) J Natl Cancer Inst 1994;86:1645—1646.

14. Stryker WS, Kaplan LA, Stein EA, Stampfer MJ, Sober A, Willet WC. The relation of diet, cigarette smoking and alcohol consumption to plasma beta-carotene and alpha-tocopherol levels. Am J Epidemiol 1988;127:283–296.

15. Nierenberg DW, Stukel TA, Baron JA, Dain BJ, Greenberg ER, and the skin cancer prevention study group. Determinants of plasma levels of beta-carotene and retinol. Am J Epidemiol 1989;130: 511–520.

16. Blot WJ, Li Jun-Yao, Taylor PR, Bing Li. Lung cancer and vitamin supplementation (letter). N Engl J Med 1994;331:614.

17. National Cancer Institute, Office of Cancer Communications Communication from the National Cancer Institute CancerFAX "Beta-Carotene and Vitamin A halted in Lung Cancer Prevention Trial", Jan 17, 1996, Bethesda, Maryland, USA.

18. Editorial, The Alpha-Tocopherol, Beta-Carotene Cancer Prevention Study in Finland, Brief Critical Review. Nutr Rev 1994;52:242–250.

19. Knekt P, Jarvinen R, Seppanen A, Aromaa A, Heinonen OP, Albanes D, Heinonen M, Pukkala E, Teppo L. Dietary antioxidants and the risk of Lung Cancer. Am J Epid 1991;134:471–479.

20. Hankinson SE, Stampfer MJ. All that glitters is not beta-carotene. JAMA 1994;272:1455–1456.

Cost-effectiveness analysis in chemoprevention of cancer: methodology

J.D.F. Habbema

Department of Public Health, Erasmus University Rotterdam, The Netherlands

Introduction

Cancer chemoprevention is potentially a rapidly evolving field of health care, with implications for resource use. Ideally, good chemoprevention programmes should be implemented and equivocal or bad ones not. The required evaluation is not easy, as we will show.

For a chemoprevention agent to have application potential, it should at least satisfy the following requirements, just as for other health care interventions:

* The agent is of proven effectiveness (effective means in this context reducing the incidence and mortality of the target cancer).
* Organisation of the chemoprevention is feasible.
* The favourable effects of chemoprevention are not outweighed by the burden and the health risks it poses to the population.
* The balance between effectiveness on the one hand and risks and costs on the other is acceptable.

The evidence for assessing these requirements should ideally be based on randomised trials, on feasibility studies of implementing a routine chemoprevention programme, and on cost-effectiveness studies or comparable evaluation research. With regard to effectiveness, a recent IARC monograph has updated the evidence on effectiveness of chemoprevention in cancer control [1].

The monograph stresses the importance of cost-effectiveness considerations. For example, one of the conclusions is that "Cost-effectiveness of chemoprevention is clearly important from a public health viewpoint, and has important implications for the implementation of the programmes. Trials exist to quantify effectiveness (if any) and provide the data upon which such evaluations can be based".

An outline of cost-effectiveness approaches in cancer chemoprevention also appeared [2] in the monograph [1]. The approach and results of this paper will be summarized in the next section. However, two important considerations were missing. First, it was assumed that the agent only acts on the target cancer. This is clearly an

---

Address for correspondence: J.D.F. Habbema, Department of Public Health, Faculty of Medicine, Erasmus University Rotterdam, PO Box 1738, 3000 DR Rotterdam, The Netherlands. Tel.: +31-10-408-7985. Fax: +31-10-436-1760.

inappropriate and too restrictive assumption for many chemopreventing agents. For example, tamoxifen, which is proposed for the chemoprevention of breast cancer, has beneficial effects not only for breast cancer but also for ischemic heart disease and spinal fractures, and risks for endometrial cancer, thromboembolic disease, retino-pathy, and maybe also for liver damage [3]. Second, the importance of the viewpoint with which the cost-effectiveness analysis is executed, was not addressed. This issue is a reason for much confusion, and will get considerable attention in the present paper. We will distinguish the societal and the individual viewpoint, and also briefly discuss other, potentially conflicting, viewpoints.

The line of reasoning in the cost-effectiveness evaluation is illustrated in Fig. 1. The boxes on the left-hand side of the figure concern background data and assumptions, and the boxes on the right-hand side concern the cost-effectiveness results.

The life table is used twice. First, it is used to determine the age-specific life expectancy. Second, the life expectancy is also equal to the average duration of a lifelong chemoprevention regimen that starts on the respective age.

We assume that cancer survival does not change after the introduction of a chemoprevention programme; only the incidence may change. We prefer to use incidence and survival rather than the age-specific mortality rates from the cancer, because application of chemoprevention is linked to a reduction in incidence, and a subsequent reduction in mortality is a consequence of a lower incidence. For a person who is just diagnosed with the target cancer there is a loss in life expectancy which is equal to the population life expectancy he would have experienced without having the cancer minus his current life expectancy as an incident cancer case.

We assume that the target population is offered a cancer chemoprevention

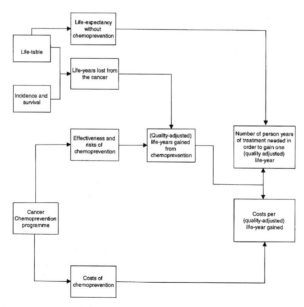

Fig. 1. The line of reasoning to be followed when assessing the effects and cost-effectiveness of cancer chemoprevention. Adapted from Habbema et al. [2].

programme from a certain age onwards. We thus assume that the intervention is lifelong (it could alternatively be assumed that the chemoprevention programme only has a limited duration). For simplicity we also assume in our calculations a 100% coverage and compliance.

The effectiveness of chemoprevention is expressed in terms of the percentage reduction in the target cancer; this may vary over time depending on the time-lag between the start of the chemoprevention and the time when the effects are realized.

The risks of chemoprevention may vary from instantaneous and limited side effects to (small chances of) serious morbidity. Rather than weighing frequent small side effects and infrequent serious risks separately, we will combine the impact of all risks into one subtraction factor to take into account a loss in the quality of life experienced by those participating in the chemoprevention programme.

We assume that the costs of the chemoprevention programme are proportional to the number of years of treatment with the agent. We thus neglect eventual fixed costs of organization, information, etc. Moreover, we will not yet consider the health care savings and costs that result from the effectiveness and the risks of chemoprevention, however, they should be included in the full cost-effectiveness studies.

Results for a hypothetical chemopreventive agent

In Habbema et al. [2], we discussed the assumptions and results for a hypothetical situation involving the chemoprevention of female colorectal cancer by an appropriate agent. The intervention was applied to an age cohort in a particular population. We quantified this intervention using data from the Netherlands. We made some idealized assumptions in order to make the interpretation of the results easier. Coverage and compliance were 100%. The chemopreventive agent has a proven favourable effect, i.e., the incidence of the cancer will be reduced by a certain fraction. We will assume that this reduction begins immediately after the start of the intervention; i.e., there is no lag-time.

We summarize some main results for a female colorectal chemoprevention programme starting at the age of 50. The loss in life expectancy due to colorectal cancer incidence from the age of 50 onwards is 0.355 years. This amount is to be gained by a 100% effective chemopreventive agent and with 100% compliance. For a 25% effective agent, which will be discussed below, the amount will be a quarter of 0.355, i.e., 0.089 life-years gained per woman. Already with rather small adverse effects corresponding to a quality of life reduction of 0.004 on a 0 (dead) to 1 (good health) scale, risks will outweigh benefits. 350 years of chemopreventive treatment are needed in order to gain 1 life-year that would otherwise be lost from colorectal cancer mortality. Costs per quality-adjusted life-year gained will be high. The cost-effectiveness ratio will be high compared to other health care services, unless the chemoprevention is very cheap and the risks are negligible. Lag-time and compliance considerations will further affect costs and effects.

Although the example is artificial, it is also realistic, and suggests that a favourable cost-effectiveness ratio is all but trivial for any chemoprevention programme. The methodology used in deriving the results is quite general. The steps in Fig. 1 can also be applied to other situations. Of course, the precision of the conclusions concerning cost-effectiveness depends crucially on the knowledge of the effects and risks of the chemoprevention. Some cost-effectiveness issues, such as discounting for time preference, have not been discussed. Hillman et al. [4] is a recent authoritative publication of cost-effectiveness analysis. Useful textbooks include Drummond et al. [5] and Warner and Luce [6]. The assessment of preventive activities is discussed in Russel [7].

Multiple effects of chemoprevention

Although chemoprevention is usually aimed at a specific cancer, effects may also be present for other diseases. We did not consider this in Fig. 1 or in our example of a colorectal chemoprevention programme. For example, as estimated in Cuzick [3], giving tamoxifen for 5 years to 10,000 women of the age of 50 with a relative risk of 2.5 for breast cancer will bring the breast cancer incidence down by 40% over a 10-year period. But ischemic heart disease will also go down by 20%, which will further improve the life table, and the 33% reduction in spinal fractures will especially increase the quality of life. On the other hand, there are risks of endometrial cancer, thromboembolic disease, retinopathy, and possibly liver damage, which will have an adverse effect on life expectancy and quality of life. Thus, the effectiveness of chemoprevention on life expectancy and quality-adjusted life expectancy cannot be assessed by addressing only the target cancer. On the contrary, a general flexible approach must be taken in which multiple effects are possible. The mortality part is illustrated in Fig. 2.

The mathematical reasoning involved is as follows: age specific mortality hazards can be thought of as a summation of the age specific mortality hazards of all possible causes of death. When chemoprevention influences these hazards favourably or adversely, they can be adjusted, and summation can take place again now including the situation of chemoprevention. Adjustments for the quality of the health status can be made in a way using the quality-adjusted life-years method.

Cost-effectiveness analysis: what perspective to take?

It is generally recommended for cost-effectiveness analysis to make an analysis using a societal point of view [4]. However, it is often relevant also to explore other perspectives. The main ones are the individual perspective, the health care perspective and other interest party based perspectives. We will consider these below.

From a societal perspective, costs are always so-called opportunity costs to society, which reflect what could maximally have been achieved with the same resources had they not been allocated to chemoprevention. When no better societal use is available, chemoprevention is a good thing to do. Apparent costs are to be distinguished from the financial prices and fees which are actually paid between parties involved. In some cases these fees and prices reasonably reflect societal costs, but in other cases

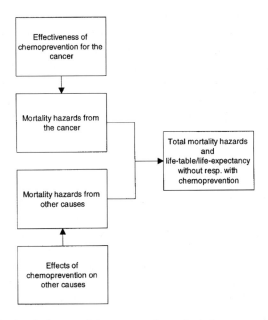

Fig. 2. Flow-chart reflecting the impact of chemoprevention on both the target cancer and on other causes of death. Life-years gained are calculated as the difference between the life expectancy with chemoprevention and the life expectancy without chemoprevention. This figure is an extension of the left upper part of Fig. 1 which considers a mortality impact only on the target cancer.

they do not correspond at all. The differences between the two are called "transfer payments". This means that they do not produce value for society; only money is shifted between parties. Concerning these effects, the public health effects are calculated. This means that an aggregation over effects on all the individuals takes place. Of course, only individuals for whom the chemoprevention has potentially a beneficial expectation should be recommended to take it. This gives rise to the concept of "indication", which means that population groups are identified — including age/sex characteristics — which have sufficient risk of the cancer to justify the chemoprevention programme.

When we take the individual point of view, indication will be further specialized to the individual risk profile of the person involved, i.e., it should be calculated given the personal characteristics, the risk for all diseases that are affected by the chemoprevention, and what the expected risks and benefits of the chemoprevention are for the particular person. An important concept which is also differently dealt with in this respect is compliance. In the societal perspective, one should make an estimate of what percentage of the indication groups will be covered by the chemoprevention programme and what the compliance within these groups will be. For the individual on the other hand, choices are based on statements like "what will be the risks and benefit of chemoprevention for me, in the case where I adhere to the programme for the full duration?" The decision for participation will subsequently also depend on the individual's personal estimate of whether he will comply. So again no aggregation over individuals, but a particular condition for the individual is involved. As far as costs are concerned, for the individual viewpoint there is a direct interest in what resources have to be paid extra — time and money when the chemoprevention is not covered by health care insurance — for the chemoprevention programme. But there may also be future costs and savings to the individuals from the effects and risks of the chemoprevention, and these future cost components should in principle also be covered.

When the perspective of the health care services is taken, the concern is mostly about extra costs incurred to the health care system by the chemoprevention programme, and also about future costs and savings induced by the effects and risks of chemoprevention. Economic implications outside the health care system are not considered. For other interest group perspectives, like insurance companies, pharmaceutical companies, and physicians in charge, economic analyses can be made which reflects the interests of these parties. The "external costs", i.e., costs not considered in the analysis, are usually far more important when considering the point of view of an interest group, rather than in a societal analysis.

It is clear that quite different conclusions may result from the different perspectives, i.e., the different valuation of the way in which the benefits and costs of the chemoprevention is distributed over different parties in society. Thus, the effectiveness issue is an essential ingredient of the societal and individual perspectives, but unfortunately not always for the other perspectives. We will not elaborate on the issue any further, but one should be aware that conflict of interest may arise. In our opinion, decisions concerning chemoprevention should be based on a societal point of view, and in practice refined according to the individual point of view. Thus, a chemoprevention programme should only be considered when it has a reasonable cost-effectiveness ratio from a societal point of view. The subsequent individualization of starting chemoprevention and deciding to comply, is left to the individual person and his or her advisors. But again, the organization of health care and society should be such that indeed all these individuals have the opportunity for an informed choice about their participation.

Conclusions

From this paper, the following conclusions can be drawn:
- A methodology for cost-effectiveness analysis (CEA) of chemoprevention is available. In a CEA, the effects on the target cancer should not be considered in isolation. The analysis should include all the diseases affected by the agent.
- CEA can help to organize and analyze knowledge and lack of knowledge concerning benefits, risks costs and savings of chemoprevention.
- CEA not only gives cost-effectiveness ratios, but also all kind of insights from intermediate, less aggregated results.
- CEA can help to decide on indication setting, i.e., the level of (high) risk for the target cancer above which chemoprevention is indicated.

- The conclusions from the CEA may depend on the point of view taken during the analysis. The two pivotal viewpoints are the societal one and the individual one.
- In view of the available evidence at this moment, a careful CEA of tamoxifen could help in the discussion on its use. For some other chemopreventive agents, exploratory CEAs could be considered in order to get a preliminary idea about their possible value.

References

1. Chemoprevention in cancer control. In: Hakama M, Beral V et al. (eds) IARC Scientific Publications No. 136. International Agency for Research on Cancer, Lyon, 1996. ·
2. Habbema JDF, van der Heide A, van den Bosch JMH, Bonneux L. Cost-effectiveness considerations in chemoprevention of cancer. In: Hakama M, Beral V et al. (eds) Chemoprevention in Cancer Control. IARC Scientific Publications No. 136. International Agency for Research on Cancer, Lyon, 1996;131–138.
3. Cuzick J. Chemoprevention of breast cancer with tamoxifen. In: Hakama M, Beral V et al. (eds) Chemoprevention in Cancer Control. IARC Scientific Publications No. 136. International Agency for Research on Cancer, Lyon, 1996;95–110.
4. Hillman et al. Task force on principles for economic analysis of health care technology. Economic analysis of health care technology. A report on principles. Ann Intern Med 1995;122:61–70.
5. Drummond MF, Stoddart GL, Torrance GW. Methods for the Economic Evaluation of Health Care Programmes. New York: Oxford University Press, 1987.
6. Warner K, Luce B. Cost-Benefit and Cost-Effectiveness Analysis in Health Care: Principles, Practice and Potential. Ann Arbor, MI: Health Administration Press, 1982.
7. Russel L. Is prevention better than cure? Washington, DC: The Brookings Institution, 1986.

Ethical issues of intervention trials in cancer*

H. Sancho-Garnier[1] and R. Joseph[2]

[1]Hôpital G, Doumergue CHU, Nîmes, France; and [2]Medical College of Pennsylvania, Philadelphia, USA

The objective of cancer prevention is either a reduction in the incidence of the disease through direct action against its causes, or a reduction of its morbidity and mortality.

Chemoprevention trials are not innocuous. They involve healthy subjects. As a consequence, careful ethical consideration must be given to such programmes. In particular, when calculating the risk-benefit ratio one must take into account not only the physical but also the mental and social wellbeing of people whose lives will be "medicalized" as a result of such intervention. The primacy of collective benefit over individual interest demands that preventive intervention be based on voluntary informed consent of the target population. The numerous consequences of the extrapolation of results of chemoprevention trials to the general population must be considered. Finally, the classical contract between patient and doctor is altered in this novel situation. The promotion of research into the psychological and social consequences of chemoprevention of cancer is essential.

Ethical issues

Cancer prevention aims to produce either a reduction in the incidence of the disease through direct action against its causes, or a reduction of its morbidity and mortality, by attacking the process leading to clinical expression of the cancer [1].

Prevention strategies include:
- elimination or reduction of exposure to risk factors, e.g., smoking cessation strategies;
- elimination of the effect of these exposures by the use of protective factors, e.g., vaccination, diet;
- treatment of precancerous lesions which have a high probability of evolution into cancer, e.g., colon polyps, cervical dysplasia; and
- screening and treatment of cancers at a stage of maximum curability, e.g., breast cancer.

The first type of action uses only public information, education and legislative methods. All the other strategies include diagnostic and therapeutic medical procedures.

Address for correspondence: H. Sancho-Garnier, Hôpital G, Doumergue CHU, Nîmes 3000, France.
*Reproduced by permission of the Director, I.A.R.C. from I.A.R.C. Scientific Publications No. 136, International Agency for Research on Cancer, Lyon, 1996, pp. 121–122.

Preventive medicine is not innocuous, particularly when such actions are based on medical interventions [2]. Preventive efforts should not lead to an impairment of the physical, mental or social wellbeing of the individual concerned. Furthermore, prevention generally applies to healthy subjects, i.e., those not needing medical care and for whom, in the majority of cases, there will be no direct benefit. Because of the haphazard and delayed nature of the benefits of intervention trials, the risk-benefit ratio of such actions must take into account not only their physical effects but also their psychological and social consequences.

The undesirable effects of preventive interventions are often poorly recognized. The attendant risks are run by the entire healthy population, while the target disease only affects a (usually small) portion of the individuals constituting this population. Even if the intervention brings a slight advantage to a reasonably large number of subjects, a significant risk of undesirable effects, even for a minority of them, is difficult to accept. An intervention trial should not be undertaken unless the expected benefits outweigh the potential risks.

Benefits are represented by a decrease in incidence and/or mortality rates of a disease, which may or may not be associated with an improvement in the quality of life. Interventions trials should be conducted under conditions that are most likely to give reliable results, e.g., scientific rationale, correct methodology, careful choice of target population, correct treatment doses and duration, good quality control, etc. Unless these criteria are met the interventions must be considered unethical.

Potential ill-effects are numerous and varied. On the one hand, any toxicity of preventive agents is usually carefully observed and documented even when unexpected, while on the other hand, the potential psychological and social consequences, such as those described below, are generally ignored.

Taking medication daily and/or submitting to repeated testing may lead healthy subjects to consider themselves as potentially or actually ill, or at least to be constantly conscious of the possibility of getting cancer. Preventive intervention leads to false hopes for those who will get the disease despite compliance with the suggested programme. As a result, these patients and their relatives may experience serious disillusionment with standard medicine [3]. Study subjects who forget to take their medication or who drop out of a trial prematurely could develop chronic anxiety as to the possible risks of their behaviour. Development of cancer in patients who decline to participate in, or who do not comply with, chemoprevention trials may engender profound guilt. Initiation of large-scale trials is often followed by major media coverage. This may lead a proportion of the population to self-prescribe the medication involved in the trial before any efficacy has been proven. Such publicity may also engender mass cancerophobia. Ethical reflection necessitates going beyond the evaluation of the risk-benefit ratio of an intervention, as already advocated by many authors [4] in the 1970s. The probability of benefit to the individual is low, and the benefit is uncertain (random) and late. The individual participant must therefore accept the primacy of collective benefit over individual interest. These considerations thus necessitate that this type of intervention be based on voluntary informed consent of the target population. It is in this context, where the interest of the research itself and the interest of the subjects almost inevitably come into confrontation, that the principle of informed consent is most important. One must also consider the consequences of extrapolating results of chemoprevention trials to the general population [5]. If the results are in favour of chemoprevention, will this type of intervention be applicable to millions of people? For example, is it imaginable that a large part of the population will swallow a handful of various medications (vitamins, microelements, ASA, hormones, etc.) everyday for the rest of their lives to avoid various illnesses? Where will we stop? Furthermore, will it be possible with such a mixture of agents to determine the contribution of each to the desired effect or to predict toxic interactions? Will toxicities, whose low frequencies are acceptable in the context of a clinical trial, become unacceptable given the large denominator of the general population? Will not the economic cost of such intervention be prohibitive? Finally, the ethical problems inherent in intervention trials cannot be resolved in the framework of the classical contract between patient and doctor. Traditionally, the patient comes to the physician seeking care. On the other hand, in chemoprevention it is the physician who proposes the intervention. This basic difference from usual medical practice demands that, before instituting such trials, the collective rather than the individual consequences of the trial should be seriously considered. Measurement of the effects of preventive interventions on the lifestyle and mental health of the population subjected to them necessitates the development of specific tools adapted to such situations. The promotion of future research in this area is essential.

References

1. Buiatti E. Intervention Trials of Cancer Prevention: Results and New Research Programmes. International Agency for Research on Cancer, Lyon (IARC Technical Report No. 18), 1994.
2. Maheu E. La Prevention Entre Responsabilité et Coercition. In: Idéologies de la prevention. Revue AGORA — Ethique Médecine Société 1994;30:3–7.
3. Bouvier P et al. Aspects Éthiques du Dépistage: Réflexions à Partir de L'Exemple du Cancer du Sein. In: Cahier Médico-Sociaux. Médecine et Hygiène 1994;38:1.
4. Jeanneret O, Raymond L. Aspects Éthiques des Études D'Intervention. Rev Epidem et Santé Publ 1981;129:269–279.
5. Lazar P. Vaut il Toujours Mieux Prévenir que Guérir? La Revue du Praticien 1994;44:2533–2534.

Chairman's summary and conclusion

C.G. Schmidt
Klinikum Essen, Essen, Germany

A new direction of cancer prevention is dealing with chemoprevention which is regarded as a promising new strategy for reducing the rates of cancer morbidity and mortality. Chemoprevention can be defined as the use of specific natural or synthetic chemical agents to prevent, suppress or even reverse carcinogenesis before the ultimate development of invasive malignancy has taken place. Recent advances in the understanding of the molecular and genetic mechanism of carcinogenesis have been crucial to the progress of our overall understanding of cancer. Several papers have pointed out that cancer is initiated and promoted through a progressive, multistep process involving multiple genetic challenges. The involved initiation, promotion and progression genes have been mentioned including cyclin D, p53, RAS and TGF. This evolving understanding of the molecular mechanism of carcinogenesis is creating new opportunities for advances in cancer prevention based on identification of specific molecules and the targeted modulation of these effects.

The original proposed definition of chemoprevention by SPORN and NEWTON refers to the prevention of cancer by the use of pharmacological agents which inhibit or reverse the process of carcinogenesis. We should therefore keep in mind that chemoprevention is different from primary cancer prevention which refers to the avoidance or removal of exogenic factors which correlate with a high risk of cancer development, e.g., tobacco, some occupational hazards, ultraviolet radiation, etc. Since the multistep progress includes an initiation step (or steps) followed by a number of promotion and progression steps, opportunities exist for intervention at early as well as later stages of the process. In general, inhibition of carcinogenesis may be defined by the point at which the intervention to the carcinogenic process takes place. This includes:

1. Compounds which prevent the formation or absorption of carcinogens (initiation).
2. Blocking agents that prevent carcinogens from reaching or reacting with cellular targets (initiation).
3. Suppressing agents that suppress the expression of neoplasia in cells exposed to doses or durations of carcinogens which otherwise would cause cancer (promotion).

Some substances have both blocking and suppressing capabilities.

Our understanding and moreover the transfer of knowledge to the health care system depends on the scientific basis of prevention. In session No.1 the present information upon the role of oncogenes and suppressor genes, the relation between genetic stability or instability and carcinogenesis have been discussed. With the understanding of genetic defect in the DNA repair disorders (e.g., Xeroderma pigmentosum), prevention measures can be undertaken to reduce cancer incidence in individuals. The DNA repair-deficient syndromes may be rare, but give view to the inside processes which underline these deficiencies. Studies have now shown that there is a link between defective DNA repair mechanism and abnormal expression of normal regulatory genes — both oncogenes and suppressor genes.

A characteristic feature of carcinogenesis is the long latency period. In humans the time interval is usually decades. The time interval may reflect subsequent mutations in the DNA up to the clonal expression after many repetitive cell cycles have taken place.

During this meeting it has been mentioned that the long latency period would offer numerous opportunities for intervention before the final step of fully developed malignancy has been reached.

The first part of our symposium focuses on targeting genetic mechanism of cancer. The activation of oncogenes from the normally occurring proto-oncogenes or the inactivation of tumor suppressor genes may cause the loss of control over cell replication. Some of the genes, e.g., RAS, MYC or especially p53, are found in a variety of tumors, indicating that a common set of genes may trigger or play a central role in the process of cancerogenesis. With regard to chemoprevention research preventing mutations in these or other cancer genes is of great interest. To date, several agents such as retinoic acid, carotenoids, vitamin E, A and D may promise the modulation of the effect of genetic alterations. Several of them are able to decrease oncogene expression or mutation in vitro or in animal models (MYC, RAS). A common genetic alteration detected in many tumors (especially in animal tumors) refers to the mutation of RAS-proto-oncogene.

Because the effect of acquired genetic changes may occur at several points within the carcinogenic process, the case of colonic cancer can contribute to our understanding. The correlation between stepwise occurring histopathological changes and genetic alterations have been described. The case of colonic cancer demonstrates the progressive accumulation of definable genetic changes including the activation of oncogenes and inactivation of tumor suppressor genes. The neoplastic progression from normal, healthy epithelium to cancer, from cellular hyperproliferation via small, benign adenomas to dysplastic larger adenomas that can become cancer, including the later step of metastatic capabilities, are seen to be a process that can take decades, involving early deletions as well as alterations, such as the loss of the p53 tumor suppressor gene on chromosome 17 and other deletions, and mutations on the RAS oncogene which occur rather late. This sequence of events over a long period of time could offer several possibilities for intervention. Because the majority of colorectal cancers occur in individuals aged 40–70 years, chemoprevention in the middle-age group may present an opportunity to reduce the incidence and mortality of these very common cancers.

To improve the preclinical evaluation of chemoprevention the development of rodent models which allow testing of several compounds at different stages of carcinogenesis have been performed and discussed at this meeting. The models allow testing of chemoprevention under standard dietary conditions, using natural products and pharmaceutical compounds as well (Lipkin). The rodent models make it possible to study individual etiological factors contributing to the development of colon cancer. The results of these studies could be the start of new clinical trials.

In identifying groups for chemopreventive agents the contribution of epidemiology is important. Due to the concept of a rather long latent period for carcinogenesis it is necessary to define the precise endpoints and the interval between exposure and outcome. Dr John Bailar referred to this complex subject with wide variation from one proposed use to another including several complexities between individual and population latent period and acute vs. continued exposure.

Epidemiology and molecular biology can help to identify cancer risk factors. One important task of chemoprevention research is the validation of early risk factors, identifying specific groups for chemoprevention. This task is easier when certain genes for family history of cancer are involved, such as BRCA 1 and 2. The genetic susceptibility includes chromosome instability, loss of carcinogenic detoxification and more.

Within the context of epidemiology I also refer to studies for the identification of several naturally occurring chemopreventive agents such as vitamin A, β-carotene (provitamin A), vitamins B 12, C and E, folic acid and the minerals calcium and selenium. Two papers, the ones of Dr Soffritti et al. and Dr E. Buiatti referred within their presentation to these studies. It should be noted that the consistency of data vary considerably. For example, former studies indicate that individuals who consume large amounts of carrots and green and yellow vegetables — all rich in vitamin A and β-carotene — have a reduced risk to develop lung cancer and esophageal and/or gastric cancer. Following these publications several clinical trials are being undertaken to evaluate the efficacy of β-carotene and retinol, alone or in combination with other chemopreventive agents, in preventing or modulating precancerous lesions in the oral cavity and in other epithelial organs as well. For some substances used in chemoprevention good epidemiological evidence is lacking, and high expectations were not fulfilled (van't Veer). Dr Soffritti's paper mentioned that application of vitamin A has no effect on survival but in the animal experimental program, vitamin A causes an increase in the incidence of mammary cancer in the three groups with the highest level of vitamin A in their diet.

The β-carotene and Retinol Efficacy Trial (CARET) for chemoprevention of lung cancer in population at high risk including former heavy smokers and males with extensive occupational asbestosis exposure should give us results at the end of this decade. The results of the Linxian trials performed by the Cancer Institute of the Chinese Academy of Medical Science and the NCI as a randomized, double-blind trial to determine whether daily ingestion of specific vitamins and minerals or multiple vitamins and mineral supplements would reduce incidence and mortality of cancer indicate a significant benefit for those receiving the β-carotene/vitamin A/selenium combination largely due to the reduction in stomach cancer incidence and mortality. Since the situation and life style in the Western countries differ from the Linxian community especially with regard to the deficiency in multiple micronutrition these results — encouraging as they are — may not be applied directly to the Western world.

The α-tocopherol, β-carotene Cancer Preventing Study (ATBC), a randomized double-blind placebo control prevention study conducted in Finland by the NCI and the National Public Health Institute of Finland, demonstrated a minimal reduction in lung cancer incidence in men who received vitamin E but in contrast an 80% higher incidence of lung cancer among men who received β-carotene. Men who took both vitamin E and β-carotene showed an increase in lung cancer similar to those with β-carotene alone, indicating no significant interaction between these supplements. Vitamin E reduces prostate cancer incidence by 34% and colorectal cancer by 16% (not significant). β-carotene seems to reduce only the incidence rate of lung cancer, giving little or no effect on other cancers.

The results of this study, lack of benefit from β-carotene together with the possibility of harm, are not only surprising but also questioning the large body of epidemiological evidence that suggests dietary β-carotene is associated with a lower risk of lung cancer. There are several explanations under discussion to explain these results including the time interval which might have been too short to inhibit lung cancer. Other suggestions point to the possibility that other constituents of food high in vitamin E or β-carotene may be responsible for the protective effect observed in several epidemiological studies. Further studies including different supplements and longer follow-up will be needed.

Tools for identifying agents for cancer prevention require in vitro and in vivo studies. Agents which are regarded as promising compounds are tested by in vitro screening systems and the ones with chemopreventive effect in the preliminary tests are chosen for further in vivo studies dealing with a set of different animal tumors. It is reasonable to assume that results observed on normal epithelial cell transformation can be expected to be seen in the malignant process of this tissue type as well.

With regard to the clinical application randomized intervention trials based on the results of analytical epidemiology and in vitro and in vivo animal screening tests have been designed to evaluate the efficacy of measures for cancer prevention. The main methodological problems have been discussed at this forum. Within the last 10–20 years many randomized controlled clinical intervention trials have been designed; some of them have reached preliminary or final results. A positive result means a reduction in cancer incidence of one or more sites in the treated group vs. placebo. Such positive results could justify a possible large-scale application of the preventive measure to the population at risk.

The clinical trials are closely related to the public health aspects of chemoprevention. These must include some general principles, e.g., the national history of the disease must be known and there should be a clear definition of risk factors.

Chemoprevention trials have to be safe, acceptable and if possible inexpensive. That means we should estimate the harm/benefit ratio carefully as well as the cost/efficiency rates. With regard to subjects for chemoprevention these include high-risk groups (acquired or genetic factors), and those with previously treated cancer.

Furthermore, the problems of recruitment and compliance which are important especially for long-lasting trials have to be considered carefully.

Given the case of a proven positive result, the strategy of cancer chemoprevention should aim to achieve a significant reduction in cancer incidence or mortality, to improve life expectancy and quality of life of the population at risk. Considering the difficult and slow-going improvement of cancer therapy this effect could be much greater and probably working even within a decade.

The rather complicated methodological, logistic, ethical and financial problems of interventional trials are of specific nature and have been discussed. One of the major problems refers to the identification of high-risk groups which are of course different for different tumor sites. There are some problems, e.g., results from experimental studies do not always give information on the effective dose, the best mode of application and the target organ because they can be species specific; on the other side epidemiological studies are normally reflecting a complex exposure and mostly do not point to a very specific agent.

The evaluation of endpoints and outcome is a specific problem for chemopreventional trials because of the long and natural history of the disease and a long latency period which has to pass before we can see definite results. Very large trials and long follow-up periods would be needed to overcome these limitations. They increase the cost and the number of drop-outs of involved subjects.

Several speakers have pointed out that the definition of interval endpoint is of utmost importance to shorten the time interval between start of the trial and availability of valuable results. Several ongoing trials are using endpoints other than the ultimate cancer incidence rate with indicators of the prevention effect, e.g., cell proliferation, labelling index, different methods of DNA damage, DNA adducts, p53 mutations, RAS mutations, progression or regression of precancerous lesions and new risk biomarkers. It is clear that intervention trials compared to clinical trials are characterized by some unique features which imply specific problems.

One of the major efforts of chemoprevention is concentrated on the prevention or intervention of breast cancer, because this is one of the most challenging tumors of all. The problem of identification and selection of high-risk groups has been discussed. This holds true for the intervention trials on dietary fat and breast cancer as well as on the latest discussion on the chemoprevention of mammary cancer with tamoxifen. The high-risk group may include women with suspected precancerous lesions of the breast (follicular or ductal hyperplasia) or women with personal characteristics such as being 60 or older, or having a family history of breast cancer, nulli parity, age 30 or older at first delivery and so on.

Germ line mutations (BRCA 1 and 2) may account for about 10–15% of all breast cancers. By definition all the subjects who have been diagnosed as carriers of these germ line mutations must be regarded as high-risk people.

The etiology of breast cancer is believed to be strongly related to estrogen activity and metabolism. The most important trials in this direction are concentrating on the inhibition of estrogen carcinogenic activity with antiestrogen compounds such as tamoxifen. The well-documented effects of tamoxifen in the treatment of advanced breast cancer as well as in the adjuvant setting are the basis for the present development. Several clinical trials of tamoxifen vs. controlled breast cancer patients showed a 35% reduction of risk of contralateral breast cancer after an average treatment duration of 2 years. We have learned during this meeting that the protection can reach even up to 50%!

Tamoxifen has been tested in three large chemopreventive trials on high-risk women (the US-Canada trial, one in the UK and one in Italy). Since tamoxifen is under question for a possible carcinogenic activity on endometrial tissue in the Italian study only hysterectomized women are admitted.

The experimental study on the chemopreventive effect of tamoxifen focuses on the mechanism of its action and its ability to suppress appearance of chemically induced as well as spontaneous breast tumors in laboratory animals. So far in vitro studies suggest that its antiestrogen action results from direct binding to the estrogen receptor leading to conformational changes in the receptor, alter RNA-transcription, decrease cell proliferation and partial estrogen agonist activity. These properties of tamoxifen correlate well with its observed ability to reduce the incidence of primary breast tumors, while leaving unanswered the question about how tamoxifen brings about these effects.

Animal experiments on the effect of tamoxifen on breast tumor suppression have been demonstrated by Prof Maltoni and his coworkers from the European Ramazzini Foundation of Oncology using spontaneously developed mammary cancer which can be regarded as human equivalent. Using different doses schedules and different timing of the tamoxifen application and different age to begin the chemoprevention tamoxifen, given for the life-span at a rather high-doses results in a complete inhibition of the onset of mammary cancer, whereas only a borderline increase in the incidence of hepatomas and uterine malignancy was observed. It was demonstrated that tamoxifen is working over a wide variety of doses, even able to protect on a very low-dose scale. The important question to be transferred from laboratory animal studies to clinical practice relates to the duration of treatment. One of the crucial point is related not only to the duration of the protective effect after the cessation of tamoxifen therapy, but also to the safety of protection which might have been reached. After the treatment is stopped and the animals are controlled until their spontaneous deaths, the chemopreventive effect remains. The protective index was even reached by a very low tamoxifen dose.

Altogether the evidence to support the use of tamoxifen for the prevention of breast cancer is substantial. Dr Costa referred to the ongoing trials on the chemo-prevention of mammary cancer with a special reference to the Italian study showing the feasibility to run the chemoprevention trials in hysterectomized women.

In summary, the positive effect of tamoxifen can be described as follows: Tamoxifen prevents or delays the appearance of virally or chemically induced breast cancer in animals, it reduces by more than 30% the risk of second breast cancer in women with a first primary breast cancer. It also has a favorable effect on lipid profile of postmenopausal women and it reduces the number of deaths from myocardial infarction and cardiovascular disease in breast cancer women without a significant increase in the risk of thromboembolism and finally has an estrogenic effect on bone which might be able to reduce the risk of fractures in those women as well.

Beside these positive effects there are still controversial discussions going on over the scientific basis of the trial and of course the risk vs. benefit effect of the drug in healthy women with a high risk for developing breast cancer must be carefully assessed. Some concern is related especially to premenopausal women within the chemoprevention trial, since their calculated risk of developing breast cancer during the 5 years of tamoxifen administration is such that more than 90% of these women will not develop breast cancer during the drug administration. The possibility of late side effects must be considered carefully. Some speakers have given figures regarding the great number of healthy women who must be treated who would never get this cancer just to protect a comparatively low number of subjects from breast cancer.

With regard to the discussion on the late effects of tamoxifen it cannot be excluded for the time being that under tamoxifen treatment a negative selection from hormone-dependant to hormone-independent tumors, which means to a more aggressive form, may take place. Other papers referred to experimental chemopreventive studies of medroxyprogesterone and retinamide compounds (HPR).

Under the experimental condition using female rats with spontaneously developing mammary cancer MPA showed a strong chemopreventive effect HPR failed to show a protective effect within the dose schedule used.

The translation from experimental data to ongoing clinical chemoprevention studies with HPR is interesting but results are not yet available for final conclusion. So far no difference could be demonstrated, but follow-up is still needed.

Before embarking on rather large multicenter, long-lasting chemoprevention trials the assessment of the cost-effectiveness of these trials should be carefully considered, some examples have been demonstrated. Furthermore the ethical issues of interventional trials especially for breast cancer prevention not only for recruitment and compliance but also with regard to the "medicalization" of life have been discussed.

In conclusion so far several hundred potential chemopreventive agents have been identified and approximately 30 of these agents are presently being tested in humans. There is indeed a great heterogeneity of these compounds which belong to very different chemical classes. We are dealing with micronutrition, food additives, nonnutritive food molecules, industrial reagents, pharmaceutical compounds, hormones and antihormones. It should be mentioned that ascorbic acid and tocopherol are acting by a prevention of formation of nitrosating agents which seem to be in close relation with cancer of the upper gastrointestinal tract. The principal compound is of course ascorbic acid (vitamin C). The main action refers to the fact that ascorbic acid can inhibit the formation of nitroso compounds both in vitro and in vivo. Probably the same may be seen for α-tocopherol (vitamin E) which is also able to inhibit the formation of nitroso compounds.

The retinoids include all natural and synthetic analogues of vitamin A. It is interesting to see that vitamin A was long known to influence normal cellular differentiation. Since the development of cancer is fundamentally a process of loss of cellular differentiation the chemoprevention of cancer with retinoids represents an interesting physiological step arresting or reversing the process of carcinogenesis. There is still a controversial discussion with regard to the chemopreventive effects of vitamins; solid experimental, epidemiological, clinical information is lacking or controversial.

With regard to the clinical application there has been a rapid expansion over the last years which means we should not forget that before the introduction of clinical trials phase I pharmacological and toxicological studies and phase II dose-intensity investigations of new chemopreventive agents are mandatory to select the least toxic effective doses for long-term trials in humans.

The chemoprevention of tumors is increasingly attracting the intention of oncologists but it still has a long way to go before reaching a consolidated status in cancer medicine. We have an increasing number of experimental data pointing to various possibilities of inhibiting the multistep carcinogenic process but we do lack important background information with regard to the molecular level of chemopreventive action. That means further research in molecular biology with regard to the biological complexity of carcinogenesis and the action of chemopreventive agents are necessary. The application of in vitro screening systems improves the selection process and opens the door for animal models to be used before clinical interventional trials can be designed with rather less toxicity under long-term application.

Since clinical chemoprevention is dealing with the administration of agents over a long period of time in healthy groups of individuals the problem of acute and chronic toxicity is of utmost importance and should be dealt with before clinical chemoprevention can be regarded as safe. We need patience because the trials are expected to take a long time before a significant result can be expected. Chemopreventive intervention trials in human beings must include several thousands of subjects, not to forget that the duration of interventional observation may exceed 10 years. The cost of chemoprevention trials are very high, the evaluation of complicance is extremely difficult, thus only well-organized and rather great trials with a sound financial background can have the chance to answer the very important questions before some chemical compounds can be recommended for chemoprevention in practice.

Altogether, chemoprevention is a promising new strategy for reducing the rates of cancer morbidity and mortality. Further research both on the level of molecular biology and clinical investigation is needed before a recommendation for practical use dealing with the great number of subjects can be given.

This meeting is considered to be one within a series of follow-up meetings and it is to be hoped it will give us further information on this interesting project.

Index of authors

Keyword index